*Laughing Mad*

# Laughing Mad

## THE BLACK COMIC PERSONA IN POST-SOUL AMERICA

BAMBI HAGGINS

RUTGERS UNIVERSITY PRESS
*New Brunswick, New Jersey, and London*

Material used Chapter 1 and 2 was originally published, in a much abbreviated form, as "Laughing Mad: The Black Comedian's Place in Post–Civil Rights Era American Comedy," in *Hollywood Comedians: The Film Reader*, ed. Frank Krutnik (London, New York: Routledge, 2003).

Excerpt from "It's Bigger Than Hip Hop," written by Lavonne Alford and Clayton Gavin, published by War of Art Music (BMI)/Walk Like a Warrior Music (BMI), performed by Dead Prez. Reprinted by permission of The Royalty Network Inc.

Excerpt from "Harlem Literati" from *The Big Sea* by Langston Hughes. Copyright © 1940 by Langston Hughes. Copyright renewed 1968 by Arna Bontemps and George Houston Bass. Reprinted by permission of Hill and Wang, a division of Farrar, Strauss and Giroux, LLC and (for publication in United Kingdom and British Commonwealth) Harold Ober Associates Inc.

LIBRARY OF CONGRESS CATALOGING-IN-PUBLICATION DATA

Haggins, Bambi, 1961–
    Laughing mad : the Black comic persona in post-soul America / Bambi Haggins.
       p.    cm.
    Includes bibliographical references and index.
    ISBN-13: 978–0–8135–3984–3 (hardcover : alk. paper)
    ISBN-13: 978–0–8135–3985–0 (pbk. : alk. paper)
    1.  African American comedians—Biography   I. Title.
    PN2286.H34   2007
    792.702′8092396073—dc22
    [B]                              2006015371

A British Cataloging-in-Publication record for this book is available from the British Library.

Manufactured in the United States of America

*For my mother, Pearl Haggins*
*In loving memory of my father, John R. Haggins*

# CONTENTS

# ACKNOWLEDGMENTS

IT TAKES A VILLAGE to finish a book, and *Laughing Mad* could not have been completed without the generosity and support of colleagues, friends, and family. I would like to thank the University of Michigan's Department of Screen Arts and Cultures, Gaylyn Studlar, and the Rackham Summer Fellowship program for fiscally facilitating my westward trek to do archival research. The staffs of the UCLA Film and Television Archive and the Museum of Television and Radio in Los Angeles allowed me to see hours of footage capturing the performances of comics discussed in this volume. I am beholden to Kristen Whissel, David Rider, Liz Weston, Ellen Scott, and Amy Kett, my earliest readers (listeners) for this project; and to Philip Hallman for his multifaceted personal and professional support (and for making sure that the Donald Hall Collection remained well stocked with black comedy). Many thanks to the Ugly Mug in Ypsilanti for providing a little writing haven (that reminds me of home) and my Black Comedy class at the University of Michigan in the winter of 2005 for keeping me honest and open to myriad interpretations of black comedy—at the lectern and in this volume. The "phraseology" and audio aid of Aaron Dresner and Jeff Navarre, respectively, and the sustenance (physical and emotional) provided by Reina Leber and Michael Thomas Griffin were greatly appreciated. Thanks to Scott Olin and Anna Jonsson for attending to the detail work that I could not have managed on my own and to Connie Ejarque and Sue Kirby for providing far more than administrative aid. The advice, guidance, and support of Daniel Bernardi, Robin Means Coleman, Susan Douglas, Herman Gray, and Catherine Squires (my scholarly sister since the summer of 2005) were invaluable at pivotal times in the drafting of the manuscript. The eleventh-hour labor and support of my de facto research assistants—Megan Biddinger, Takeshia Brooks, and Stephanie Wooten—and the tireless, ongoing efforts of Emily Chivers Yochim and Sarah B. Crymble were more vital than I can possibly express. As always, I am indebted to Teshome Gabriel and John Caldwell: there would be no *Laughing Mad* (nor scholarly career) had you not acted as my advisers, advocates, and most cherished mentors. Special thanks to the Joseph and Bolinda Kahr Scholarship Fund, which has undoubtedly saved this academic more times than I care to mention, and Kevin Hayes, my hip-hop sensei, who gave guidance and cred to a scholar who came late to the rap game. My deepest gratitude to Beretta Smith-Shomade, Jennifer Skulte Ouaiss, Whitney Haggins, Val Frederick, Bo Kahr, Kat Albrandt, Kristen Haggins, and Alena Wilson, my sisters/editors/audience/cheerleaders/confidantes. Finally, I thank my mother, Pearl, for the strength and fortitude to face and surmount obstacles, in work and in life, and my late father, John, for the belief that each of us, in our own way, can make a difference—and for his mild smile that assured me that there was always some goodness to be found in laughter.

*Laughing Mad*

# Introduction

*"MY JAW WAS TIGHT."* I can't remember the first time I heard this phrase but I'm sure that it was my father who spoke it—whether in response to a slight on the job, an injustice in the world, or a blatantly bad call made by some person in a position of authority. When recounting the incident, which in a different man might have elicited either a stream of obscenities or other exclamations of anger and frustration, my father would say with a mild smile, "I wasn't angry, but my jaw was tight." Decades later, when I heard Richard Pryor say, in a sketch on his short-lived television series, that his jaw was tight—expressing his resentment that the then Los Angeles Rams had released their first and only black quarterback, James Harris—I was struck by the resonance of those words. Arguably, there have not been two more different black men on the planet than Richard Pryor and my father—one a comedy icon who profanely and profoundly gave voice to the black experience and lived life with operatic bravado, the other a strong, gentle working man, who was raised in the segregated South, served in World War II, a former sailor, whose idea of "hard" language was "hey, fella," and who, along with his wife of forty-nine years, struggled to make sure that his six daughters attained a larger piece of the American Dream. Yet the phrase ties them together—and me to both of them. What does it mean when "your jaw is tight"—the physical reality of teeth clenched, unable or unwilling to speak, biding your time, holding your tongue, not saying the things that you yearn to say. And what do you mean when you say, "My jaw was tight," and how does one respond to the African American legacy of enforced silences: with covert conversations, with sly stories embedded in trickster tales, with kitchen-table witticisms and wisdom. The antithesis of one's jaw being tight has been performed in monologues on the Chitlin' Circuit, on comedy club main stages, and on myriad screens, large and small: mouths open, laughing mad is a liberatory act.

Rooted in a history where commentary and critique had to be coded for *the folks* (to borrow Zora Neale Hurston's oft-repeated moniker for African American communities), black comedy is tied inextricably to the African

American condition. As the annunciation of laughing mad, black comedy also supplied laughter for (white) mainstream audiences when constructed through the narrowing and diminishing lens of minstrel tropes. Nonetheless, the function of humor and the therapeutic value of the accompanying laughter, inside safe, communal black spaces—whether Granny's front porch or center stage at the Apollo—spoke to specific black experiences. As Langston Hughes notes in the autobiographical prose of *The Big Sea*, the laughter was, more often than not, the weapon used to fight the pain. Providing emotional paraphrasing of lyrical blues sung by "an old beggar with a guitar," Hughes writes:

> You don't know,
> You don't know my mind—
> When You see me laughin'
> I'm laughin' to keep from cryin'[1]

Black comedy, in its literal and literary construction, has always overtly *and* covertly explored the trials, tribulations, and triumphs of African American communities. Yet, as Wil Haygood aptly notes, crossover complicates by the manner in which black humor has been produced and consumed: "The Negro comic's trajectory has gone from minstrel shows and outdoor tents, from honky-tonks to Greenwich Village saloons, from amphitheaters to the big screen. Laughter washing over them like brittle sunshine. Sometimes the laughter is of a confused sort, owing to misinterpretation, the joke merged with history and the ears of whites placed at awkward angles."[2]

This book's aim is to examine the circulation of the black comedic social discourse by focusing on black comic personae that have become firmly ensconced in contemporary mainstream American popular consciousness. By offering detailed analyses of different personae (in their movement across mediums) and the varying ideological and pedagogical imperatives in their comedic discourse, *Laughing Mad* explores the place of African Americans in mainstream American comedy and popular culture and how, by performing myriad notions of blackness, they do or do not speak of and to multiple black experiences. In addition, by interrogating the nature of the laughter fostered by these comic personae, I hope to explore why "crossover" still plays a role in both interracial and intraracial discussions of race within the problematic genre of comedy.

In the years prior to the civil rights movement, the black comic persona occupied clearly delineated spaces for black and white audiences. Crossing over, while possible for a few, required strict adherence to codes of conduct that did not transparently challenge the race relations of the day. The path from America's first black crossover star, Bert Williams, who, in burnt cork, on the vaudeville and theater stages of the late-nineteenth century and early twentieth, managed to humanize the dim "darky" and dig deeply into the *actual* pathos of the minstrel trope as fodder for his humor while never threatening his mainstream audience, to the cinematic frightened physicality of Mantan Moreland's "cooning" and televisual iterations of the misspeaking "Sambo"-like dandy of Tim Moore's Kingfish on *Amos 'n' Andy* is long and circuitous. Yet the conception and reception of black comedy on this trek, which varied widely, depending on the audience, illustrates how black comic personae, like the African American condition, were diffused and often distorted in mainstream popular consciousness.

The civil rights movement not only transformed multiple black ideologies—social and political practices, as well as black thought—but it also changed the nature of black comedy. By 1963, the centennial of the Emancipation Proclamation, the African American condition could not be ignored as the battles for civil rights were waged on multiple fronts—and this part of the revolution was televised. The media coverage of the civil rights struggle forced the recognition of racial inequality into American popular consciousness and acted as a catalyst for growing the movement. Moreover, as television news programming brought the images of Birmingham (peaceful protestors being beaten, sprayed by high-pressure fire hoses, and attacked by dogs at the order of Police Commissioner Bull Connor), as well as Washington, D.C. (the historic march that culminated with Dr. King's famous "I Have a Dream" speech), into living rooms across the country and across the world, race was placed squarely on the discursive table in a highly visible way.

Dick Gregory was there—in Birmingham and in Washington. In 1960 the clean-cut comic, dressed in the conservative manner that replicated the civil rights protestors of the era (a dark suit and tie), had broken the color line when he brought sociopolitically charged black humor to the comedy club mainstream. By 1963 Gregory, whose comedy confronted racial inequality, was using his celebrity to bring attention to the struggle: Gregory was on the front line, leading the first wave of black teens and children in the Children's Crusade of the Birmingham protest. On May 20, 1963, after being released from jail, the comic addressed the nonviolent protestors congregated at St. John's Baptist Church: "One of [the] greatest problems the Negro has in America today is that we have never been able to control our image. The man downtown has always controlled our image. He has always told us how we're supposed to act. He has always told us a nigger know his place—and he don't mean this, because if we knew our place he wouldn't have to put all those signs up."[3] One of many truisms spoken that day to a congregation of the civil rights faithful, this humorous statement was also emblematic of the content of Gregory's comedy. Strong, declarative statements elicited knowing laughter from this audience as it did from those who watched Gregory onstage at The Hungry I in San Francisco or The Playboy Club in Chicago—as well as those who were introduced to the comic via the electronic hearth. As part of the "New Comic" movement, in which Lenny Bruce challenged social and cultural mores and Mort Sahl contested intellectual and political complacency, Gregory challenged everything—and, in so doing, changed the nature of the laughter in black comedy.

No longer was the laughter solely to keep from crying; the civil rights moment marked the beginning of black humor's potential power as an unabashed tool for social change, for the unfiltered venting of cultural and political anger, and for the annunciation of blackness. The humor, as conceived and received within the community, spoke to a deep cultural impulse, extending beyond articulating suffering in muted tones to howling about oppression and subjugation, as well as the victories in survival and amidst strife. Comics and audiences were laughing *mad*.

Over the past forty-five years the black comedian and African American comedy have become progressively more central to *mainstream* popular culture. Just as other forms of black cultural production, such as music—from blues to jazz to soul to funk to hip-hop—that have been sampled (literally and figuratively) and embraced by those on the cutting edge of hipness (or those endeavoring to position themselves there), the black comic emerged as a player in post–civil rights era American comedy. Then as now, the black comic's access to the mainstream pool is restricted by both industrial and taste-cultural imperatives that reflect the sociohistorical moment. Whereas Bill Cosby and Pryor are icons in American comedy, Eddie Murphy, Whoopi Goldberg, Chris Rock, and Dave Chappelle represent new breeds of black comedy for the latter half of the twentieth century and the beginning of the new millennium—the black comedic A-list actor with crossover appeal. Although the term *crossover* carries with it the problematic baggage of liberal-pluralist notions of inclusion and industrial imperatives of market share and box office, one cannot ignore the fact that the number of black comics who consistently engage audiences across lines of race, class, culture, and region are relatively few. The process of crossover— and the extension of both humor and influence beyond black communal spaces—adds a problematic twist to the already Byzantine task faced by the African American comic: to be funny, accessible, and topical while retaining his or her *authentic* black voice.

In *Laughing Mad* I offer a cultural theory–informed analysis of a small swath of this rich comedic history of black comic personae as products of the "post-soul era." The term *post soul*, coined by cultural critic Nelson George, refers to the period after the black power movements. George's assessment of the post-soul babies' experience positions them in a time of extreme changes after an era of *great* change:

> They came of age in the aftermath of an era when many of the obvious barriers to the American Dream had fallen. Black people now voted wherever and whenever they wanted and attended integrated schools. They . . . hurried toward a future with a different set of assumptions from any minority kids in American history. . . .
>
> . . . As they grew up, both the black middle class and the black lower class expanded; they grew up with Wall Street greed, neo-con ideology, Atari

Gameboys, crack, AIDS, Afrocentricity, and Malcolm X as movie hero, political icon, and marketing vehicle.[4]

While George names the group from whom both the buppie and B–Boy emerged, Mark Anthony Neal narrows the chronological framework for those he terms "children of soul," born between the march on Washington in 1963 and the Supreme Court decision in *The Regents of the University of California v. Bakke* case (although I would extend the framework back in time to include the late boomers—those born after the beginning of the sit-in movement in Greensboro and the election of JFK in 1960).[5] Regardless of the term (or which exact time line, for that matter) one prefers, one can discern what forces impacted the processes of identity formation for those whose coming of age coincided with the burgeoning post-soul era. As Neal states, these were the black folks "who came to maturity in the age of Reaganomics and experienced the change from urban industrialism to deindustrialism, from segregation to desegregation, from essential notions of blackness to meta-narratives on black-ness, without any nostalgic allegiance to the past . . . but firmly in grasp of the existential concerns of this brave new world."[6]

Understanding the sociohistorical positioning of this group is vital to this study because the most significant voices in contemporary black comedy are— either chronologically or spiritually—post-soul babies whose comic personae are inflected by complex tastes and cultural practices that emerged in the post–civil rights era, as well as by race, class, gender, and region. Those practices are experiential, based on individual and communal experiences of the African American condition, but they are also mediated: post-soul babies are media babies. The comic persona of the post-soul baby may, albeit rarely, reflect a view of black cultural productions and sociopolitical discourses through rose-colored glasses; but more often than not it is with jaundiced eyes—and this kind of hopeful cynicism (or cynical hopefulness) permeates contemporary black comedy and the construction of the black comic persona.

The comic persona is the performance of the intersection of multiple ide-ologies and lived experiences. My choice to focus on the persona, which is con-structed by acculturation, individual choice, and industrial imperatives—rather than the person—allows for the close examination of the inherent tenuousness of the black comic's place in contemporary American comedy. By probing the disparities between the stand-up comedian's comic persona and the one con-structed for cinematic and televisual consumption, I investigate the tensions between contemporary representations of blackness and the dichotomies embed-ded in the term *crossover* (whether achieved by homogenization or as a result of shifts in taste cultures). Given that *Laughing Mad* is not intended to be a "star" study, the autobiographical details that often inflect the content of the comic's act will be included only when necessary to understand how this background is utilized in the construction of the comic persona. This book teases out the ways that the black comic persona provides the lens through which sociocultural and sociohistorical shifts in notions of race might be observed—both within the African American community and within mainstream popular culture.

One might be tempted to assert that the edges of the African American comic's rant are trimmed to fit into the construct of a movie star's shtick, with the comedic social commentary—along with the critical bite—left on the cutting room floor. While there are instances when this is undoubtedly true, this volume will illustrate that the trade-offs are far less transparent when complex processes of aesthetic, ideological, and industrial compromise cloud notions of complicity and culpability. Historically, the black comic has retained the ability to get the audience laughing while slipping in sociocultural truths. The boundless promise of the African American comedic actor in social screen comedy, however, remains for the most part unfulfilled as the performance of blackness continues to be made more culturally digestible for mass consumption.

One could argue that the stand-up material of a majority of the aforementioned A-list black comics has placed them on the critical cutting edge of black comedy—as comedic cultural critics with unique insights on the African American (and American) condition. "The comic-as-cultural-critic-and-social-commentator does not merely celebrate or valorize the culture from which he or she emerges. Such comics enable us to understand our culture as they honestly explore it and thus help explain black culture's internal contradictions, stress its positive features and acknowledge its detrimental characteristics."[7] Michael Eric Dyson eloquently presents the ideal comedic cultural critic as one not only clear on his or her ideology and pedagogy but also unflinching and unmerciful in his or her comedic critique. This description is reminiscent of Mikhail Bakhtin's definition of the role of the rogue, the fool, and the clown in the novel. These figures have, says Bakhtin,

> a privilege—the right to be "other" in this world, the right not to make common causes with any single one of the existing categories that life makes available; . . . they see the underside and the falseness of every situation. . . . Their laughter bears the stamp of the public square where the folk gather. They re-establish the public nature of the human figure: the entire being of characters such as these is, after all, utterly on the surface; everything is brought out on to the square. . . . This creates that distinctive means for externalizing a human being, via parodic laughter.[8]

Given that the stand-up comic's persona might arguably be a conflation of the three (the rogue, the clown, and the fool), Bakhtin's assertion that the clown is constructed in opposition to "everything that is conventional and false" (162) seems to capture the essential directive of the comic as cultural critic. According to Bakhtin the laughter elicited by the comic is "of the public square"— understood and defined collectively by and directed to the very community, which the comic (necessarily) lampoons. Consequently, this definition, which extols the comic's conflation of the insider's knowledge of the community and the outsider's objective view, is part of what empowers the comedic cultural critic to expose the "internal contradictions" within myriad aspects of black life for "us" (African Americans), while still speaking to the multiple forms of hegemony one experiences while living as a black person in America. In order for the comedic discourse produced by the black comic to be effectively edifying, it must be self-aware *and* self-reflexive—able to illicit thought along with the laughter. Given industrial limitations, as well as the "ideas" regarding audience expectations of the comic persona as filtered through primetime network (or netlet) television or mainstream Hollywood film comedy, it appears that following this pedagogical directive becomes progressively more problematic as the comic moves from one medium to the next.

Interestingly, discussion of the African American comic is frequently segregated into discourses around a specific medium—television comedy, film comedy, and stand-up comedy—or a specific genre or subgenre—the interracial buddy film, the ghetto sitcom, or the "black block" sitcoms on Fox, the WB, or UPN. In terms of television history, J. Fred MacDonald's *Blacks and White TV* and Donald Bogle's *Primetime Blues* provide definitive surveys of televisual representations of blackness. While each author grapples with the roles played by depictions of blackness in television and their impact on and reflection of popular culture, the African American comedian is discussed in relationship to specific televisual texts (Jimmie Walker on *Good Times*, Bill Cosby on *The Cosby Show*, Martin Lawrence on *Martin*). MacDonald addresses the connections between the medium's practices, its representations, and their impact on the televisual spectator, acknowledging that because of the limited number of African Americans on prime time, "each performance by an African-American is regarded as a chance to make a statement about realities, [and] each appearance takes on additional weight."[9] Bogle traces the repetition of black stereotypes from the moment of television to the present and underscores the significance of the black "star" to African American audiences: "Black viewers might reject the nonsense of the scripts on some episodes of *Sanford and Son* or *The Jeffersons* or *Martin*. . . . But they never really rejected a Redd Foxx or a Sherman Hemsley or Martin Lawrence."[10]

In *Revolution Televised: Prime Time and the Struggle for Black Power*, Christine Acham skillfully melds historical and textual analysis of significant black-oriented television programs, including *Tom Brown's Journal*, *Soul Train*, *The Flip Wilson Show*, *Sanford and Son*, and *The Richard Pryor Show*. Acham brings to light the "social, political and industrial factors brought about in [the] shift from invisibility to hyperblackness in the late 1960s and 1970s."[11] By supplying detailed biographical and performance background on black comics such as Flip Wilson, Redd Foxx, and Richard Pryor, Acham situates programs within a rich sociopolitical and sociohistorical context of televised black experience in the post–civil rights era.

In *Watching Race* Herman Gray explores the manner in which "blackness" is "played out" in contemporary televisual narratives and endeavors to reveal how these narratives "push [African Americans] towards an imaginary center."[12] Gray asserts that the discourse of race is informed by "the key cultural and symbolic figure in American politics in the 1980s, the 'sign of blackness' [which] circulated in a conservative-dominated discursive field, where it continually served to galvanize, articulate, and mobilize the central issues facing frightened, angry, and resentful white Americans. From the Willie Horton political ads and nightly news representations of black criminality, which stirred and fed white fears, to *The Cosby Show*, which quieted them," Gray traces the industrial shifts that seem to run counter to the ideological imperatives of Reaganism.[13] Gray asserts that television programs like *Julia* and *I-Spy* can be seen within the context of "assimilationist discourse," with an ethos of invisibility (where specific social-political issues and racism are constructed as "individual problems"), while series like *The Jeffersons* and *The Cosby Show* fall into the category of "Separate but Equal" (pluralist) discourse, where black characters live and work in hermetically sealed social milieus that are approximately equivalent to their white counterparts. In the shows of the pluralist discourse cultural difference is explored without ever coming into direct conflict with "mainstream" America by "critiquing the hegemonic character of (middle-class constructions of) whiteness or, for that matter, the totalizing constructions of blackness."[14] The final category of discourse, "Multicultural/Diversity," is exemplified by the short-lived series *Frank's Place*, *A Different World*, and *In Living Color*, which "seldom, if ever, adjusted its representation of African American cultural experiences to the gaze of an idealized white middle class audience."[15] These discursive categories (assimilationist, pluralist, and multicultural) correspond to iterations of comic personae whose humor is purposefully designed to serve much the same function as the aforementioned comedies (from *Julia* to *Frank's Place*): to speak for and to very specific audiences.

Like *Watching Race*, Beretta Smith-Shomade's *Shaded Lives* examines televisual representations of blackness from the eighties to the present; however, Smith-Shomade's interrogation of the representations of African American women across genres (situation comedy, talk show, music videos, new programming) reveals inherent disparities between the essentialized constructions of black womanhood as televisually realized and the lived experiences of black women. Smith-Shomade's examination of the construction of black women in the situation comedy is particularly instructive in its systematic analysis of these representations as inflected by class and sexuality, as well as race. Smith-Shomade speaks directly to the narrative marginalization of black women's voices in comedy, which most certainly extends beyond the fictions of the small screen. Astutely observing that sitcoms of the nineties often "excavated stereotypes of White women and superimposed them on Black ones," Smith-Shomade also notes that "the greater proportion of Black women's representations remained in supporting, mammified, and one-dimensional capacities."[16] *Shaded Lives* sheds light on the unsettling tendency for the normative elements of dominant culture to seep into black comedy. Perhaps more significant, however, Smith-Shomade examines the plethora of ways that black women's place in comedy is limited by conflicting media images (each of which purports to capture the essence of a singular black female subject), generic conventions, and narrative biases that continue to inflect the stories that are told about black women and that they, in turn, tell about themselves.

Black comedy, and by extension the black comic, often receives "limited" attention when included in film histories that discuss the genre within the larger rubric of contemporary black film. According to Thomas Cripps's *Making Movies Black* these messages were delivered in dramas but not in film comedy. Donald Bogle's *Toms, Coons, Mulattoes, Mammies, and Bucks* provides a historical look at a select group of black comedy "stars" to emblematize the relationship between the comedian as comic force and the context of trends in black and white film of their respective eras. While Bogle also touches on the lives and filmic careers of Whoopi Goldberg and Eddie Murphy, his analysis of the *cinematic* constructions of Richard Pryor is the most expansive, rooted in both comedic and industrial shifts of the seventies and eighties. Bogle traces Pryor's progress as comedic actor through the "crazy nigger" incarnations of *Richard Pryor: Live in Concert* (1979) and *Uptown Saturday Night* (1974) to the diluted version of that comic persona in the role that brought him "co-starring" fame in *Silver Streak* (1976). Bogle ends this analysis with the eighties' cinematic iteration of a Pryor who was disconcerting in pedestrian comedic roles like *Superman III* (1983), in which, Bogle notes, "he looks like a terr'fied Willie Best wandering through the haunted house with Bob Hope in *The Ghost Breakers*."[17] The use of textual analysis of these film roles in Bogle's de facto "star" studies and Ed Guerrero's analysis of Richard Pryor and Eddie Murphy's stints in the biracial buddy oeuvre of the late seventies and eighties (with Gene Wilder as Pryor's white counterpart, and various Anglo actors, including Nick Nolte and Dan Ackroyd as Murphy's) gives rich narrative and character detail that justifiably complicates the quasi-integrationist "We Are the World" rhetoric that informs this subgenre.

Mel Watkins's *On the Real Side*, which explores the roots and routes of black comedy, most assuredly informed the post–civil rights era analysis in this study. As the title suggests, Watkins's exhaustive and insightful history of African American comedy traces the multiple facets of the performance and reception of African American humor. The subversions of minstrel narratives—the little "victories" necessarily "hidden" in character construction, plot, and performance that went unseen by white audiences—to the bold sociopolitical critique of Dick Gregory, whose politically informed and socially aware comedic discourse acted as a model for Pryor, his contemporary, and Rock, his comic progeny, Watkins celebrates the expansiveness, resilience, and ingenuity of African American comedy.

Unlike studies that focused predominantly on either a single medium (stage performance, film, or television), individual televisual or cinematic texts or the comic star, or Watkins's work, which endeavors to span the breadth of black comedy's history, this volume traces the movement of individual black comic personae across media in the latter part of the twentieth century and early twenty-first. In order to determine how the culturally and industrially determined construct of the black comedian's persona is in conversation with both his or her era and the African American condition, *Laughing Mad* provides detailed and nuanced readings of the acts, the televisual and cinematic roles, and the extratextual presence of four post-soul comics, whose arrival in the promised land of crossover came early in their careers and for whom keeping it "real" has been an ongoing struggle, with varying levels of success. Before one can understand where these post-soul comics were (and are) going, it is necessary to understand who had made that comic middle passage before them.

The first chapter provides the requisite background to this cultural study by examining the comic televisual and cinematic personae of four comedians who came of comic age during the sixties and early seventies: Dick Gregory, Bill Cosby, Flip Wilson, and Richard Pryor. As the comic equivalent of the Talented Tenth, their presence in comic mainstream expanded the possibilities for the black comic's success. Examining the paths of these comics reveals how they set the stage for black comedy in the next four decades and how the progression of their comedic trajectories acted as ideological and pedagogical models for the black comedians of the post–civil rights era. The progressively controversial nature of Gregory's comic discourse acted as a de facto decision for him to abandon the quest for crossover success. For Cosby and Pryor the easy move from stand-up stage to television and film, respectively, corresponded to both the historical moment and the "suitability" of their comic personae to the medium into which they sought entry, whereas for both Gregory and Wilson the movement (or lack thereof) was determined as much by individual agency as by the cultural and/or medium specificity of their comedic styles. If there is, indeed, a correlation between ease of entry and mainstream friendliness, it is more circuitous than direct—particularly when one considers that Pryor's "crazy nigger" persona (which was extremely marketable in concert films but entirely unpalatable to prime-time television) could be tailored to fit into the interracial buddy offerings, whereas Cosby's incarnation as comic for *all* audiences brought him the status of televisual icon but never allowed him to emerge as the star in a successful mainstream film comedy. Nonetheless, the career trajectories of these comics, as well as the ways in which their contributions to both black and American comedy have been valorized, vilified, or forgotten, provide both template and cautionary tale to the post-soul generation.

Chapters 2 and 3 examine the comedic development and transformation of Eddie Murphy and Chris Rock as emblematic of the first and second waves, respectively, of post–civil rights era African American comedy. Just as the issue of crossover success was problematic for their civil rights era predecessors, Murphy and Rock navigate the tumultuous waters of the entertainment mainstream with varying levels of success. The examination of the incarnations of Murphy's and Rock's comic personae—as constructed in stand-up and on television in chapter 2 and as realized cinematically and industrially in chapter 3—reveals the changing parameters for what it means to be crossover-friendly. Clearly, their brands of stand-up audaciousness differ—Murphy's "blue" bad boy rap (sexually explicit and socially irreverent) versus Rock's scathing comedic critique (simultaneously radical and reactionary in sociopolitical terms). Both of their comic personae, however, have been "reframed" and "retooled" for mainstream consumption in ways that replicate some of the transformations made by their comic predecessors.

While the changes in Murphy's filmic persona—from Axel Foley's sexualized savvy in the *Beverly Hills Cop* oeuvre to John Doolittle's affable and harried "every-dad-ness" in the *Doctor Doolittle* movies—may seem more extreme than Rock's comic alterations—from cultural critic to new millennial populist hero in classical Hollywood-informed films *Down to Earth* and *Head of State*, both sets of transformations speak to the place of the black comic actor in mainstream comedy. Although no longer de facto second bananas (as in Pryor's roles with Gene Wilder), neither are they exactly comic leading men or direct cinematic iterations of their stand-up personae. When one examines the cinematic translation of Murphy's and Rock's comic personae for mainstream consumption, the questions about the cost of crossover in terms of comedic content and cultural specificity are brought into relief. In keeping self-aware and self-conscious in construction, Murphy's and Rock's comic personae provide partially translated enunciations of blackness that speak to various audiences on variable registers. Thus, for the first and second waves of the post–civil rights era, the emergent black comic persona is necessarily culturally and stylistically hybrid—borrowing, losing, keeping aspects of black experiences that can be utilized as "accessible" material in temporally relevant, medium-specific performances of blackness.

In chapter 4 the intersecting issues of gender, crossover, and sociocultural politics are revealed as integral to Whoopi Goldberg's comic persona. From her Mike Nichols–directed Broadway debut in 1984 to her revised revival of her one-woman show in 2005, from her Oscar-winning turn as Oda Mae Brown in *Ghost* (1990) to her short-lived stint as the spokesperson for Slim-Fast, the comic actor has been consistently engaged in the practice of crossover. Furthermore, with the possible exceptions of Chitlin' Circuit veteran and mainstream sensation Moms Mabley and Pearl Bailey, the "down-home" diva of the stage (Broadway and nightclub), no black female comics have been able to gain the access and success in the entertainment mainstream that Whoopi Goldberg has attained. Yet, as a black woman in American comedy, Goldberg has had to confront gendered notions of "how to be funny," as well as those tied to the function of racial and cultural specificity in stand-up comedy, in the theater, and on the big and small screens in the post–civil rights era. Understanding Goldberg's emergence as a crossover diva requires that one look to the past and future of crossover and the black female comic. Through the exploration of the comic kinship between Bailey, Mabley, Goldberg, and diva-in-training Wanda Sykes, one begins to discern how these crossover divas play with and against the cultural politics of sexuality, gender, and race. Moreover, when one examines the correlations between the constant and shifting aspects of Goldberg's comic personae and those of her black female comic predecessors and progeny, the intersections between the extratextual construction of their personae and the impact of the openly espoused politics of each woman on both the mediated construction of her persona and its degree of mainstream acceptance offers fascinating commentary on the position of the black female comic in the second half of the twentieth century and the beginning of the twenty-first.[18]

Chapter 5 explores the emergence of Dave Chappelle as a new millennial comic wunderkind. By tracing the comic lineage of the sketch/variety show from Richard Pryor's series in the late seventies through *In Living Color's* netlet era birth in the early nineties, one can discern how and why *Chappelle's Show* marks a point of rupture *and* a point of convergence for conflicting ideological impulses. One can also begin to see how the de facto crossover appeal of the series problematizes the series' and the comic's unique status as industrial and cultural phenomena. Furthermore, the tensions between the comic's stand-up persona and those of his series in terms of the internal and external pressures of widespread de facto crossover success (from the comic himself and from the black community, as well as from his audience, black and white, and from industrial forces, respectively) also must be probed when exposing Chappelle's status as a comic provocateur extraordinaire. Thus, this volume concludes by raising new questions about the presence of emergent black comic voices—across media—that might direct future studies on African American comedy to interrogate further the significant impact of the post-soul baby throughout black and mainstream American popular culture and consciousness. "The post-soul imagination . . . has been fueled by three distinct critical desires, namely, the reconstitution of community, particularly one that is critically engaged with the cultural and political output of black communities; a rigorous form of self and communal critique; and the willingness to undermine or deconstruct the most negative symbols and stereotypes of black life via the use and distribution of those very same symbols and stereotypes."[19]

The comic personae and sensibilities of the post–civil rights era comedians examined in *Laughing Mad* resonate with this rumination on the post-soul imagination. By using the microphone as a weapon in comedic discursive combat, Murphy, Rock, Goldberg, and Chappelle have interrogated myriad social and political maladies, including issues of race, and have spoken to multiple articulations of blackness. Yet their comic critique of black communities, social practices, and media representation, whether in their acts or their televisual and cinematic endeavors, have drawn praise and condemnation from the entertainment mainstream, as well as disparate segments of the very communities they are purported to represent. Whether one considers Goldberg and Murphy, whose comic emergence took place in the eighties, on the cusp of the post-soul era; Rock, in the nineties; and Chappelle, in the new millennium, firmly embedded in a post-soul aesthetic, their comic personae are all in contentious conversation with the sociopolitical milieu of contemporary American society. No doubt excavating these discursive processes and the historical, industrial, and social factors that inflect them will provide an instructive base on which further sociohistorical cultural study on black comedy can be constructed. Without underestimating the significance of my theoretical goals, my most sincere wish is that this book provides insight into how these performers make us laugh when dealing—or not dealing—with race.

My thoughts return to the conflation of emotions and histories in the phrase "my jaw was tight"—those words that, with poignant playfulness, serve to concretize a response to social, political, and economic realities of oppression . . . for my father, for Pryor, for me. Exposing the subtext—the sociohistorical and industrial factors that inform both the material and our reception of it—and discerning the nature of the laughter that the joke, the act, the episode, or the film representation elicits are key to understanding whether the multiplicity of African American identities and black cultural productions are able to resonate with enough force to register not only in mainstream American comedy but in American popular consciousness. But nagging questions remain. How are these comic black voices being acknowledged and constructed—as comedic discourse or as easily dismissed light entertainment without either critical or ideological bite? And what of the laughter? Is it nervous laughter or patronizing laughter? Or are the comic players themselves, like many of us in the audience, jaws still tight, laughing mad? In the end I hope these questions will not be rhetorical.

# CHAPTER 1

# From Negro to Black

## COMING OF COMIC AGE
## IN THE CIVIL RIGHTS ERA

BILL COSBY'S *WONDERFULNESS* was the first comedy album I ever heard. I remember the feeling of anticipation as I watched my older sister lift the center panel of the huge walnut Philco stereo console and place the LP on the turntable. With the static crackle, as the needle hit the vinyl, I listened to Cosby recount, for a generation at least once removed from radio days, his experience of listening to the Lights Out presentation of "The Chicken Heart Who Ate New York City." Even though in this early routine the young Cosby torched a couch and smeared Jell-O to deter the radio-generated "Chicken Heart" monster, his material was always seen as acceptable fare for kids trapped inside on smog-alert days or, on occasion, as after-dinner family-time entertainment. In the mid-sixties Cosby's comedic style and persona represented "ideal" and "idealized" aspects of American Negro life (although by 1966, in our family in Pasadena, California, we were already "black"). This was my introduction to black stand-up comedy.

Fast-forward to 1975. I sat with a bunch of kids in the basement of a friend's house waiting to watch *Saturday Night Live* because Richard Pryor was hosting. I had listened to *That Nigger's Crazy* in the back office of my high school's journalism room. My folks preferred the "old, clean" Richard to the "crazy nigger," with whom I was enthralled, whose act was raw and real and spoke to a black experience that had previously gone fundamentally unspoken. Pryor's monologue was strong—working the edgier side of the drug culture material so popular back then—but it was the "Job Interview" scene, often referred to as the "Word Association" sketch, with Chevy Chase that was both hilarious and, unexpectedly, provocative. As a personnel director interviewing Pryor for a job, Chase asks Pryor to do a word association exercise—which degenerates from a harmless verbal test into an exchange of racial slurs:

CHASE: Colored.
PRYOR: Redneck.
CHASE: Jungle Bunny.

PRYOR: Peckerwood.
CHASE: Burrhead.
PRYOR: Cracker.
CHASE: Spear-chucker.
PRYOR: White Trash.
CHASE: Jungle Bunny!
PRYOR: Honky.
CHASE: Spade!
PRYOR: Honky-honky!
CHASE: Nigger!
PRYOR: Deeeead honky!

It seemed that we were all laughing uproariously at first, but then I noticed a difference in our laughter. I caught one friend steal a quick guilty look at me—to make sure I was laughing, too. Another surveyed the room and didn't laugh at all until she was sure that everyone else thought it was *really* funny. While this could easily be written off as an example of peer-pressure-induced paranoia or just a puzzling memory, the truth of the matter is that I was the only black person in the room. The exchange of looks seemed fairly insignificant at the time, but the change—the difference—in the laughter stuck with me.

The names *Cosby* and *Pryor* have iconic currency in the world of American comedy—yet there are other black comics of the civil rights era who gained both access and success in significant pockets of the American entertainment mainstream. For me, and I fear many other post-soul babies, the name *Dick Gregory* was associated more with political activism (from marches to hunger strikes), dietary zealotry, and conspiracy theories than his revolutionary position as a black comic who used the microphone as a weapon. During my undergraduate research on celebrities in the civil rights movement I saw Gregory, as a "comic/political activist," on news programs, at rallies, and in documentaries: being beaten and arrested in Birmingham, Alabama, marching on Washington, and having been shot in Watts trying to quell the rage amidst the 1966 riots.

Dick Gregory was a pioneer in the politicization of American comedy. Clad in suit and tie (a Brooks Brothers suit), Gregory replicated in his appearance the visual construction of the legion of civil rights volunteers from SNCC and CORE seen on the nightly news in the early sixties. The comic's persona exuded sophistication and provided a black cultural position that was unapologetically urban and urbane. Gregory brought socially conscious racial humor to the main stages of the premiere comedy-club circuit and, later, the couches of late-night television talk in a time when, as Juan Williams said, "the Civil Rights movement forced America to confront its very unfunny history of racism."[1] Gregory's contribution to changing the nature of American comedy, which should have positioned him alongside Lenny Bruce as a twentieth-century comedy pioneer, had a marginalized space in my consciousness simply because

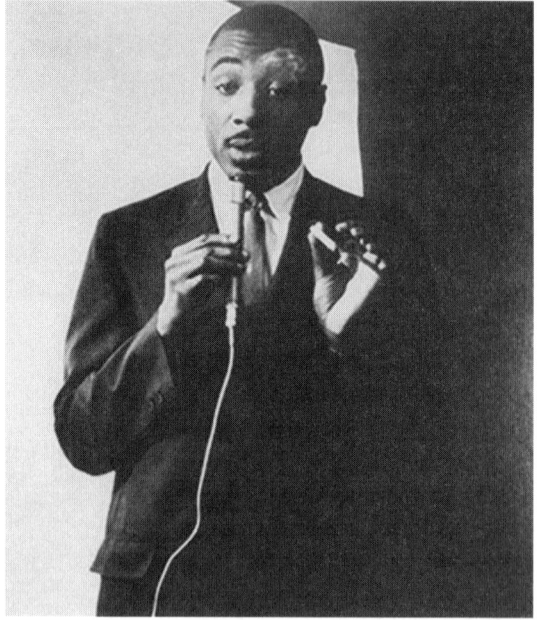

1. In the post–Playboy Club press photos, mainstream America was introduced to the urban and urbane Mr. Gregory (1961). Photo from Photofest.

I did not realize how the content of Gregory's comedy and the strength of his politicized character continues to reverberate through African American comedic discourse. Like other (personally unsubstantiated) legends from a previous era, Gregory was a figure I respected, but prior to this study my reverence was mitigated by my lack of knowledge.

I did, however, know that Flip Wilson, like Cosby, had been a television star. Wilson's fame was at its pinnacle during the early adolescence of this particular post-soul baby. For the first two seasons of his series our family, like millions of other Americans, watched the immensely "likable" Wilson strut his comic stuff. At the peak of the show's popularity it came in second in the Nielsen ratings to the social sitcom omega of Lear-Yorkin's *All in the Family*. *The Flip Wilson Show* "arrived just as America was slowly exploring its hipness—and its blackness. His humor was steeped in inner city traits, yet it was non-threatening enough for mainstream consumption."[2] *The Flip Wilson Show*, family fare for black and white America with a black cultural flare, owned its Thursday night prime-time slot—until *The Waltons* tapped into the nostalgia for a mythical vision of America in economic depression (which was fundamentally without folks who were poor, disgruntled, and of color) during the second half of the series' run.

Wilson, whom *Time* declared "the first Black television superstar" in 1972, created a bevy of unmistakably black characters: from the mod yet modest self-proclaimed sex symbol Geraldine Jones to the sly, evangelical huckster Reverend Leroy of the Church of What's Happening Now and, of course, the persona who was "everybody's friend," Flip. One could become enmeshed in arguments about whether the "throwback" qualities of Wilson's characters can be posited as part of progressive or regressive forces in seventies black televisual representation. Nonetheless, the fact that Wilson's presence on network television (like that of Cosby, Pryor, and Gregory) brought Negro-ness—and then blackness—into American living rooms is undeniable. Thus, in its very "likable" way Wilson's series demanded a degree of recognition for both comic diversity and multiple iterations of black identity.

Cosby and Pryor came of comic age during the era of civil rights and black power. Their comic personae, like those of Dick Gregory and Flip Wilson, can be seen as setting the stage for later black performers seeking to move from stand-up to screen; they emblematized distinct sociocultural and sociopolitical threads in black comedy during this time. Gregory's comic activist preceded Cosby's assimilationist observer, just as Wilson's affable jokester's foray into the televisual mainstream coincided with the evolution of the kinder, gentler Pryor into the "crazy nigger" cultural critic. These initial forays into the comedic "performance" of blackness would exert considerable influence on subsequent black comedians like Eddie Murphy, Chris Rock, Martin Lawrence, and Dave Chappelle. Besides the impact of their carefully cultivated personae, these four performers also provided crucial lessons in the logistics of crossover through the ease or difficulty of their transformation from comic to comedic actor—across medium and across audience, as well as across both their externally and internally defined ideological and pedagogical imperatives.

The style and content of Gregory, Cosby, Wilson, and Pryor's stand-up acts (as well as the iterations of their comic personae across mediums) mark different positions on the comedic spectrum. Each comic persona represents a differing depiction of African American identity, which, in turn, is tied to changing notions of blackness during (and after) the civil rights era. Although the careers of this quartet may have begun on the same comedic trail as Dewey "Pigmeat" Markham, Redd Foxx, Jackie "Moms" Mabley, and Slappy White, and although their humor was inflected (to varying degrees) by a comic lineage that stretched back to the original Chitlin' Circuit with the Regal in Chicago and the Apollo in Harlem as its twin capitols, the trajectories of all four personae and their comedic discourse followed a course into *mainstream* American popular consciousness. Each in his day spent time comfortably ensconced on the comic A-list and was widely embraced for his craft—whether this privileged position occurred only for a pivotal moment (Gregory's breaking the color line on main stages with socially relevant humor while utilizing his celebrity to draw attention to the picket line during the sixties) or extended through the latter half of the twentieth century and into the twenty-first (the stereotype-shattering televisual constructions of Cosby's evolving comic persona).

Nonetheless, Gregory, Cosby, Wilson, and Pryor exemplify multiple, albeit interconnecting, trajectories during times when both black humor and black cultural production were becoming progressively more central to the style and function of American comedy; thus, these four comics played significant roles in the articulation and understanding of blackness in American popular culture and society as a whole. *Laughing Mad* does not chronicle their story, although one could easily dedicate a volume to precisely that endeavor. Rather, my aim is to provide, albeit elliptically, a frame of reference requisite for mapping the trajectories of the post-soul comics and for understanding how the evolution of the black comic personae of the A-list in the next generation continues to be in conversation with the comic discourse and pedagogies of those who occupied those prized, "crossed over" spaces before them.

### DICK GREGORY: USING THE MICROPHONE AS A WEAPON

Dick Gregory, one of the first black comics to bring the critique of race relations into his act, stopped only briefly on the Chitlin' Circuit. Unlike other veteran black comics like Nipsey Russell and Slappy White (who began on the circuit and slowly worked into the white comedy clubs), Gregory went from playing Chicago's Esquire Theater to *The Tonight Show with Jack Paar* after his highly successful gig as a replacement for Professor Irwin Corey at the Chicago Playboy Club in 1961. Gregory tells that he had learned from watching others "kill" in black clubs (sometimes with integrated audiences) and "die" in whites-only clubs. Since the earliest days of his stand-up career, he had been eyeing the white comedy clubs—"where the bread is"—and was painfully cognizant of what it would take to cross over, which was the key to fiscal success and mainstream exposure: "I've got to go up there as an individual first, a Negro second. I've got to be a colored funny man, not a funny colored man. I've got to act like a star who isn't sorry for himself—that way they can't feel sorry for me. I've got to make jokes about myself before I can make jokes about them and their society—that way they can't hate me. Comedy is friendly relations."[3] Perhaps a result, in part, of his short time on the Chitlin' Circuit, his routines were a departure from either the jokester comic patter of White or Russell or the sexually explicit banter of Redd Foxx or Moms Mabley.

Yet in his breakthrough stint at the Playboy Club he complicated his "friendly relation" to the white audience by openly blasting the injustices and hypocrisies of racial inequality and, as a result, became famous for his in-your-face social and political critique.

> Good evening, ladies and gentlemen. I understand there are a good many Southerners in the room tonight. I know the South very well. I spent twenty years there one night. . . .
>
>      . . .
>
> Last time I was down south I walked into this restaurant and this white waitress came up to me and said: "We don't serve colored people here."

I said, "That's all right, I don't eat colored people. Bring me a whole fried chicken."

About that time these three cousins come in, you know the ones I mean, Klu, Kluck, and Klan, and they say: "Boy . . . anything you do to that chicken, we're gonna do to you." So I put down my knife and fork, and I picked up that chicken, and I kissed it.[4]

Gregory's triumph on white main stages quickly yielded fiscal rewards—from $5 per gig in 1961 to $6,500 per appearance in 1962. Lauded as one of the "new comics" like Mort Sahl, who left behind mother-in-law jokes in favor of humorous discourse on the American sociopolitical condition, Gregory was featured on *Bell and Howell's Close Up*, which described the humor of the new comedic cadre as "Post War humor—irreverent, biting and deliberately controversial . . . recogniz[ing] no sacred cows and few divinities."[5]

Gregory's direct engagement in racial discourse—and his very public commitment to the  civil rights movement and social justice—separated him from the rest of this "new breed" and made an indelible mark on the history of American comedy. The calmly confrontational style of Gregory's comedy was designed to provoke his audiences; as Gregory himself stated during a series of gigs at the Hungry I in San Francisco, "If I've said anything to upset you, maybe it's what I'm here for. Lenny Bruce shakes up the puritans; Mort Sahl, the conservatives; and me—almost everybody!"[6]

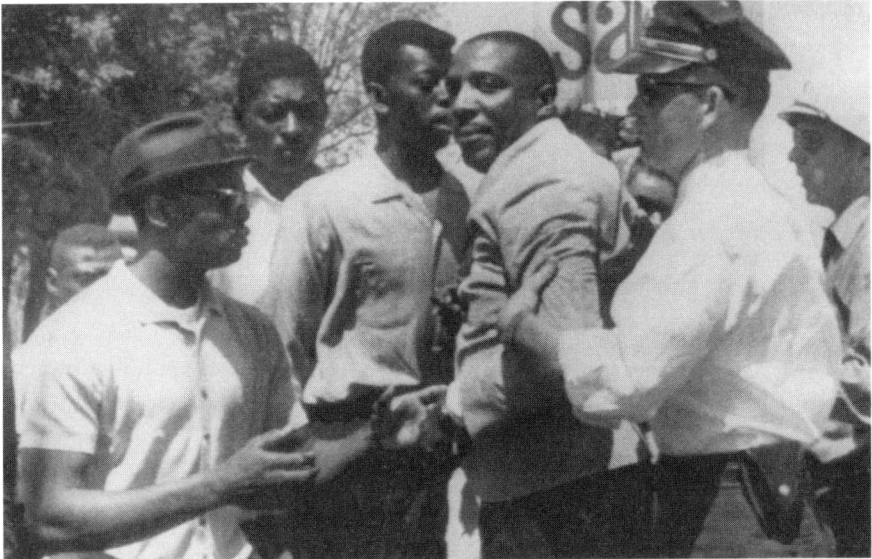

2. Dick Gregory brings star power to the civil rights struggle. Gregory (center) is arrested at a voter registration examination in Greenwood, Mississippi (April 2, 1963). Photo from Photofest.

Gregory's awareness about the power of celebrity to pull the focus of media attention (in order to get issues to the American mainstream) and his willingness to put his body where his ideology was made him an (often unsung) asset to the movement and separated him from his "New Comic" brethren. As he noted on *The Steve Allen Show* in early 1964, "To be honest, I'm so glad to be out of jail for a change."[7] In his act Gregory pondered, with self-reflexive precision and ease, the space and place that he (and, by extension, the American Negro) occupied in American society. Even though one might argue that Gregory's persona exemplified what the comic described as "the new Negro" in one late-night talk show set—"Ivy League suit, short haircut, Brylcreem— 2 dabs—but it's Brylcreem"—the comic payoff of the joke series problematized the public conception of the "good ones" by implying that there was more to the requisite performances of idealized assimilation than met the mainstream's eye: "You see us everyday: *Wall Street Journal* under one arm, *New York Times* under the other and *Jet* and *Ebony* tucked in between them."[8] Just as the mention of the additional "dab" of Brylcreem required to keep black hair smoothed down (one more than the product's jingle prescribed) in the era prior to the emergence of "the natural" or "the Afro" acts as a semantic wink to the black audience, Gregory uses the black magazines, hidden inside of periodicals associated with white intellectualism and capitalist prosperity, to slyly complicate the notion that "assimilation = uplift" by attesting to the fact that these "New Negroes," to use the vernacular of our day, were still "keeping it real." During his frequent appearances on *The Steve Allen Show*, as well as on *The Jack Paar Program* in the early sixties, Gregory used his eight minutes of stand-up and his time on the couch to disseminate information about the movement and the struggles it faced. After doing a particularly well-received set (which included the aforementioned "New Negro" material), Gregory used his couch time with Allen not to pitch a film or his next club date but to reflect on why legislation (the Civil Rights Act) could not eradicate racial inequality (particularly when institutions remain racist)—explaining to the attentive host how on every third Thursday of the month in Mississippi the names of registered voters were printed on the front page of the paper, "intimidation disguised as recognition for good citizenry." Nor did Gregory shy away from exposing that racism was not confined to the American South, as exemplified by a 1963 guest spot on Paar's series, when Gregory reflected on the state of race in his hometown of Chicago. In a time when the focus of media and popular discourse on race centered on the violence faced by those on the southern front of the struggle, Gregory's comic aside in this very public forum called attention to the fact that racism existed above the Mason-Dixon Line. With a wry, world-weary delivery, using long drags on his ever-present cigarette as punctuation for the beats of the joke series, the comic asserted that the frigid weather yielded a warming trend in race relations: "Oh yeah, the morning it was like 22 below, I was standing on the corner freezing and this guy came up to me, very cold and very angry, he said 'Why don't you go back to Africa where you belong and take me with you.'"[9] In discussing the comic persona of Gregory, it becomes progressively more difficult to separate his *act* from his *actions*. Malcolm X, who, like Martin Luther King Jr., was a personal friend of Gregory's, expounded on the comic's use of the microphone and his celebrity as a tool of revolution:

> Dick is a revolutionary. . . . Dick is one of the foremost freedom fighters in this country. I say that in all sincerity. Dick has been on the battlefront and has made great sacrifices by taking the stand that he has. . . . Whenever you see a person, a celebrity, who is as widely known and as skilled in his profession as Dick, and at the same time has access to almost unlimited bookings which provide unlimited income, and he will jeopardize all of that in order to jump into the frontlines of the battle, then you and I will have to stand behind him.[10]

By the early seventies a shift in comic pedagogy away from the "New Comic" ethos made Gregory unpalatable to the entertainment mainstream, in general, and Hollywood comedy, in particular, despite an urgent media agenda to promote blacks on television. During the same period Gregory, who had ceased performing in spaces that were not smoke and alcohol free, expanded the content of his comedy and the commitment of his activism to issues of social justice across the nation and across the world. This new content did not always receive the same warm reception that his earlier discourse on southern racism had gotten. In a 1970 appearance on the very mainstream *Ed Sullivan Show*, after the musical cut-off cue, Gregory continued the final joke series in his monologue that tied together the Black Power movement and the "troubles" in Northern Ireland. The advice that he provided for Irish Catholics of the North reverberates with a degree of cynicism and disdain for the pervasive wisdom that encouraged blacks to "go slow" as the civil rights era drew to a close and the ills of economic recession that would rack urban America for decades to come was just taking hold: "[The Irish Catholics] need to be more like black folks. Stop all the looting and burning. Pull themselves up by their bootstraps. Go out and get themselves jobs—work ain't never hurt nobody. Most of all, they must learn one thing: be patient. They're moving too fast. Harlem wasn't built in a day, baby. . . . [There were] no riots this past summer because all of the black leaders were in Ireland as technical advisers."[11] The audience response was somewhat muted, as was Sullivan's, who remarked simply, "Quite a performance."

Whether or not the content of Gregory's comedy was making him less a factor in the burgeoning world of black comedy as it moved into the mainstream, the comic's activities offstage progressively took him out of the entertainment mainstream—from his literary efforts (including his autobiography, *Nigger*) to his civil rights and social justice activism and stints as a 1967 Chicago mayoral candidate and the 1968 Freedom and Peace Party candidate for the presidency).[12] By the late sixties Gregory was calling himself a "social commentator who uses humor to interpret the needs and wants of Negroes to the white community, rather than . . . a comedian who happens to deal in topical social material." He spent so much time being jailed for protesting, however, that he virtually stopped scheduling stand-up gigs: "In fairness to the nightclub owners, my loyalty was to the movement. And so if you invested your money to advertise that Dick Gregory was coming . . . and then there was a big battle in the South I was going to be there. And so you had the right to say, 'Wait a minute now' . . . [and] my agent, who was white . . . [would have to say]—'Well, we can't guarantee he will be there.'"[13] Between 1967 and 1971 Gregory also turned to hunger strikes as a form of nonviolent protest—fasting forty days (starting on Thanksgiving) to protest the war in Vietnam in 1967, forty-five days in solidarity with the burgeoning American Indian Movement (AIM), and eighty-one days to raise awareness about the growing drug problems in urban America in 1970. Gregory's comedian contemporary Dick Davy summed it up: "[There was a] big rush to give Black comedians a push on television. . . . To keep Black people from rioting, let's put them on television but not controversial Black faces . . . not Dick Gregory."[14]

Gregory's practice of putting his body where his ideology was extended beyond his presence at marches and his many hunger strikes. After he became a vegetarian, a marathon runner, and an expert on nutrition, his dietary zealotry became deeply rooted in his ideological convictions. His business venture with his nutritional product, the "Bahamian Diet," around which he built Dick Gregory Health Enterprises, Inc., targeted the lower life expectancy of black Americans, which he attributed to poor nutrition and the use of alcohol and drugs. Although Gregory's advocacy and his voice have progressively faded from mainstream entertainment and political venues, his voice continues to be heard, particularly in black-oriented venues: talk shows of black talk radio, whether as frequent guest on WVON's *The Cliff Kelley Show* in his native Chicago or the weekly BlackElectorate.com program on Matsimela Mapfumo's "Make It Plain," broadcast on XM (satellite) radio. Gregory returned to performing stand-up in theatrical spaces in the late nineties (and did a 2000 date at the Apollo Theater with Paul Mooney), but he continues to use his humor and wit in service to political advocacy: whether from the podium at the 1995 Million Man March, where he commented on this being a great day for the black family because "1 million black women knew where their husbands were,"[15] or from his desk, where he "created" the Committee for a Formal Apology in 2003 and, as a "representative" of that body, appealed to Virginia Republican senator George Allen to be the resolution's advocate on the right side of the aisle. ("There was no committee," the comic later explained; he simply wrote a letter to Allen and copies of James Allen's *Without Sanctuary: Lynching Photography in America* were mailed to all one hundred senators.)[16]

In the past decade Gregory's conspiracy-theory-informed commentaries, often framed and inflected with humor, have received mixed responses from audiences inside and outside the black community. Nonetheless, his declarations continue to resonate with the comic activist's deep, abiding convictions about speaking truth to power. In the wake of the 1996 "revelations" about the CIA's counterintelligence program (COINTELPRO) role in the crack epidemic in black urban America, Gregory, along with Congresswoman Maxine Waters of South Central Los Angeles, called for governmental accountability—even after the newspaper that published exposés on the "Dark Alliance," the *San Jose Mercury News*, responding to the CIA's systematic rebuttals of the stories, withdrew its support from the conclusions drawn in the series.[17] In October of 2001 Gregory expressed his wariness of the (then new) post-9/11 patriotic fervor, urged the audience to remember that "the truth does not have to be validated by ignorance" at the Black Spectrum Theatre Company in Queens, New York, and joked about the ties between the Bush and Bin Laden families long before Michael Moore had a draft for *Fahrenheit 9/11*. While one sees Gregory in contemporary media as an activist, a dietary guru, and conspiracy theorist, his calmly confrontational humor continues to resonate for the post-soul comics (who are actually aware of his work), as exemplified by the fact that his comments at the Million Worker March in October of 2004, which labeled Bush and his administration a bunch of "thugs," whose tactics were those that one would expect of thugs, seemed to be televisually realized in the "Black Bush" segment of the second season finale of *Chappelle's Show*.[18]

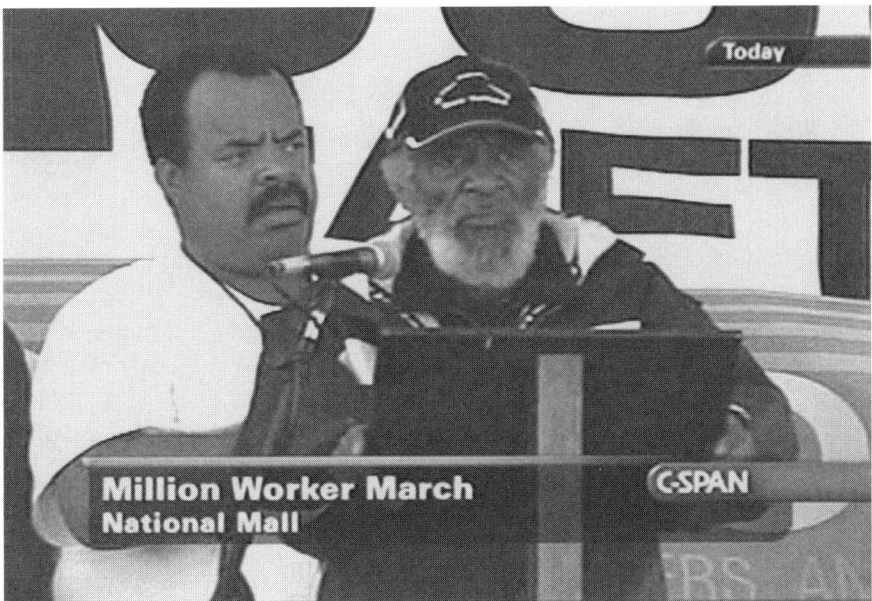

3. Dick Gregory (wearing hat) remains committed to multiple struggles for human rights. C-SPAN coverage of the Million Worker March (Oct. 17, 2004).

Although Gregory's is not a household name to contemporary audiences, recognition of his significant contribution to comedy and to the African American community has come to him in the past decade, although it has not been given (or accepted) in the most conventional ways. In 2004 the University of Missouri, which the young Dick Gregory had not been allowed to attend because of segregationist practices, awarded the comic/activist son of St. Louis an honorary doctorate. Gregory described the conferral with typically sardonic humor: "My opening line to them [that day] was 'I never thought I'd see the day, having been born and raised in the state of Missouri, that I'd grow up and let some old white men with robes on put a hood around me—that's progress.'"[19] Even a very public, impromptu tribute was paid by Chris Rock during an evening when another comic pioneer, Richard Pryor, was being honored; Rock, a presenter, suddenly reached into the crowd and pulled Gregory onstage in order to celebrate this other black comic force.[20] In 2000 the tribute to the comic featuring important figures from black arts, culture, and politics, including Isaac Hayes, Ossie Davis, Ruby Dee, Coretta Scott King, and Sonia Sanchez, was organized by a private organization known as "The Friends of Dick Gregory" at New York's Kennedy Center. His civil rights era brother, Bill Cosby, who acted as the master of ceremonies for the tribute, spoke passionately about the comic/political activist's contribution to the craft and the country on NPR's *Talk of the Nation* broadcast during the week in October of 2000: "Dick Gregory is history, man. Lenny Bruce wasn't on the line in the Civil Rights march. Mort Sahl didn't march. Mort Sahl didn't get his head whipped by the police. Mort Sahl didn't give up, nor did Lenny Bruce, nor did Bill Cosby give up salary to go down and spend two days in jail after facing dogs. Dick Gregory is not over there with those people. Dick Gregory is standing alone."[21]

### BILL COSBY: EVERYBODY'S ALL-AMERICAN

Unlike Gregory, whose ideological imperatives prevented him from maintaining and furthering his acceptance in the comic mainstream (much less the Hollywood comedy), Bill Cosby became and continues to be a comedic darling of American television. Cosby embodied the optimism of the integrationist New Frontier—his squeaky-clean likability and universalist comedic approach won over audiences regardless of race, creed, or color. When Cosby came onto the stand-up scene, he occupied a unique space as a comedian whose humor was observational and assimilationist. At the peak of the civil rights movement Cosby would not use race as a subject in his comedy. "I don't think you can bring the races together by joking about the differences between them," he said. "I'd rather talk about the similarities, about what's universal in their experiences."[22]

Although one clearly sees the convergences between the physical constructions of Cosby and Gregory—the clean-cut Negro in a conservative, yet stylish, suit with a style of delivery that reveals (but does not flaunt) the comic's college-educated status—the divergence in terms of the content of the comedy becomes immediately obvious. Whereas Gregory's act, beginning with his Playboy Club appearance, was always contesting mainstream conceptions of contemporary cultural and racial politics, Cosby's comedy was fundamentally soothing, regardless of the audience. In one of his earliest television appearances, on *The Jack Paar Program* in 1963,[23] the material that Cosby chose was a decidedly contemporary (but also uncontroversial) take on the Bible, Noah, and the Great Flood. Constructing Noah as a modern everyman, who looks incredulously at both the Lord's choosing him (replying, with the coy smile of one fearing he is the butt of a joke, "Right . . . Am I on *Candid Camera?*" to the initial visitation) and God's subsequent requests affords Cosby the opportunity to reveal his considerable talents as a storyteller who skillfully uses language and pop-culture inflection to position himself with his audience (a hallmark in the comic's humor). Cosby, with the gestures and intonation of the flustered everyman (with which audiences will become familiar over the course of his career), acts out Noah's plight, ridiculed by his neighbors for his ark-building activities, his animal wrangling, and, of course, the fact that his efforts are divinely directed: "I told one of my friends I'd been talking to the Lord and he laughed so hard he wet his pants. Do you know I'm the only guy in town with an ark in his yard? People are picketing and calling the health department. Strangers walk up to me and say 'How's it going, Tarzan?'" The comic's inclusion of references to the original reality show, *Candid Camera*, the iconic (if not unproblematic) Tarzan, and visions of an apolitical picket line place the bit in conversation with the early sixties social milieu (the year of the famed march on Washington); at the same time, however, the eliding of any sort of ideological commentary positions the comic's as the friendliest of relations. Within the safety of this biblically informed bit, Cosby's comic persona simultaneously offers a vision of the new American Negro while not pushing the audience to acknowledge the newness of the construction. No cultural translation is required for the audience to empathize with Noah, when, despite his frustration and hardships, he abandons his short-lived rebellion and acquiesces to his Higher Power's inscrutable master plan—after it begins to rain: "This isn't a shower is it? [sigh] Okay. All right, it's me and you, Lord; me and you, all the way."

Jack Paar described Cosby as "something other young comedians sometimes neglect . . . [being] darn funny," thus acknowledging (and helping to inscribe) a separation between Cosby and his comic brethren (black and white). His comedy, unlike the rapid-fire joke telling of the comics of the previous era (whether Henny Youngman or Slappy White), is rooted in constructing commonalities of experience rather than exploring difference.[24] This sense of universalist humor was furthered by a majority of Cosby's early routines, which

revolved around nostalgic visions of growing up in his Philadelphia neighborhood. His comic bits on his friends and family are inflected with semiautobiographical detail, but specific issues of race and/or black culture are notably
absent. Unlike Gregory or, later, Pryor, Cosby excised from his storytelling the
arduous aspects of his particular Negro condition: the darker realities of growing up in the projects in Philadelphia, the alcoholic and fundamentally absent
father, and his mother's fiscal struggles as a de facto single mom were afforded
only a tertiary space in his comic universe and only as impressionistic asides
made sunnier for inclusion. "Tonsils," one of the most widely known of his early
comic bits, recounts his tonsillectomy-driven quest for the bottomless bowl of
ice cream.[25] Cosby gives voice to his mother, the doctor, and his fellow patients
and explains the comic details of his treatment, such as the doctor's explanation
of his malady: "Your tonsils, which we're going to have to take out, guard your
throat. They're two guards who stand there with hand grenades and bazookas
and everything. And anything bad that comes into your mouth, they fight it off
[making artillery sounds]. Well, in your case, your tonsils have lost the war. In
fact, your tonsils have gone as far as to join the other side." The promise of "all
the ice cream in the world that you can eat" wins his trust, and he joyfully sub-
mits himself to the doctor's care. Revealing the unique ability to convey the
voice and the logic of his childhood self, he describes the glee with which he
and his roommates (on the children's ward) awaited surgery and ice cream: "And
we sang, Ice Cream . . . we're gonna eat ice cream. And we'll eat it everyday . . .
in the middle of the night. . . . You know what I'm gonna do with my first bowl
of ice cream. I'm not gonna eat it or nothin'. I'm just gonna smear it all over
my body, and then I'm gonna put a cherry in my navel. I'll be the most beautiful chocolate sundae you ever saw."

   "Tonsils," like much of Cosby's stand-up material, was not rooted in the
social turmoil of the era but rather in a sanitized and universalized depiction of
growing up poor in an urban setting. There is a "kid solidarity" that informs this
world: bonds form quickly (like those between Bill the younger and his ward
mate, Johnson, as they discuss postoperative ice cream consumption). On one
level this kid kinship, which Cosby will explore further in his *Fat Albert* material, seems to simply operate on a type of childhood logic that lacks real contentiousness. Even the theft of baby carriage wheels for go-cart construction in
"Go-Carts" and the disobedience and small-scale living room destruction in
"Chicken Heart" are presented in such a way that they cannot be seen as anything other than childhood hi-jinks.[26] This also speaks to the overall amenable
tone of Cosby's stand-up material. Designed for a mass audience, his routines—
and, in particular, the childhood material—simply did not threaten anyone.
What Elvis Mitchell described as "a trace of streetwise sensibility beneath lum-
bering affability" may inform both Cosby's comic persona and his performances
(particularly in terms of the "sanitized-street" inflection of the Cosby kids'
voices in *Fat Albert*), but it is the "timeless" quality of the routines (never fixed

in relation to a sociohistorical moment) that allows the humor to stand up almost forty years later. That same quality also served to assuage late twentieth-century fears about social change in the dominant culture and, most certainly, in the entertainment industry.[27]

As Cosby moved from behind the mike to in front of the camera in the breakthrough role of Alexander Scott in the buddy-"Bond" series, *I-Spy*, his character (and, by extension, the actor's persona) was the embodiment of the well-dressed, well-educated, and extremely articulate "Super Negro." Cosby's affable and accessibly hip comic persona reflected and refracted the mid-sixties "Camelot" moment in style if not substance. The apolitical nature of Cosby's material and the cold warrior "superiority" of Scott provided an ideological match with the liberalism of New Frontier/Great Society rhetoric.[28] Yet the significance of Cosby as comedian, comic actor, and televisual icon cannot be underestimated. Whether during the civil rights era or in the present day, Cosby exemplifies how the stand-up comic's persona is a part of, yet remains apart from, the historical moment in which it is produced. His coming of comic age during the civil rights era is addressed, quite literally, by his presence and (almost) never by the content of his words in either his act or his television roles. His stand-up success translated into small-screen stardom and popular culture icon status: first as the televisual construction of the "Super Negro" in the sixties, Alexander Scott (*I-Spy*, NBC, 1965–68), and then as the Saturday morning television translator of a pastoralized view of black urban life in the seventies (*Fat Albert and the Cosby Kids*, CBS, 1972–79). Despite his status as a televisual icon, Cosby's television outings have not all been unmitigated successes. Unlike *I-Spy*, *Fat Albert*, and, of course, *The Cosby Show*, the comic's foray into television variety, *The New Bill Cosby Show* (CBS, 1972), after the cancellation of his first sitcom, and the child-oriented version, *Cos* (ABC, 1976), were short-lived. The seventies was an era of an edgier Cosby, when the bearded, mustached Afro-ed comic was making appearances on PBS children's show *The Electric Company* (1971–81), doing guest spots on other variety series (frequently *The Flip Wilson Show*), and producing more adult comedic entertainment fare like *Bill Cosby on Prejudice*, an independently produced project cowritten by the comic. The filmed one-man show featured Cosby as a self-proclaimed bigot who regales the audience with a litany of racist, xenophobic, and sexist commentaries.[29]

By mapping the salient features in the sitcom iterations of Cosby's comic personae, from Chet Kincaid (*The Bill Cosby Show*, NBC, 1969–73) to Dr. Heathcliff Huxtable (*The Cosby Show*, NBC, 1984–92) and, finally, to Hilton Lucas (*Cosby*, CBS, 1996–2000), from the civil rights to post-soul era, one can see the trajectory of the ideological and pedagogical dimensions of his comedic discourse. As Chet Kincaid, the hipster teacher and coach in his first sitcom, the comic presented a single black man, in a community (coded as inner city), who espoused the same pragmatic view of middle-class values that would become

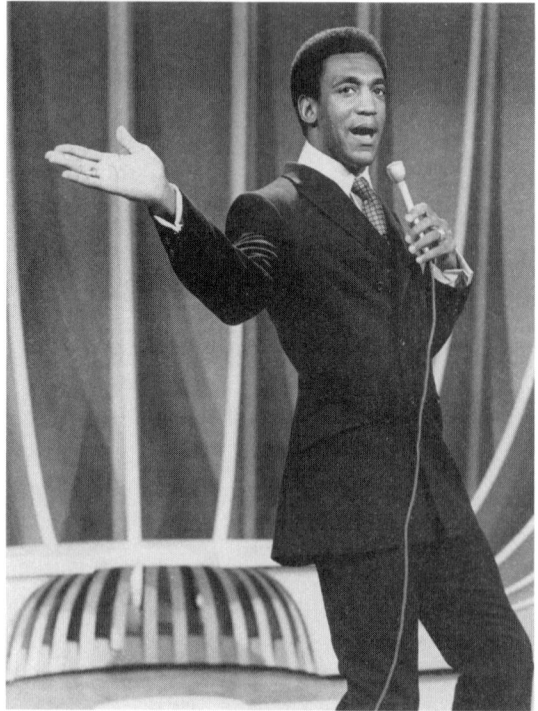

4. Everybody's all-American: Bill Cosby. *The Second Bill Cosby Special* (NBC) (April 9, 1971). Photo from Photofest. Reproduced with permission from NBC.

the staple of the chronicle of the Huxtable clan. As the series followed Kincaid's maturation (as teacher and coach, from single man to young married) and the challenges he faced engaging his students, their parents, and his colleagues, the sitcom presented a world that was neither idyllic nor problematic—which, when depicting an actually integrated milieu in 1969, was no small feat.

Like his hipster contemporary Mr. Dixon on *Room 222*, Kincaid presented an educated black everyteacher, who was afforded a personal life (with an attractive colleague as the love interest) and a sensibility far closer to the students (and the popular culture mainstream) than his colleagues. Unlike history teacher Mr. Dixon, however, who dealt with pressing social issues as best one could in the twenty-two-minute precursor of the dramedy, Chet Kincaid rarely offered *direct* socially relevant, ideologically informed prescriptions. Through Chet, the audience learned object lessons that spoke across rather than to the times. In "The Longest Hookshot in the World" the issue of prejudice is addressed, with Coach Kincaid being accused of being prejudiced (against short people) by his perky, white liberal colleague (played by Joyce Bulifant)—although Chet contends that "some of [his] best friends are short people." The episode ends with a chastened Chet, walking off the court after a last-second loss with two of his players: the previously underestimated short black teen and the overestimated, tall, white one thus providing a simple morality tale about judging individuals by their merit, not one's preconceptions. Like the moral of this episode, his reactions speak to and draw empathy from a broad audience: whether his jealousy over a Ferrari-driving black doctor vying for the attentions of his fellow-teacher love interest ("He bought that car with American sick people money") or his rejection of a wealthy donor's request to include children in an activity only if they look like his old gang ("I'm not running Central Casting, this is a community center, you help one kid, you help them all").

As one might argue would be the case with *The Cosby Show*, the significance of the series was not necessarily the content of individual narratives but the construction of both Cosby's sitcom persona and the televisual milieu in which he existed. "In most episodes," as Bogle observes, "Cosby was interested in expressing—without simplifying—the important values, outlooks, and norms of an emerging new Black middle class," thus depicting "Black Americans who in many respects were no different than white Americans."[30] During its run, *The Bill Cosby Show*, despite its aversion to directly addressing the sociopolitical milieu of the late sixties and early seventies, was not viewed as an extension of the Super Negro televisual representations of either Cosby's first television outing, *I-Spy*, or the series' sitcom contemporary *Julia*. I would argue that this construction of a black everyguy was achieved by making efforts to call subtle attention to blackness in the series' milieu and its politics of representation, whether in Kincaid's commitment to the inner-city community center where he volunteered, his eligible black bachelorhood and then happily married status, or the insertion of moments that depicted "very real and important differences that existed in the Black community, even if it merely be an aunt and uncle [played by Chitlin' Circuit veterans Moms Mabley and Dewey "Pigmeat" Markam] shooting the dozens."[31] While Cosby as Chet Kincaid played on the already likable and accepted aspects of his comic persona, the less than "Super" construction of the character failed to garner the widespread acclaim of his previous television stardom or the monumental success that would follow with his trek into stand-up, literary, and televisual ruminations on fatherhood.

In the eighties Cosby gained television icon status as the father who knew best in a colorized American Dream. Dr. Cliff Huxtable on *The Cosby Show* was a role that very directly corresponded to his stand-up persona.[32] In the aptly titled *Bill Cosby: Himself* (1983), possibly the quintessential example of his stand-up skills, Cosby's performance represented the fully evolved incarnation of his comedic persona—the product of the previous two decades onstage and on the small screen.[33] *The Cosby Show* established Thursday evening on NBC as "Must See TV" and, with it, established for Cosby another significant place in television history. Throughout his comic career Cosby has occupied a unique position in which his comedic articulation of blackness was viewed as both representative and idiosyncratic. In many ways he has achieved the "friendly relation" of which Gregory spoke early in his career: Cosby is an African American funny man with an unquestionably original comic voice that "transcends" issues of race—which is never an unproblematic space to occupy.[34]

Although, given the wealth of material written about *The Cosby Show*, the inclusion of this analysis seems a bit like the scholarly equivalent of reinventing the wheel, one would be remiss not to discuss the character that made Cosby a television icon: Heathcliff Huxtable. "The series depiction of the Huxtable family continued the 'movin' on up' trend of Blacks in sitcoms of the late seventies and early eighties (*The Jeffersons, Different Strokes, Benson*). However, unlike its predecessors, for whom 'movin' on up' meant moving into a fundamentally White world, the world of the Huxtables was primarily Black, and the series began with the family as long-standing members of the upper middle class."[35] In many ways the series was a direct reflection of the universalist sensibility that has informed Cosby's stand-up from his first appearance on *The Jack Paar Program* in 1963 to his 2004 stand-up tour. The picture of upper-middle-class success, Cosby's obstetrician-father, Cliff; lawyer-wife, Clair (Phylicia Rashad); along with their three (then four) daughters and one son constructed a new poster family for the American Dream, one easily embraced by the viewing public because, as Herman Gray states, "it is a middle class family that happens to be black."[36]

The series' premiere was one of the most successful translations of a comic's stand-up act into the sitcom format. Cliff and the kids, particularly Vanessa (Tempestt Bledsoe), the middle child, labeled "the Informer" in Cosby's stand-up, spoke dialogue cribbed from the *Himself* performances. Just as significant, from its first episode, in 1984, *The Cosby Show* forwarded the traditional "family values," the catchphrase of the era, and a civil rights era informed notion of uplift, conveying it more as individual wisdom than as ideological agenda in much the same way that, until recently, Cosby, both onstage and in other public venues, had espoused. Throughout the series' run he retained tight creative control. Cosby brought psychiatrist and cultural critic Alvin F. Poussaint, a longtime friend, onboard as a consultant because he "wanted the show to be real, the psychological interactions of the family to be real. And he wanted the issues to be real issues, universal to families."[37] The black bourgeois setting of the series did not preclude dealing with social issues facing the African American community, but it facilitated a presentation of *situations* common to the domestic comedy and far more closely akin to the family Stone in *The Donna Reed Show* than to the family Evans in *Good Times*.[38] Arguably the most direct narrative tip of the hat to class disparity came early in the series: in one episode from season 3 Vanessa gets into a fight with a girl who calls her "rich"; Cliff explains, "Your mother and I are rich, you have nothing."[39] Furthermore, Cosby, as creative producer of the series, as well as its star, remained adamant that sociopolitical issues (namely, race relations) need not be a part of the narrative: "It may seem that I'm an authority because my skin color gives me a mark of a victim. But that's not a true label. I won't deal with the foolishness of racial overtones on the show. I base an awful lot of what I've done simply on what people will enjoy."[40]

"And So We Commence," the series finale, which culminated with Theo's graduation from NYU, aired on April 30, 1992, with news coverage of the LA uprising acting as its lead-in. While the irony of the televisual saga of the country's most fully assimilated African American family (with its depiction of African American access to the American Dream) ending at the same historical moment when images of the explosion of racial tensions and Los Angeles burning is lost on no one, one must also question how much the "*positive imagined* of the Huxtable world had to do with the actual state of race relations in the United States."[41] Nevertheless, the televisual translation of Cosby's comic persona transformed him into America's Dad—a position that continues to endow the television icon's voice with immense cultural cachet (and attract immense media attention). Within that function as America's Dad, Cosby/Cliff passed on a particular value system—the familial guidelines for access to the Dream—within the trials and tribulations of the televisual families. In addition, great pains are taken to make sure that the next generation learns these lessons and lives by them: assuring that their post-soul-era offspring knew what was expected of them and what was desired for them was a dominant theme, with object lessons drenched in ideologies of education, uplift, personal responsibility, and pragmatism.

Since *Bill Cosby: Himself* and the publication of *Fatherhood*, Cosby's comic persona has been tied to the purveyance of fatherly wisdom, which is in conversation, albeit circuitously, with the notion of "getting a piece of the Dream." In his return to the sitcom after a four-year hiatus (and two unsuccessful non-sitcom television outings) in CBS's *Cosby*, the series' premise offered a far less idealized notion of African American life—in mitigated struggle rather than unmitigated success. The situation of this television comedy was in conversation with the specific historical period of airline deregulation and the beginning of the industry's economic downward spiral. Inspired by the British series *One Foot in the Grave*, Cosby starred as Hilton Lucas, a thirty-year employee of an unnamed airline, who has been unceremoniously "retired" and struggles with his place in a world where hard work and perseverance did not yield the rewards he had envisioned (not even a gold watch and a retirement party). The pilot episode even begins with a reference that frames the Dream as a nightmare. Hilton tosses and turns violently in bed, waking Ruth (Phylicia Rashad, again, stars as his television spouse), who shoves her flailing hubby off the bed.

HILTON: I had a dream I was fired.
RUTH: It's been three weeks, Hilton. Get a good night's sleep.

Their exchange is decidedly un-Cliff and Clair, with Hilton's dejected curmudgeon facing off with Ruth's exasperated pragmatist: her response to his "My

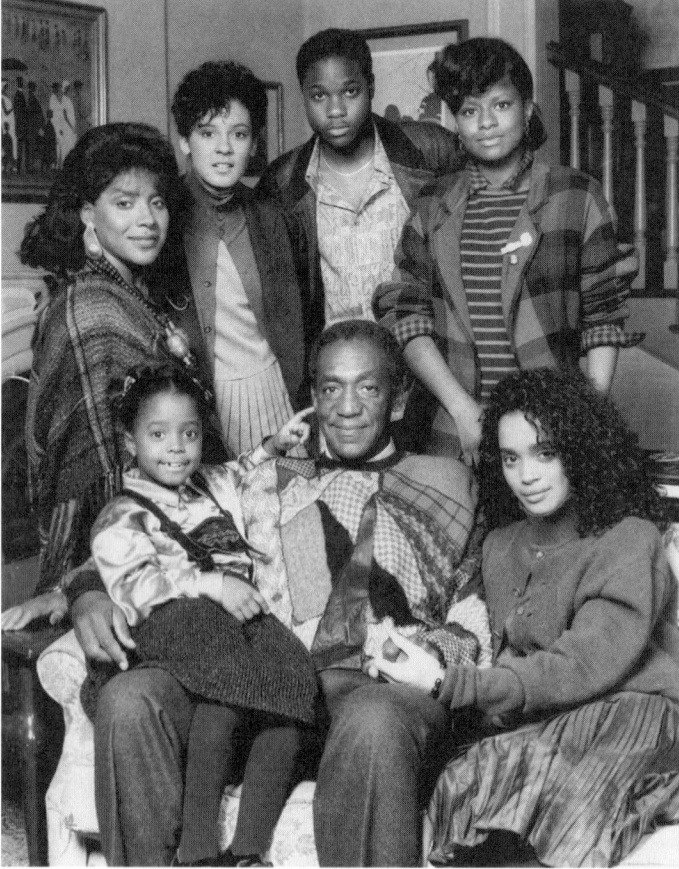

5. The Huxtables: The Dream has been colorized. *The Cosby Show* (NBC), season 3 (1986-87). *Clockwise from bottom left*: Keshia Knight Pulliam (as Rudith Lillian "Rudy" Huxtable), Phylicia Rashad (as Clair Olivia Hanks Huxtable), Sabrina Le Beauf (as Sondra Huxtable Tibideaux), Malcolm-Jamal Warner (as Theodore Aloysius "Theo" Huxtable), Tempestt Bledsoe (as Vanessa Huxtable), Lisa Bonet (as Denise Huxtable Kendall), Bill Cosby (as Dr. Heathcliff "Cliff" Huxtable). Photo from Photofest. Reproduced with permission from NBC.

life is over" histrionics is "You're not dead. You were just downsized." From the moment that we see this new image of Cosby and Rashad in bed together (an image tied to a plethora of televisual memories of the idealized Huxtables and their ideal life and lifestyle), it seems clear that a different vision and version of both Cosby's comic persona and the Dream are at play here. Although it would be an overstatement to cast Hilton as a sitcom Lear raging against the tempests, one does get the sense that, for this character, the ground beneath him is not quite solid. Furthermore, the varying shades of bitterness in his oft-repeated variations of his claim, "I didn't lose my job. My job was taken from me. I know where it is. If I were to go there, they could give it back," is cut by Cosby's delivery, but there is more darkness in the amiable bluster. In fact, the pilot provides moments that recognize that the American Dream appears to hemorrhaging: from Hilton's postlayoff nightmares to the mistaken assumption by Ruth's best friend and business partner, Pauline (played in New Age-y splendor and great aplomb by the late Madeline Kahn), that the suicide note of a former shop patron was penned by Hilton (and includes her giving CPR to a soundly sleeping Hilton). Although these almost slapstick moments in the series, as well as his exchanges with Griffin (played by Doug E. Doug), in which Cosby treads familiar ground as incredulous patriarch dealing with the lack of pragmatism and/or forethought of his (in this case, "surrogate") child, resonate with earlier and more familiar aspects of Cosby's televisual presence, both the series and Cosby as Hilton are far less amenable to the world in which they live. The construction of Hilton (and the rest of the Lucas family) speaks less to a sense of realism than to a de-idealization of the comic's America's Dad persona and an African American familial milieu untouched by recession. However, given that the loss of Hilton's job is never a fiscal issue for the family, the thwarted hopes or unforeseen misfortune of the Dream unfulfilled is still not a part of this televisual iteration of Cosby either.[42]

Nonetheless, both Hilton and Cliff, like Cosby's post-*Himself* comic persona, presented clear notions of individual agency and familial responsibility in their American Dream–inflected directives to their children, which were clearly articulated in the pilots for each series. The outcomes for the televisual fathers and their children differ, but ultimately the message does not. The central story line of *The Cosby Show*'s pilot is the parental reaction to son Theo's abysmal report card and Cliff's and Claire's desire to change their son's view of education's importance. After Cliff points out the impossibility of getting into college with D-filled report cards, Theo invokes his desire for a sort of working-class normalcy because college is not required to be like "regular people." Cliff provides an object lesson on the fiscal travails of "regular people" when the stack of Monopoly money wages given to Theo disappears as Cliff subtracts the costs of living. "Regular people," Cliff remarks to his now penniless son. "Although the situation is handled with pragmatic humor, the class-based expectations built into the Huxtable world (and the fictive world of the sitcom, in general) are clearly revealed here and differentiate this middle-class milieu from the world of 'regular people.'"[43] Theo's attempt to counter his father's pragmatism is framed as a treatise on acceptance:

THEO: You're a doctor; Mom's a lawyer—you're successful. Maybe I was born to be regular people. If you weren't a doctor, I wouldn't love you any less.

I love you because you're my dad. And so maybe instead of acting disappointed because I'm not like you, maybe you can just accept me for who I
am and love me anyway because I'm your son.

After a beat (and a smattering of audience applause), Cliff replies, "Theo, that is
the dumbest thing I've ever heard in my entire life." Although the discussion
closes with kinder, gentler reasoning (Cliff to Theo: "I just want you to do the
best you can, that's all"), Theo's rejection of a middle-class ethos (and its accompanying education-based work ethic) is subsumed by humorous, patriarchal
correction in which Father (Cliff) knows best and directly communicates the
values embedded in the American Dream.

When the ideological equivalent of this moment is replicated in the pilot
of *Cosby*, the comic payoff is diminished, given that both the father's pragmatism and the child's rebellion are more deeply rooted in two conflicting value
systems. Amid his struggle with being unemployed for the first time in thirty
years, Hilton is confronted by his daughter Erika's identity crisis. One can easily
imagine that Erika received the same talk about "regular people" that Theo
received in the pilot of *The Cosby Show*. Unlike Theo, however, whose rejection
of a professional path was greeted with a full-court press of civil rights era ideological directives, Erika's rejection of her legal career in order to follow her
bliss (reminiscent of Denise's leaving Hillman to find herself in the chronicles
of the Huxtable family), while depicted humorously, plays like an affront not
just to Hilton but also to Cosby's televisual ideological paradigm, which forwards a vision of the American Dream that promises that through hard work,
education, and steadfastness the next generation will be able to surpass the
achievements of those who came before them:

HILTON: I worked thirty years with the airlines to send you through law school
     and as soon as you did that, you got a job at the airlines to work another
     thirty years. There is something missing in the middle.
ERIKA: But I'm happy, Daddy. Isn't that enough?
HILTON: No, I want my money back.

Despite this contentious beginning, that seemed to recognize a generational
divide, by series end Erika has married, is out of the house, and is teaching high
school, thus reinscribing the values of education, giving back to the community,
individual responsibility, and, of course, the nuclear family. As was true throughout Cosby's career, the gender politics of his sitcom personae are characterized
by a sort of revisionist traditionalism: respectful to women (almost reverential at
times) and never involved in even light blue forms of objectification but still
viewing them, for the most part, in relationship to their roles as girlfriend, wife,
and mother—even though she might also be a doctor, a lawyer, or an educator.

While *The Cosby Show*, which was an unmitigated network success, was
decried by some critics for providing an idealized vision of African American

life, which, in turn could be (and was) mobilized as evidence (a sort of race-based fairy tale/object lesson) by the Reagan Right (and the neoconservatives to come) that anyone—regardless of race, creed, or color—could get his or her piece of the Dream, the less than idyllic vision of *Cosby*, in which the ideological directives yielded mixed results for the black family, was not embraced by the same cross-racial and cross-generational audience.[44] By the premiere of *Cosby* in the mid-nineties, the sociopolitical climate had changed significantly: the bloom was off the rose with the Clinton administration, as the promised "nationwide dialogue on race" had yielded little but rhetoric, the gap between rich and poor (black and white) continued to widen with systematic cuts labeled as "welfare reform," and the neoconservatives (black and white) stood waiting in the wings. In this climate the portrait of a black family, which *should have been* struggling, living without struggle was not particularly popular with any audience: while everybody loved "Raymond," audiences were not crazy about Cosby.[45]

In an interview in *Jet* magazine prior to the premiere of *Cosby*, the comic repeated the question that many people were asking when he chose to return to the world of the sitcom: "Can I make a 20 year old laugh along with 65 year old people?" Were one to judge solely by ratings, the answer would be "no." Had I not seen the multigenerational, multiracial crowd at Cosby's performance at Detroit's Opera House in January of 2004 (before his much-publicized commentary at Constitution Hall), I might have agreed.[46] Cosby's act sampled pieces of his literary outings (most heavily from his recent endeavor on the perils of having indulged in the banquets of life, *I Am What I Ate . . . and I'm Frightened!!!*), but his meandering storytelling style and his frequent engagement with the audience made the material seem both personal and personable. As Teresa Wiltz noted in her review of his performance at Wolf Trap on the Washington leg of the tour: "[Cosby] is above all a storyteller, a man who seems more comfortable traipsing through a past cast with a relatively rosy glow. Race is an aside; growing up in the projects is mentioned only in passing. Instead, fodder is found in the humor wrought from the big little moments: first kisses, puberty, parents who aren't afraid to say no—or administer a whack when the moment warrants it."[47] Regaling the audience with truisms about the power dynamics in marriage ("The longer you stay married, the farther ahead mentally [wives] are. You cannot compete."), both parenthood and grandparenthood (his wife loved becoming a grandmother, because having to rear all those babies would pay their daughters back for what they did to her), and his increasingly age-induced health consciousness (the loss of his beloved stogies and chili-dogs), Cosby segued from being America's dad to being America's grandfather.

Inasmuch as Cosby's act offers snapshots of his worldview, it also speaks to the ideological directives in his comedy: the privileging of the pursuit of a middle-class, civil rights era–informed American Dream. Not only has Cosby's comedic discourse given instruction on the pursuit of *that Dream*; through his life, his art, and his philanthropy he has become its embodiment. Having reviewed the content and context of his sitcoms, which televisually codified both the comic's persona and the ideologies embedded therein, is it all that surprising that Cosby would bemoan behaviors within the black community that did not adhere to his de facto directives? In his now famous remarks at the anniversary of *Brown v. Board of Education*, Cosby, speaking as black America's grandfather rather than America's dad, expressed with vehemence his frustration with generational as well as class-inflected constructions of black cultural practices. His words seemed rooted in a deep personal disappointment, as though the inadequate efforts of the next generation (Erika and Theo's generation), as well as the underclass for whom the Dream has been indefinitely deferred, had let him down.[48]

### WILSON: THE CHITLIN' CIRCUIT MADE HIM DO IT

Whereas Bill Cosby broke down representational boundaries on television with comic personae clearly informed by ideological directives of the civil rights era, Flip Wilson's "greatest contribution was the introduction of a distinct black voice to mainstream comedy" with an ideological agenda that was far less transparent.[49] Flip Wilson was (arguably) the "nicest" of the comic's to emerge in the civil rights era. Pryor maintained that "Flip was the only performer when he comes out onstage, the audience hopes that [he] likes them." Normally, the word *nice* rings hollow, an innocuous adjective describing something or someone who is mildly pleasant, someone you don't mind having around; however, for Wilson "niceness" functioned as a tool in his comic arsenal and facilitated the embrace of mainstream audiences. Given that his comic personae embodied both a departure from and a return to disparate strains of black comedy in the sixties and mid-seventies, the "niceness" was like the heaping spoon of brown sugar in the (decidedly) black coffee that was Wilson's act. The comic blended the trickster and the jokester, the easy embellishments of humor in African American oral tradition with the broad physical humor (mugging and movement) of the juke-joint comedian, in his tales of black folks.

As Redd Foxx wrote in his *Encyclopedia of Black Humor*, "[Wilson] was known for his ability to tell a story. . . . When Flip tells a story, you almost wish he wouldn't end it. He doesn't rely on monologues paced with one-liners. . . . His phrases are emphasized with body motion, facial expressions and funny voices. He acts out the entire story, character by character."[50] Thus, it makes sense that Wilson, who had arguably spent more time on the Chitlin' Circuit than Pryor, Gregory, or Cosby, would blend the voice of a truly old-school black humor (and a patina of minstrelsy) with a sensibility that celebrated cultural specificity in his comedy. What made Wilson unique was the lack of either overt judgment or direct sociopolitical contextualization of the aspects of black life he presented. Wilson's style—mischievous rather than sly, cheerfully cheeky but (not necessarily) irreverent, and never insolent—enabled the comic to bring material that had previously been reserved for the Chitlin' Circuit and black communal spaces onto main stages and, later, into America's living rooms. Long before the height of the comic's popularity in the early seventies, Wilson's comic personae could be clearly delineated from his civil rights era brethren: "[Wilson] does not have the slashing wit of a Lenny Bruce, the angry bite of a Dick Gregory, the satirical punch of a Godfrey Cambridge or the intellectual edge of a Bill Cosby. His approach is at once older and newer than the others."[51]

In many ways his comic persona, formed during his years in black juke joints and the Chitlin' Circuit, was arguably more akin to his Chitlin' Circuit predecessors (like Russell) than his civil rights era brethren, Gregory, Cosby, and Pryor. Like his contemporaries he presented the clean-cut, suit-and-tie image of the young Negro comic pioneered by Gregory. Unlike Gregory, however, for whom race and racial inequality and the movement became a comic staple, or Cosby and early Pryor, for whom race and the specific articulation of blackness (then, Negro-ness) was essentially absent, Wilson's act was inflected by a decidedly black urban hipster vernacular, and his engagement of the sociopolitical ramifications of contemporary race relations was engaged amiably, thus distancing him from accusations of any form of social or political extremism. Nonetheless, Wilson's comic personae were embodied in a cast of characters conveying black experiences and anchored by the voice of an exceedingly likable emcee. Wilson's humor was unabashedly culturally specific: urban street humor, downhome humor, black humor. Thus one must also recognize that the construction of Wilson's comic persona (as well as the style of his delivery and content of his act) has roots *very literally* in the humor of the minstrel show.

When Wilson was asked about his comic inspirations at the Museum of Television and Radio's 1993 celebration of *The Flip Wilson Show*, part of the museum's Tenth Annual Television Festival, Wilson told a story about where his comedy came from and about his quick-witted uncle, his "hero" who was "faster than Groucho":

> "You want to get rich," [he said]. . . . I said, "Yes." He said, "You meet me here tomorrow at 5 o'clock." My uncle had had a stroke. . . . [At] 5 o'clock I saw him a block away—coming up the street dragging, dragging [the comic imitates his uncle's labored passage across the small stage]. He gave me this little book. He said, "You want to get rich, what's in this little book will make you rich." . . . And I started glancing through it. It was old slave plantation humor—that dis, dat, dem and dos [humor]. . . . I said Wow . . . Uncle said this would make me rich but this is terrible. But he came all that way struggling and he said that it was in that book and he's my hero. It must be here so I must find it and I found my blackness.

Like many of Wilson's more personalized stories, it mixes notions that seem pragmatic, earnest, and, given the civil rights historical moment in which he came of comic age, more than a touch conflicted. It does, however, directly make clear why and how Wilson would cull any material to find the funny—without judgment and without hesitation. His humor was driven by the desire to find and widen his audience, and his decisions, which one could argue were idiosyncratic, were in actuality tied to utilitarian notions of success and a notion of uplift that was about the results rather than the perception of the process. Although Wilson carried this comic legacy (including his uncle's advice) throughout his professional career, his act conveyed that it was far less about where he came from than where he was going.

Like Cosby's, Wilson's act was never mean, nor were the difficulties of his upbringing (childhood poverty and bouncing around the foster care system in pre–civil rights America) ever engaged as more than brief, beautified asides. Wilson was a "clean" comic, who, again, like Cosby, avoided both profanity and sexually explicit jokes, except for the occasional use of double entendre in bits that, at worst, can be deemed a pale "blue." On the whole his sexual humor fit somewhere between the comic patter of a Chitlin' Circuit jokester (such as the bawdier Nipsey Russell's couplets) and the lunchroom of a middle school. On *Flip Wilson: Live at the Village Gate*, after doing a setup that deals with the surgeon general's report on the dangers of smoking (men are more likely to get cancer than women), the comic segues into the payoff: "90 percent of women who have breast cancer got it from men who smoke." The comic pauses as the laughter slowly swells; you can see the devilish smile as he adds, "Takes a little time, a little time."

At least initially, the hipness factor was a large part of his comic appeal. Wilson used a bit of his double entendre in his sort of anti-Reefer Madness, cool jazz, quasi-Beat construction of drug culture. On *Live at the Village Gate* Wilson incorporates this sensibility into the story of Private Jenkins, one of the most amiably constructed drug users in contemporary comedy.[52] When Jenkins is assigned to work with the outfit's chaplain, he states, "Private Jenkins reporting for duty, Chap baby." Jenkins thus establishes his brand of hipster cred, which is further elaborated on in the subtle signal that reefer madness is probably not the private's problem. After the chaplain agrees to give Jenkins a chance to redeem himself, saying, "I'll give you another shot at this," the "zonked" private perks up significantly, "Y'say shot?" Thus, although not specifically stated in the story, it is a safe bet that Jenkins was a junkie.[53] Although the material is later excised from the television constructions of Wilson's comic persona, through some of his characters (including "The Mack" of the small screen, Freddy, the playboy), the quotidian kind of cool of Wilson's drug material, albeit through inference, makes its way into the televisual mainstream. When Private Jenkins advises a fellow serviceman to "be cool" (in terms of just staying where he is), it also provides an indication of how, in his act (and, later, on his show), Wilson naturalized the use of black slang, ushering it into the mainstream televisual vernacular. In much the same way that Martin Lawrence would take phrases like

"Whazzup," "You Go Girl," and "You So Crazy" out of the neighborhood and into the televisual entertainment niche (and, later, mainstream), Wilson's catchphrases, including, "What you see is what you get" and "the devil made me do it," would ease a certain kind of jokester black cool into the American living room without drawing particular attention that the freshness and difference of language and style was rooted in blackness, in race.

That is not to say that Wilson did not engage issues of race. He did so—with a light touch and, as one might expect given his skill as a storyteller, an indirect discursive style. On his debut album, *Cowboys and Colored People*, Wilson plays with expectations about comedic social discourse by replacing the discussion of the Negro in America with that of another oppressed people. In so doing Wilson establishes dual (and, arguably, conflicting) credibility, forwarding and undermining the comedy's role in sociopolitical critique: "I asked myself, 'Should I do any racial material in my set?' and a voice in the back of my mind said, 'No.' Then another voice said, 'One more time.'" As Wilson conveys this internal struggle and his ultimate decision to state his opinion, the audience is set up for a discussion that does not *directly* take place. "The Indians are not ready," the comic states flatly. His assessment of their "lack of readiness" addresses the threat of integration and property values (a wigwam next to a $50,000 home) and deflects the accusation of an anti-Indian bias: "There are Indians I admired, guys I looked up to, fellows who, in my opinion, didn't let the fact they were an Indian hold them back. Guys like Tonto." Wilson plays it absolutely straight and, as a result, the satirical bite of his displacement of white justifications for black exclusion, as well as the delineation of the "good ones" from the "troublemakers," is read as being malice free.

The same technique was utilized in his early show captured on *Live at the Village Gate*, when his conversation about "riggers" in the audience becomes both a play with words and audience expectations and a means of positioning himself as Negro comic during the civil rights era. Wilson explains, with righteous indignation, how managers attempt to "rig" audiences when live performances are recorded, a process he cannot abide. Despite his protestations, he believes that there are "riggers" in this audience. Given that The Village Gate in New York's Greenwich Village is not a primarily black venue, the wordplay takes on a deliberately racialized tone. "That's right—there are riggers all over. [As he pauses, there are titters of laughter.] When I came in, two riggers followed me in here. [Laughter begins to swell as the comic waits a quick beat.] The guy on the door said he saw a whole carload of riggers pull up out front." By this point everyone in the audience has "gotten" the joke—which is further underscored by his tally of how many of the folks *working* at the club are "riggers." The joke's denouement takes place when Wilson focuses on one particular patron: "You see that guy? He's a rigger. He doesn't look like it but he is. I could show you a lot of 'em but I won't [Wilson takes a long pause as if to signify the crowd could say this last line with him] because you've seen one rigger, you've seen them all." Interestingly, Wilson ends this segment of his set with a reflection on what some might have considered a politically questionable issue: "I'm taking a helluva a lot of liberty doing this. I might be banned from the [civil rights] movement. They might get equality for everybody but me." In many ways this sentiment seems consistent with Wilson's desire not to be viewed as affiliated with any group or movement: "I never affiliated with any group because I'm a group. I'm for what I represent and I try to be what I represent."[54]

One might consider Wilson's persona (as well as the characters he inhabited) to be representational counterpoints to Super Negroes Julia Baker and Alexander Scott and, thus, threatening the civil rights era's pervasive images of idealized Negro-ness of the mid-sixties. Yet Wilson's presence as a Negro comic in high profile mainstream venues—particularly on television—represented significant strides for black performers. Furthermore, Wilson seemed to deliberately shun the notion of directly confronting either the existence or the roots of racial strife in America, as exemplified in a review of Wilson's performance as the inaugural comic act at New York's Rainbow Grill during the long, hot summer of 1968. Critic Dan Sullivan marvels at Wilson's willingness to engage material that "the average [read white] nightclub patron would not be expected to find amusing— race riots, looting, police brutality," including the characterization of his dapper attire (slate-blue suit, matching shirt, and white tie) as "his riot outfit," which the comic claims to have "got[ten] in last year, out of the window."[55] While Wilson goes on to draw a personal correlation between his consumerism and "looting season" ("I'm waiting until August, do my shopping in the summer"), he also quickly distances himself from the race and class anger that has acted as an impetus for these uprisings (beginning with the events in Watts in 1966 and extending beyond those after Dr. King's assassination in 1968) by reassuring the audience: "Just kidding, folks. The suit is from J. Press. I don't dig riots either."[56] Just as these joke series simultaneously acknowledge the state of race relations and refuse to comment on them, Wilson contended with criticism throughout his career regarding the overtly apolitical nature of his humor. "My racial message and my political point of view is my humor. My funny is my defense and my offense. Either you like it or you don't. . . . I'm a comic—all of my experiences and my emotions and hard times—I have reflected in what I do."[57]

By 1965, when Redd Foxx sat on the couch with Johnny Carson and hailed Wilson as the new young comic to watch, he had already established an extremely successful act as a headliner at the Apollo Theater and had begun to garner the top spots in mainstream (white) comedy clubs across the country. Actively endeavoring to expand on his "friendly relation" with mainstream audiences, Flip Wilson and his management carefully sought to maximize his crossover potential. As Monte Ray, Wilson's longtime manager, stated, "We set our sight on television but first we had to prove that Flip could play to white audiences. So we did Playboy Clubs to test material on a white middle class audience. It worked fine and we got a booking on *The Johnny Carson Show*."[58]

His set on *The Tonight Show*, later the same year, featured a routine that had already appeared on his debut album and featured the character types that would become staples for the televisual Wilson, the story of Christopher Columbus. Like Cosby's choice to use the Noah routine for his television debut, which managed to have a contemporary sound with material that was fundamentally noncontroversial, Wilson's take on Columbus showcased the multiple black voices in his comic arsenal without making blackness an issue. The highlight of the routine was Columbus appealing to the Queen, "Isabelle . . . Isabelle Johnson. That was the Queen's name":

> Chris tells her, "If I don't discover America, there's not going to be a Benjamin Franklin or a Star Spangled Banner or a home of the free and a land of the brave. And no Ray Charles." When the queen heard no Ray Charles, she panicked. [Wilson slips into the sassy falsetto and the hip swishing sashaying that will be associated with his most famous character, Geraldine.] The Queen say, " . . . You're gonna find Ray Charles." Chris says "Damn right, that's where those records come from." So the Queen's running through the halls of the castle screamin', "Chris gonna find Ray Charles, honey. . . . What you say."

Through this hilarious form of historical disjuncture, racial displacement (by racializing both the hipster aspects of "Chris" and his queen, "Isabelle Johnson," in speech and motion), and ratcheting up the hipness quotient (by referencing the widely revered—and crossed-over—musical artist Ray Charles), Wilson colorizes a white milieu in the least threatening way possible—by fictionalizing and colorizing it. Even in Wilson's small-screen debut, what Watkins describes as the comic's "frank reflections of typical black attitudes and flamboyant use of the timbre and resonances of black street language" was presented in a way that allowed him to move easily into the televisual mainstream.[59]

It was only a matter of time before Wilson was able to master the medium: the intimacy, the immediacy, and the amiability of his performance style would enable American audiences to welcome him into their homes via the electronic hearth—at least for a little while. In the late sixties Wilson made frequent appearances on the talk/variety show circuit doing guest spots on *The Merv Griffin Show*, *The Andy Williams Show*, *The Ed Sullivan Show*, and *Rowan and Martin's Laugh In*, as well as acting as guest host on *The Tonight Show with Johnny Carson*. After two moderately successful television specials and a pilot (that was viewed as "too satirical" by network brass), veteran television producer Bob Henry was brought onboard along with a concept for a series that would truly be focused on Flip. In the waning days of the variety show format, *The Flip Wilson Show* premiered on NBC in September of 1970 as a retooling of the genre (with a greater focus on comedy) and became an instant success.

The new variety series was truly Wilson's show: the comic was directly involved in every aspect of the series: from the design of the round stage (that

he felt afforded greater intimacy with the audience) to the writing of the
sketches (over which the comic had close oversight). Wilson's vision of the series
was extremely clear, and as producer Henry stated, "I told [the writers, makeup
and costume staffs, and the crew] the best thing we could do was keep out of
Flip's way."[60] In many ways Wilson's degree of creative control and comic
agency was unprecedented: "I've got all the freedom I could want in this show.
If it doesn't work, I won't have anyone to blame but myself."[61] But it did work.
One of the keys to the series' success was that it had something for everyone.
His guest stars appealed to the older generation (black and white) with main-
stream Hollywood film and television stars (including Lucille Ball and Bing
Crosby), as well as black entertainment stars known by white audiences (Lena
Horne and Louis Armstrong), and those who had not necessarily crossed over
(Mahalia Jackson and Billy Eckstine). For the boomers (black and white) there
was a wide range of stars with significant popular cultural cred from the world
of sports (including Muhammed Ali and Joe Namath), music (such as Aretha
Franklin and The Temptations), and comedy (including Cosby, Pryor, George
Carlin, and Lily Tomlin). Even Big Bird from Sesame Street and British broad-
caster and satirist David Frost were guests on Wilson's first show. The biggest
appeal of *The Flip Wilson Show*, however, was Flip Wilson, who *Los Angeles Times*
critic Robert Hilburn hailed as "one of the hottest comedians in the country"
on the eve of the series' premiere.[62]

Often the pilot episode of a series gives the clearest picture of what the creator's intentions for the series are (a sense of what they would like the series to
be) before the reviews, the first set of ratings, and the network notes based on
the ratings can begin to mold the show in a different image. Such was the case
for *The Flip Wilson Show*. The comic subscribed to the belief that the success of
the series depended on his "tenets of comedy": "First, I'm a friend. The audience likes me. . . . The second thing is that they like my characters. . . . The third
thing is that I talk to an audience honestly. I don't waste their time. I do my act
with everything I've got every second I'm on camera."[63] Wilson, their friend,
emerges from the audience and bounds onto the stage in the round setting. The
comic exudes hipness in his gray flared suit, magenta shirt, and gold and paisley
tie. Smiling broadly and making little bows to the audience, Wilson makes clear
that this is all about them. Even his opening monologue situates him as both
"one of them" and someone "sharing" something real with them—even if it is
being done while just telling them a story. Regaling the crowd about how
everyone has been asking him "What's *The Flip Wilson Show* gonna be like?" The
question is repeated several times in reference to the folks calling him at home
"all hours of the night," stopping him on the street, and even resorting to running into his car in order to ask the comic, "What's *The Flip Wilson Show* gonna
be like?" With the slightly exaggerated gestures accompanying casual speech, the
comic maneuvers the audience into his confidence—he lets the audience know
what's going on with him. Both the energy level of his delivery and the broad-

ness of his gestures move up a level as he answers the oft-repeated question: "I decided to put in a way to be as explicit as possible. . . . The best way to put it would be to say (Wilson pauses for a little James Brownesque backward strut step), 'Watch out!'"

Smiling, clapping, assuring the audience that they are going to "dig it," Wilson continues developing his bonding with the "everyfolk" in the audience by explaining his decisions about the show's opening—that his initial desire to do a big production number with great scenery and dancing girls (the comic sashays to a tune of his own making) seemed a great idea until he saw the $104,000 price tag. Determining that the cost was just "ridiculous" and that "this show is gonna start off in the hole if you do it like that," he comes up with a solution that again positions him with the crowd: instead of the celebrity performing for them: "Everybody's seen those fancy production numbers on the other shows but how many people have actually seen $104,000? You know. I decided that we'll open the show by showing you what $104,000 actually looks like. May I have the envelope please?" A trumpet flourish accompanies the entrance of a tall, white, slightly stern looking guard in uniform carrying a large envelope, which he hands to the comic. He stands, at ready, next to the comic. As Wilson takes cash out of the envelope, does a quick double take in the guard's direction, "What are you doing with your hand on the gun? People can't relax and enjoy looking at the money with you standing there with your hand on the gun." Playfully, making a little move toward the guard (as though he is going to try to get past him), the comic says, "I bet if I tripped you and ran, you couldn't catch me." The crowd laughs and even the stern guard smiles slightly. Everybody likes Flip. As he fans the cash for the audience, Wilson states, "This is it, ladies and gentlemen, $104,000—[pauses slightly, again, as if letting them in on the joke] $500 is actual cash. Now wasn't that better than watching girls jumping on the stage." The audience laughs and applauds as the comic replaces the money in the envelope. Again, the mischievous Wilson emerges as he twice fakes a handoff to the guard, the way a child on the playground would play "keep away" with a ball, saying, in a slightly higher pitched timbre, "Yea-ah, Yea-ah." Finally he hands it over to the guard with the parting phrase, "Here you go brother." Wilson's clever opening is hardly revolutionary comedy. However, the opening, like the Alphabet song duet with Sesame Street's Big Bird that follows, exemplifies his "friend" tenet and the strategic mobilization of his likability in service to making his audience both broad and loyal—as one would want friends to be.

Wilson's second tenet regarding the likability of his characters speaks directly to his ability to create a universalizing appeal with culturally specific material. With Wilson's Reverend Leroy in black tailcoat, white dickey, black string tie, and spats, he is clearly visually constructed as a figure from a different era, further accentuating the Calhoun-like (*Amos 'n' Andy*) aura of the character. Offering a visual contrast to his "backups," the Deacons, four black men (roughly Flip's age and younger) dressed in plain contemporary black suits and ties, white shirts, and gloves, and wearing white flowers on their lapels, the Reverend, a visual throwback, makes clear that this church is all about the present: "Welcome to the church of what's happening now. We don't tell you what happened a long time ago or what happened in the future, we tell you what's going on now." Strutting around the stage, à la sixties black evangelist Reverend Ike, with a few quick-stepping moves more reminiscent of a soul (rather than gospel) performer thrown in, the Reverend Leroy blends the old school Baptist preacher, the Chitlin' Circuit comic endman (who delivers the punch of the joke), and the black hipster humor of his contemporary persona. The little growl in his voice as it deepens and rises for emphasis, the rhythmic patter of his sermonettes, and the didactic one-liners act as homage to the past while the little self-satisfied chuckles, smiles, and glances to the audience act as a signal to the viewer that Wilson knows exactly what he is doing—a de facto wink to one segment of his broad audience. Certainly, black audiences understood the inter- and extratextual sampling he utilized—the image of black hucksters (including Kingfish and Calhoun) and the personage of Reverend Ike supplied commonplace cultural references. However, the foibles of the comically arrogant reverend and his performance, which for good and ill harkens back to earlier televisual constructions of the black hucksters (*Amos 'n' Andy*), provided an uncritical celebration of a very old-school form of black humor with which white audiences were also familiar.

Reverend Leroy made his television debut in a sketch that was as benign as it was culturally specific. The character constructions and performance style in the sketch that parodied the black church were familiar in African American humor—from the ongoing appeals for funds ("Money is like blood, it needs to circulate") to indications that unimpeachable virtue and a vow of poverty were not a part of the Reverend's calling (when asked to move his blue Cadillac El Dorado blocking the driveway, he replies with a wry smile, "The 'raffles' were good to me this month"). The Reverend's debut was also unchallenging for the mainstream audience, supplying neither political directives nor nuanced cultural edification. As Acham states, "Wilson's engagement in Chitlin' Circuit humor was apparent and appreciated by black audiences raised on this type of humor. . . . [When] he brought this to a mainstream audience, he did not disguise his blackness and his routines were based in traditional African American comedy."[64] When transferred from his act onto the small screen, the flamboyant antics and broadness of decidedly black humor in Wilson's various comic alter egos were extremely popular. However, the laughter generated by Wilson's characters also proved disconcerting to those in the audience who viewed their mainstream embrace warily. Arguably, no character was more popular or more problematic than Geraldine Jones.

Flip Wilson's Geraldine Jones was part Sapphire, part Foxy Brown (and, in terms of fashion sensibility, part *That Girl's* Ann Marie). Geraldine was alter-

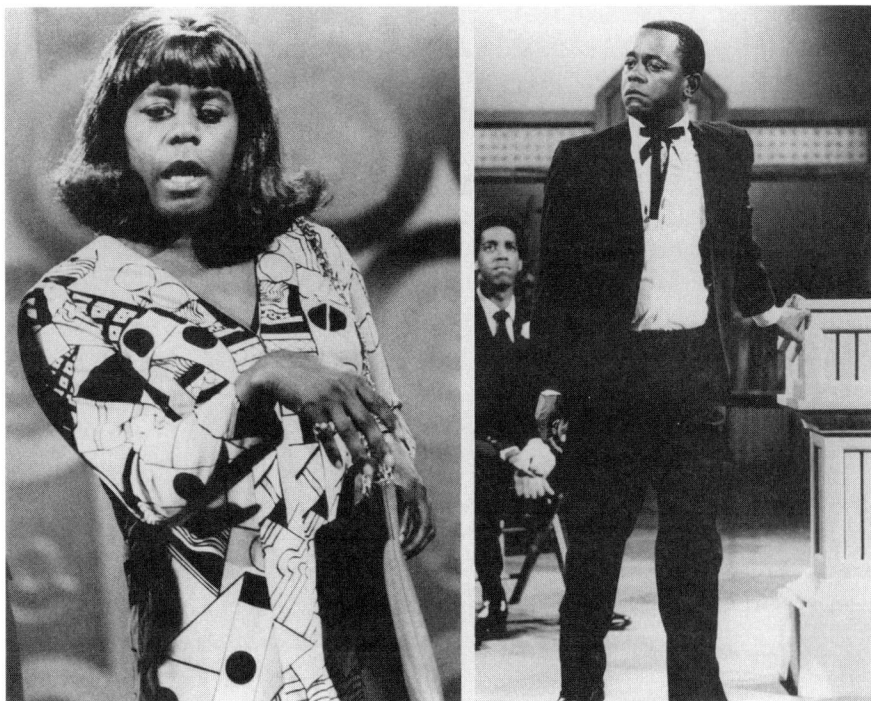

6. Flip Wilson's Geraldine and Rev. Leroy bring cultural specificity to prime time. *The Flip Wilson Show* (NBC) 1970–74. Photo from Photofest. Reproduced with permission from NBC.

nately praised as a progressive construction of a black working-class girl and vilified as a caricature of the bossy black woman. One might argue that the use of drag can be seen as either a liberating device utilized to interrogate stereotypes or as a means of rearticulating (and, arguably, recodifying) them within the context of black comedy. When Wilson did drag, it was both.

On one hand, Geraldine's perfectly coiffed hair and miniskirted designer wear were intended to look decidedly (and attractively) feminine. Geraldine's visage was carefully crafted to at least approximate the (hip) everywoman. Thus, Wilson's character was a far cry from either the lipstick-smeared, outrageously costumed vaudeo drag of Uncle Miltie (Milton Berle), from television's early years, or the frat-boy version used by Martin Lawrence in his construction of a ghetto-not-so-fabulous fly-girl wannabe, Sheneneh Jenkins, on his nineties net-let sitcom, *Martin*. In other words, Wilson attained a degree of drag credibility.[65] Audiences viewed neither Lawrence's nor Berle's characters as women because they were intended as caricatured comic devices for broad and physical humor; however, Geraldine, unlike her drag predecessor or progeny, took on a life of her own. Wilson believed that "the secret of the success of Geraldine was that she's not a putdown of women. She's smart, she's loyal [and] she's sassy. Most drag impersonation was a drag. But women can like Geraldine, men can like Geraldine, everyone can like Geraldine."[66] Much of the laughter was generated by the cherubic faced Flip, recognizable as Geraldine, completely immersed in the character—not exactly playing it straight but playing it earnestly. Thus, while there was the acknowledgment that Wilson was doing drag, Geraldine, arguably, became the iteration of black womanhood most familiar to the American television audience in the seventies.

On the other hand, there were aspects of Geraldine that not everybody liked. Although, as Watkins notes, "her trademark quips—'When you're hot, you're hot; when you're not, you're not,' 'The devil made me do it' and 'What you see is what you get'—became national catch phrases, part of everyone's vocabulary," so too did a problematic construction of black womanhood as overtly sexual, as possessing questionable intellectual acuity (at least, in academic terms), and as more than slightly assertive and outspoken. In the character's television debut in a sketch featuring British journalist (and glitterati) David Frost, Geraldine Jones is introduced as the "average woman." When Wilson emerges, clad in purple minidress with matching hose, shoes, and purse (and, of course, hair in what became her signature "flip"), Geraldine struts, dances, and poses as she makes her way down the runway to Frost. When Frost attempts to make the chivalrous gesture of kissing her hand, Geraldine pulls away, saying, "Watch what you're kissing, honey." During the "interview" Geraldine pivots back and forth in the swivel chair saucily while admiring her own appearance with the pronouncement, "What you see is what you get," punctuated with a snap and "Woooo" (a feminized, high-pitched version of James Brown's patented "lyric"). The crowd goes crazy, and Frost, who was also viewed as a notorious playboy, quips, "Promises, promises." Her responses to Frost's inquiries are laced with sexual innuendo: whether the blissful shiver and "Woooo" when first talking about her boyfriend, "Killer" (who, although never seen, resonates with the aura of the "black buck"), or her recounting that, in a childhood without television, "playing behind the couch" was her primary activity.

Interestingly, Geraldine was given more sexual agency than many black women on television: as the fried chicken (!) delivery girl she flirted shamelessly with actor/athlete/activist Jim Brown, and she encouraged and then spurned the advances of quarterback playboy Joe Namath (sending Killer to the rendezvous "in the booth in the back at the table in the dark" in her stead). In what Wilson considered the funniest Geraldine moment, Miss Jones appears as a Playboy bunny, the ultimate symbol of woman as sex object, with old Hollywood stalwart, actor/singer Bing Crosby, as a slightly inebriated conventioneer. Despite the network expressing concerns over the character's costumes getting "too skimpy" (and their desire for wardrobe approval), Geraldine makes her entrance, sauntering down a sweeping staircase, clad in a strapless one-piece, bunny ears, tail, white collar, and black tie.

CROSBY: I see but I don't believe.
GERALDINE: You better believe it, 'cause you ain't gonna see it.

While Crosby's conventioneer makes a halfhearted play for Geraldine's affections, which is staved off by her mention of Killer, one wonders if the uproarious laughter generated by "bunny drag" is also inflected by both Eurocentric notions of beauty and an ahistorical construction of black woman as sex object. Yet Geraldine's sexual agency was mitigated—particularly in terms of her primary relationship with the eternally absent Killer—in a manner that seemed to hearken back to aspects of the desexualized mammy rather than embody the sexual revolution ethos.

When Frost inquires whether she and "Mr. Killer" are engaged, Geraldine replies, "Sort of. He gave me a ring, but I couldn't keep up the payments." This exchange, as well as others that address Killer's possessiveness and a degree of his disinterest, seems akin to the dynamic between an early televisual representation of the "good" black woman waiting for the purportedly unreliable black man (the happy domestic/mammy, Beulah, and her partially committed and sporadically employed beau, Bill). At the same time, the threat of violence ensuring her fidelity (the boyfriend's name is Killer) and the flirtatiousness that informs all of her interactions (with black and white guest stars) complicate Geraldine's image of black womanhood and sexuality, which is simultaneously valued and devalued, empowered and disempowered.

This tension is further problematized by Geraldine's assertiveness, which is undercut by the limited nature of her vocabulary (which, arguably, reads as a signifier of her level of intelligence). From her assertion that she wasn't in a "relationship" with Killer, but rather they were "going together," to her admonishment of Frost's praise of her as "a couturier" because of her self-designed ensemble ("You better watch your mouth. You don't know me. . . . I'll turn this television studio out."), the responses seem to be coded by class as well as race. The notions of strong assertions (tainted with the threat of physicality) and limited understanding further play out when Geraldine is asked to comment on the state of women in America; she supplies both extraneous additional information and a patented one-liner that does not directly address the question: "Your show and the news are my favorite programs. I listen to all of them . . . and can't nobody tell Geraldine what to say. . . . The cost of living is going up and the chance of living is going down." (Again, punctuated with the snap, swivel, and "Woooo.")

Although at the end of this scene Geraldine convinces Frost to allow her to regale the audience with a lounge singer–like version of the standard "All of Me," after which he sweeps her up and carries her offstage, the banter that precedes the denouement provides yet another moment of differentiation between Geraldine and the comic personae of other black female comics of Wilson's day. When she insists on being allowed to sing, Frost quips, "I didn't have this trouble

with Moms Mabley," to which Geraldine replies, "I didn't have this trouble with
Johnny Carson either." As will be discussed in chapter 4, Moms Mabley's comic
persona, as revisionist mammy, presented one of the few iterations of black
female sexual agency in mainstream comedy that was seen as acceptable because
her artifice made it impossible for her to be seen as a sex object. Wilson's Geraldine was constructed repeatedly as sex object, although both the narrative of the
sketches and the acknowledgment of drag acted as mitigating factors. Nevertheless, during Geraldine's heyday the black man playing a black woman was
given greater comic license than actual black comediennes—as well as greater
mainstream acceptance. Geraldine's retort that she didn't have this trouble with
Carson speaks to both the comic's long-standing relationship to the king of late
night and the mainstream embrace of his image of the black everywoman.

There is still disagreement about the impact and importance of the manner
in which *The Flip Wilson Show* brought ethnic humor back into prime time.
Donald Bogle points out that for some black televisual spectators the fact that
Wilson's characters "were funny when performed within the black community"
did not assuage their concerns that once "taken out of an African American
context and put on white television . . . [they] could be misinterpreted."[67]
According to Christine Acham, critiques rooted in "the tenets of uplift, [and]
the fear of what white America might think of the black characters that Wilson
presented," were so preoccupied with the nature of mainstream (read white)
audiences' readings of the series that they often underestimated both the power
and the pleasures of the text for black viewers.[68] In actuality both assertions are
valid, particularly when one juxtaposes the Chitlin' Circuit–informed, broad
ethnic humor of Wilson's show (full of mugging, misspeaking wordplay, and
fundamentally uncritical takes on contemporary black life) and the social relevance dramatic programming emerging on network television in the late sixties
and early seventies, including *The Mod Squad*, *The Young Lawyers*, or even *Room
222* (each of which in its own right had problematic representational politics).
Wilson's series, like his act, was structured for both broad appeal and the adherence to his comic sensibility, which was driven not by social critique but rather
by his own, albeit culturally informed, notion of what was funny.

The aspects of Wilson's show that were out of sync with black culture in
the age of black power did not go unnoticed—even in the entertainment mainstream. In his 1971 *Life* feature on the comic, John Leonard asserted that "in a
time of Black Panthers and savage rhetoric," Wilson had succeeded in "tak[ing]
the threat out of the fact of Blackness."[69] Although one must process Leonard's
statement a bit warily within the sociopolitical context of an era when, as J. Fred
MacDonald stated, "Thanks to Wilson, Americans fell in love with racial comedy," it speaks to how and why Wilson's show, as well as his comic personae, had
a life span far shorter than one would have anticipated given its initial success.[70]
During the trek from Negro to black in the waning days of the civil rights and
black power era, Wilson's comic personae *showed* blackness to the mainstream—

celebrating the unique voices, humor, and cultural practices past and present—without actually engaging, *telling*, what it meant to be black in America at that historical moment. Thus, the criticism of Wilson's comedy as diffusing his blackness is inaccurate, but I would assert that the comedy was decontextualized. His series, rightfully lauded as bringing the black voice into the mainstream of American comedy, represented black humor, centering it within that one-hour time slot without relating it to the realities of blackness (on and off prime time) during the other twenty-three.

Wilson maintained "my show is my statement," and as the seventies drew to a close, the facts of blackness were beginning to be addressed *directly* in comedic social discourse, black film and music, and black popular culture at large. In popular consciousness, by the end of his series Wilson's comic persona was tied to the show and to the characters that it made famous—particularly, Geraldine. When tributes to Wilson were held at the Museum of Television and Radio in Los Angeles and New York in 1993, the comic fielded numerous questions about his most famous character, from her inspiration (named after the girl who got away in his adolescence) to his comfort with drag (dating back to his childhood performance as a black Clara Barton). As if to end discussion of Geraldine (and stave off requests for her reincarnation), Wilson stated, "Geraldine carried me longer than my mother did—and I enjoyed it. And I am always flattered and honored when someone requests and acknowledges their affection for Geraldine—and it was fun but I'm approaching 60 and I would rather always have her be that fun fresh memory that she is and I think that Mr. Wilson will go the rest of the way on his own."[71] On his own, however, Wilson's likability and the cultural specificity of his black comic voice, vital elements in his mainstream popularity, were not easily transferable after the end of his series' run, either to the Cosbyesque *Charlie and Company* in the eighties or to his medium of second choice, cinema.

In 1971, at the height of the series' popularity, Wilson articulated both his comic and his ideological imperatives: "What I'm trying to say through the show is that the Old Uncle Tom of the Negro is not necessary. That a Negro can stand up and be a man, simply by being himself—just like me."[72] The statement seems more than slightly ironic given that the comic's comedic bread and butter came from Wilson's standing up and being a "woman," Geraldine. Nevertheless, on both stage and small screen Wilson achieved that goal and, in so doing, won the battle to maintain comedy's friendly relation. Just as Wilson's "handshake" (slapping hands [in the "give me five" fashion], knocking elbows, and bumping hips), a play on physicalized greetings within the black community, was fleetingly appropriated as a sign of "down-ness" in mainstream American popular culture and later abandoned as no longer "hip," his comic's persona, tied to an individualistic notion of black representational politics, lost the war in staying in tune with the changing tides of black thought and popular culture. This does not diminish Wilson's comic legacy: by bringing black voices with inner-city vernacular and ties to traditional forms of black humor into the mainstream, Wilson provided a point of departure for a new comedic discursive strategy. He opened up the possibility for the African American condition to be both subject and object in stand-up told by an unabashedly, specifically black voice. As Bruce Britt stated in his 1998 homage to the comic, "his show was gentle, classy and soulful—the television equivalent of a Motown tune"; and by 1974 Wilson was no longer "hip" in the new age of funk and disco and the "raunchy realism" appearing on the comedic landscape. Wilson's time passed, perhaps, too quickly; Pryor's was just beginning.

### PRYOR: FROM NEGRO TO BLACK

Traces of Cosby's universalist riffing, Wilson's culturally specific cast of characters, and Gregory's social commentary can all be seen in the evolving comic personae of Richard Pryor. As Pryor himself noted, "Dick Gregory used to have stuff in *Jet* magazine. That's how I started reading his material and do[ing] it on stage. That was my first breakthrough.... Then I moved on to Bill Cosby ... [impersonating Cosby]. And I know [doing the hand gestures as well] ... I made a lot of money as Bill Cosby."[73] Indeed, early Pryor was extremely Cosbyesque—the clean-shaven rubbery-faced kid in the Beatle suit doing physical shtick on *The Ed Sullivan Show* while recounting schoolyard exploits ("Look at Richard running, but he's running cool"). In 1967, when the comic made a premature exit from an appearance onstage at the Las Vegas Aladdin Hotel Stage (he left in the middle of a performance), Pryor stated that he knew his "days of pretending to be as slick and colorless as Cosby were numbered. There was a world of junkies and winos, pool hustlers and prostitutes, women and family screaming inside [his] head, trying to be heard."[74]

Pryor spent two years in Berkeley, reading Malcolm X, engaging a group of black intellectuals (including Ishmael Reed, Claude Brown, and Cecil Brown) ensconced in the Bay Area in the early seventies and visiting bars, clubs, and street corners to observe myriad aspects of black life. During this time a transformation took place for Pryor, and when he returned to performing, first to predominantly black audiences at Redd Foxx's club in Los Angeles and the Village Gate in New York, the comic had "killed the Cosby" in his act. Having abandoned the pursuit of audience acceptance through the comic reification of middle-class norms and mores, Pryor offered his audiences characters, metaphors, and language that was earthy, profane, and true, rooted not only in the lived experiences of those he had observed during his Berkeley exile but also those who peopled the sketchy spaces of the Peoria, Illinois, brothel run by his family (his grandmother was the madam) and his own coming-of-age experiences that involved constant engagement with moral ambiguity, as well as numerous encounters with a distinctly midwestern brand of racism. Thus, Pryor began to challenge "traditional show business assumptions about the viability of ungentrified black material and an unmoderated black voice ... [and broke] with blacks' long standing tradition of subterfuge and concealment of inner community customs."[75]

After the Berkeley years the plethora of voices began to coalesce in Pryor's comic persona. However, as early as 1968 the seeds of the burgeoning persona could be seen on his self-titled first comedy album—as was indicated by the cover. Emblazoned with the image of Pryor gone "native" (almost naked in a parody of *National Geographic* photographs of African tribesmen), the album, like the cover art, offered a contentiously hilarious picture and "routines like 'Super Nigger' revealed the voice that was breaking through. A point of view was percolating beneath the surface": "We find Super Nigger, with his X-Ray vision that enables him to see through everything except Whitey, disguised as Clark Washington, mild-mannered custodian for the *Daily Planet*."[76] In this new persona one sees the uncontainable and unpredictable "crazy nigger" to come—and one also realizes that this iteration of Pryor will have almost nothing in common with the easily assimilated "Super Negro" types.

During this comic metamorphosis, spanning the end of the sixties and early seventies, Pryor simultaneously played with teasing out his burgeoning persona and, after the critical praise gained from his skillful wedding of pathos and wit as "Piano Man" in *Lady Sings the Blues*, parlaying his newfound celebrity into television and film roles. Pryor's life on the small screen reveals both the growing popularity of his profane and politicized voice and its lack of palatability in most mainstream televisual spaces—when Pryor was allowed to be Pryor. At times the comic power of his persona was simply underutilized; at others it was woefully misplaced, as exemplified in his appearance on the musical family domestic comedy *The Partridge Family*. In an episode entitled "The Soul Club" he and Lou Gossett Jr. played the patrons of a struggling Detroit club, who are saved by the family performing a street-party benefit.[77] One can almost hear the smirk in Pryor's voice when he utters the line, "We'll have the biggest party ever and go down in flames"—an interesting choice of words, given that the year is 1971 and the setting is Detroit. In this part of the televisual universe, there was simply no place for a voice as contentious, disruptive, and provocatively funny as Pryor's.

However, as Dick Gregory said, on the stand-up stage in this same era "[Pryor] did brain surgery on America's head."[78] His routines embodied both the rage and the vulnerability inherent in the burgeoning tide of heightened black awareness. As James McPherson surmised in his 1975 feature in *New York Times Magazine*: "Almost single-handedly, [Pryor] is creating a new style in American comedy, a style that some of his admirers call theater because there is no other category available for what he does."[79] The risks that Pryor took in his comedy seemed driven by the desire to articulate multiple forms of blackness—black voices—that had not previously been heard. As Pryor himself stated, "When I do characters, [I] have to do it true. . . . If I can't do it, I'll stop in the middle rather than pervert and turn it into 'Tomism.' . . . [There's a] thin line between laughing with and laughing at."[80] The divergences between Pryor's and Wilson's use of characters are worth noting, particularly in relationship to the ease with which their stand-up personae could cross over into mainstream media (namely film and television). As in Wilson's case, Pryor's characters evolved inside the comic's stand-up act and spoke to varied constructions of urban blackness. Unlike Wilson's, however, Pryor's voices more often than not lacked the amenable nature that made Wilson's characters likable to a broad audience. Furthermore, unrestrained by the mainstream sensibilities that had previously guided his comedy, Pryor challenged the audience through his use of characters although, as the comic stated matter-of-factly in 1975, "When I didn't do characters, white folks loved me."[81]

Pryor, who wrote for and guest starred on *The Flip Wilson Show*, brought a comic edge that could not easily be softened for television.[82] His stand-up (or sketch comedy) appearances on television often generated an excitement and volatility that drew audiences and scared network executives. As J. Fred Mac-Donald wrote in *Blacks and White TV*, "As seductive and popular as Pryor was with live audiences, his humor possessed a racially political quality which was foreign to network television."[83] Yet regardless of the venue, whether as a writer or a performer, Pryor brought that sensibility to the television efforts—when he had some degree of autonomy. In Lily Tomlin's 1973 comedy special, the "Juke and Opal" scene provided a seriocomic interlude with equal parts anger, cynicism, longing, and wit. Penned by a writing staff that included Pryor, the sketch featured the comic as Juke, a charming junkie, and Tomlin as Opal, his lover and coproprietor of a soul-food joint. The insightful and incisive humor was anchored in the characters' understanding of themselves and the world in which they lived—during the beginning of the post-soul era, when it became clear that the promises of the Dream had been either deferred or denied. This awareness of the urban American condition can be seen in Juke's and Opal's observations about the effectiveness of government-funded work/training programs:

JUKE:  I was doing the suit and tie thing last week. Now I learned how to do a job they don't need to.

OPAL:  Sometimes I think the only jobs from job training go to those doing the training.

Juke also encounters a young white liberal couple, survey "constituents" for the local congressman, asking invasive personal questions about a variety of issues (including addiction) with a mixture of ignorance and arrogance. (Although Juke answers he's addicted right now, he asks them not to write that down, "That's personal.") When Juke confiscates their clipboard and begins to ask them pointed but ludicrous questions, the implied mistrust of failed governmental efforts and lack of genuine concern for the underclass is palpable:

LIBERAL GUY:  We don't make up these questions.

JUKE: Gee, golly.
LIBERAL GUY: Try to understand.
OPAL: Try to understand, we *do* make up the answers.
JUKE: Press conference is over. Thank you, Mr. Cronkite.

As the sketch ends, Juke asks Opal for money, "I need it. Either I'm gonna get busted or you're gonna give me the bread." Over the objections of the Liberal Guy and Girl ("You know what he's going to do with it"), Opal acquiesces and creates a cover story—as much for Juke and herself as for the liberals—which makes it seem as though Juke can do the right thing, "I know what he's gonna do. He's gonna get me 10 lbs. of potatoes. I like the little red potatoes for my potato soup." As the liberals leave, Juke admonishes them for both their judgment and their inherent lack of understanding of his position as well as Opal's: "You wrong, man. I ain't a bad cat or nothing. [Because] you hurt me and I wasn't trying to interfere in your life."[84] The pathos and political commentary in the sketch, and the entire special, resonates with the postindustrial realities and the political disillusionment of the post–Watergate era: the comic, as part of the writing staff, won an Emmy.

Pryor's act was both topical and timeless, designed to challenge the audience, exemplified in the routine "Junkie and Wino," featured on his *That Nigger's Crazy* album, as well as on *Richard Pryor Live in Concert* (1979). After having advised the young junkie to "lay off that shit, nigger . . . shit done made you null and void," the Wino's sociopolitical advice can be found in his asides about the war on drugs ("They call it an epidemic now cuz white folks are using it"); and his final piece of advice speaks to the power dynamics between whites and blacks ("You don't know how to deal with the white man, that's yo problem. I know how to deal with him—that's why I'm in the position I am"). By depicting "the wino as a city-living country wit and the junkie as a wasted young urban zombie," Pryor, "an artist/cocaine addict himself, provided nuance to the difference between addiction to heroin and alcohol and to how it would eventually affect the entire black community," as well as the humanizing vision of cross-generational despair.[85]

As Mel Watkins states, Pryor incorporated pride in black folkways and the exuberance and joy of much black humor and thereby "completely unmasked the complex matrix of pride, self-mockery, blunt confrontation of reality, double edged irony, satiric wit, assertive defiance, poetic obscenity, and verbal acuity that finally define the elusive entity that may be called African American humor."[86] In many ways Pryor's comic personae existed in this intersection of contemporary black comic sensibility and folk humor as exemplified by the Pryor character with the greatest longevity, Mudbone. Through this sly, meandering country philosopher, whose voice (equal parts Mississippi Delta blues singer and early Chitlin' Circuit storyteller), the comic embodied the black folk construction of the trickster that also resonated within the street humor of urban black America. In his autobiography, *Pryor Convictions and Other Life Sentences*, Mudbone, who acts as the omniscient narrator for the comic's life story, tells "the truth" about the kind of comedy that Pryor was compelled to do: "See I was honest with the motherfucker. I told him comedy—real comedy—wasn't only tellin' jokes. It was about telling the truth. Talking about life. Makin' light of the hard times. Definitely not as funny as it looks . . . you start telling the truth to people and people gonna look at you like you was askin' to fuck their mama or somethin'. The truth is gonna be funny but it is gonna scare the shit outta folks."[87]

Pryor rejected the notion of deemphasizing cultural difference and economic and political disparities between black and white lives; rather, his comic persona embraced the identity of an equal-opportunity offender: everything and everyone was fair game, including himself. The tumultuous events in his offstage life fed his act, as exemplified in his depiction of his rapid romance with drugs in "Cocaine" and his recounting of how "being funny saved [my] ass," quite literally, in "Prison." Yet the personalized stories provided multiple levels of commentary: his "I Killed My Car" begins as a self-revealing description of the death knell of marriage number three (as he takes a Magnum and shoots the car in which his wife is planning to depart), and it evolves into a commentary on the mistrust of white authority: "Then the police came and I went into the house because they got Magnums, too. And they don't shoot cars, they shoot *nig-gars*." Furthermore, Pryor's espoused belief that "black people can't disassociate themselves from race because we're living in a white world" acted as a pedagogical imperative for his lived experiences as material for critiquing the differences between being black and white in America, as exemplified in the "Just Us" routine from his 1975 release *Is It Something I Said*: "I went to jail for tax evasion—I didn't know a motherfucking thing about no taxes. I told the judge, 'Your honor, I forgot.' He said, 'You'll remember next year, nigger.' [Then they] start riding on your ass. They give niggers time like it's lunch down there. You go down there looking for justice and that's what you get—just us."

From the freebasing accident, which left him with third-degree burns over 75 percent of his body, recounted with mitigated veracity in *Richard Pryor: Live on the Sunset Strip* to the terrifyingly funny material on his heart attack from *Richard Pryor Live in Concert*, Pryor still managed to shade the humor with racial specificity: "[After the heart attack] I woke up in an ambulance, right? And there wasn't nothin' but white people starin' at me. I say, 'Ain't that a bitch. I done died and wound up in the wrong motherfuckin' heaven. Now, I gotta listen to Lawrence Welk for the rest of my days.'" Likewise, his emergent black consciousness acted as fodder for the comedic discursive mill in the "black power" routine: "I was a Negro for twenty-three years—I gave it up . . . there was no room for advancement."

For Pryor the trek from Negro to black went through nigger. Beginning in the seventies, the comic's use of the word *nigger* became a hot-button issue for both his critics and his audiences. One might argue that Pryor deflated the negative power of the word by using it to describe all black folks as he incorporated characters and stories culled from his childhood among the dispossessed of his native Peoria and his stints on the Chitlin' Circuit. Nevertheless, in his act, his life, and the titles to his comedy albums (including *That Nigger's Crazy*, on which his initial observations about law enforcement appear), Pryor used the term—both casually and pointedly—to differentiate black and white experiences of American life. "Police in y'all's neighborhood 'Hello, Officer Timson, going bowling tonight?' 'Why, yes. Ah, nice Pinto you got there.' Niggers don't know 'em like that. . . . See, white folks get a ticket, they pull over, 'Hey, officer, yes, glad to be of help . . . cheerio!' Niggers be talkin' 'bout, 'I am reaching into my pocket for my license, cuz I don't want there to be no motherfuckin' accident.'" In the stand-up world Pryor was repeatedly lauded for presenting the experiences of the black underclass with startling clarity and equal candor, as Dick Gregory stated in the HBO documentary *Mo' Funny*, "articulating the [black] experience the way we hear each other do it." While Pryor's routines, undoubtedly, exposed an insider's view of multiple segments of the black community, they also illustrated how the personal was political.

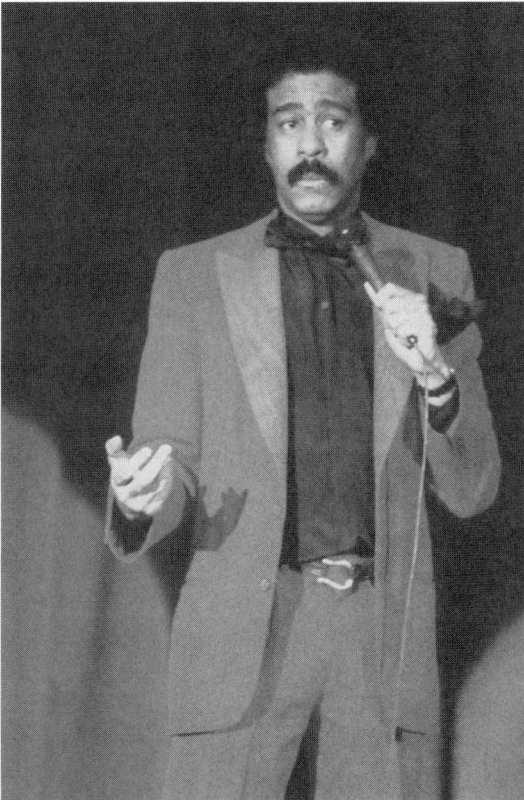

7. Richard Pryor's profane, profound, and painfully personal performance. *Richard Pryor: Live on the Sunset Strip* (1982). Directed by Joe Layton. Photo from Photofest. Reproduced with permission from Columbia Pictures.

By 1982 the comic offered an undertaking that was more than a semantic reenvisioning of previous assertions about the *N* word. However, the impetus to recuperate the word were rooted in notions of black pride and the articulation of the African American condition born during his Berkeley walkabout. Thus, it was not surprising that when *Wattstax* (1973), the film capturing the celebration of black music and culture in the neighborhood known as the site of an explosion of rage and frustration in the riots six years earlier, was released, Pryor played a prominent role. The description of *Wattstax* in *The Death of Rhythm and Blues* captures the quintessential post-soul moment: "On August 20, 1972, Bell and Jackson stood side by side in the middle of the cavernous Los Angeles Coliseum, chanted 'I Am Somebody,' and then raised their fists in the black power salute before a hundred thousand music fans. With that gesture began a long day of live music by every Stax artist to raise money for the Watts Summer Festival. It was a symbol of black self-sufficiency."[88] Pryor acted as part casual commentator/part Greek chorus in filmed excerpts between the concert performances of his fellow artists on the legendary Stax label, including Isaac Hayes and The Staples Singers. His commentaries focused on the lived experiences of blacks in California with startling candor. Long before the events that would incite a second uprising in black Los Angeles, he addressed the issue of police brutality: "California's a weird place. . . . They have laws for pedestrians. You know, like you can cross the street but they don't have laws for [black] people at night when cops accidentally shoot people. They accidentally shoot more niggers out here than any place in the world. Every time you pick up a paper: 'Nigger accidentally shot in the ass.' How do you accidentally shoot a nigger six times in the chest? [In white voice] 'Well, my gun fell and it just went crazy.'"[89] An essential element of Pryor's comic persona was its rawness in terms of its outspoken viewpoint, its language, and the vulnerability it revealed to audiences. Just as his act reflected the ongoing saga of his public and private travails, Pryor's comic persona was in conversation with the evolution of his personal and political consciousness.

In the famous Africa bit from *Richard Pryor: Live on Sunset Strip* (1982) Pryor shares a genuine epiphany that, like his early assertion about Negro-ness, speaks to both an ideological and a stylistic shift for the comic, as well as the abandonment of the word *nigger*, which had been a staple in the comic's lexicon for a significant part of his career:

> One thing that happened to me that was magic was that I was leaving, sitting in the hotel lobby, and a voice said, "What do you see? Look around." And I looked around, and I looked around, and I saw people of all colors and shapes, and the voice said, "You see any niggers?" I said, "No." It said, "You know why? 'Cause there aren't any." There ain't no niggers in Africa! 'Cause I'd been there three weeks and hadn't said it once. And it started making me cry, man. All that shit. All the acts I've been doing. As an artist and comedian. Speaking and trying to say something. And I been saying

that. That's a devastating fucking word. That has nothing to do with us. We are from a place where they first started people.

In the seventies, after the golden age of blaxploitation and before the emergence of the buppie, during an era when black nationalist mobilization of Afrocentrism was slowly transforming into an era driven by an almost marginally historicized (see *Roots*) fashion-driven cultural embrace, any comedic articulation of blackness could not help but be contingent and conflicted, and Pryor gave voice to these strong, fluid, and contentious notions of blackness.

As Jill Nelson states in her review of Pryor's autobiography, "What could we expect from this man who at his best balanced precariously on a comic edge, who used the joy and tragedy of his own life and the lives of those derisively called niggers—pre-hip-hop, before it was spelled 'Niggaz' and declared cool—to create not simply comedy, but streetwise social commentary?"[90] By extrapolation, one can see the comic lineage that connects Pryor to the post-soul comics. Pryor's direct and indirect influence (via the first- and second-wave comics like Murphy and Rock) on the Def Jam generation is inestimable. Pryor, inspired by blue comic extraordinaire of the previous generation Redd Foxx, folded aspects of his predecessor's raunch and rawness into his own particular sociopolitically informed comedic mixture. Likewise, these post-soul comics, as will be discussed in greater detail in the chapter focusing on Dave Chappelle and the Def Jam persona, created something markedly different from Pryor's comedic discourse—particularly in relation to the comic's problematic gender politics. Pryor's material often deals with women in relation to their sexual use to men. In one routine acknowledging the differences between a white and black male's response to a date ending with only a goodnight kiss, he forwards the black male's position ("Nigger spent $35—somebody's gonna fuck"), an assertion with which the hypothetical date's father agrees. In another, dealing with "your woman leaving you," the woman is given the power to deeply wound the male ego in his most vulnerable place, his sexual prowess:

MAN: I know the dick was good to ya. If it wasn't, why was you hollerin'?
WOMAN: I was hollerin' to keep from laughin' in your face.

Undoubtedly, these joke series illustrate how Pryor's sexual politics is informed by both the problematic black pride discursive that bell hooks refers to as "a dick thing" and an old-school bad-ass black machismo. Pryor, however, like his predecessor and unlike his progeny, while clearly engaging in objectification, does not exhibit the kind of *hatred* of women required to label his comedy misogynistic. Although Pryor may use the word *pussy*, he does not reduce women to the sum of their reproductive parts, the way Eddie Murphy does in *Raw*, where women are only "pussy" and "predator." One might argue that Pryor's sexual politics are inflected by a form of gender- and race-based self-awareness that alternately lauds and lampoons black masculine responses to women, as well as varying degrees of female sexual agency, which dilute the sexism in the comedic mixture. On the other hand, it might also be that Pryor, because he is Pryor, is simply given more slack.[91]

Despite the popularity of Pryor's work with young audiences (black and white) and the successes he experienced in mainstream film comedy (*Silver Streak*, 1976), Pryor was still deemed truly unfriendly to prime time, and his forays into television were marked by controversy. When *The Richard Pryor Show* premiered, it came into a network world (NBC) where LOP (least objectionable programming) was still a guiding force. Despite the fact that Pryor's humor seemed better suited for late night and his history with the network (when Pryor hosted *Saturday Night Live* in 1975—the episode that debuted the famous "word association" bit with Chevy Chase—the live show was put on seven-second delay), NBC gave the series the green light.[92] Whether inspired by the overwhelming critical and popular acclaim for *The Richard Pryor Special* (1997)—which, for the most part, allowed Pryor to be Pryor—or the belief that they could repeat the comic-centered sketch/variety show success that they had experienced with Wilson in the early seventies, it seems an understatement to say that in fall of 1977 NBC executives were anxious about what Pryor and his cadre of talented young writers (with head writer Paul Mooney) and comics (John Witherspoon, Tim Reid, Marsha Warfield, Sandra Bernhard, and Robin Williams) would do with an hour of prime-time programming. Furthermore, in a televisual landscape where *Happy Days* was the king of television comedy, *The Richard Pryor Show* was doomed.

One might hypothesize that NBC scheduled the show at the beginning of the Tuesday night prime-time lineup—and during family viewing hours—in an attempt to set clear parameters in terms of content. If indeed this was the case, the strategy was unsuccessful, and it placed Pryor in an untenable position. The battle with network Standards and Practices began with the first show and ended after the fourth and final episode of the series. In fact, the battle that signaled the end of an amenable relationship between Pryor and NBC involved the series' opening. The sketch, which never aired, codified the contentious tone of the rest of the series—the closing bit of three of the four episodes involved the "network" somehow trying to control Pryor's ability to leave: in the first episode bars slammed across his dressing room door; in the second he emerges from the swamp set, with broken shackles on his wrists and the sounds of barking dogs in the background; and in the third he is, literally, backed into the corner, guarded by a lion.

The long-lost opening clearly annunciated what would be the series' undoing and why Pryor would walk away after four episodes.[93] In medium close-up a shirtless Pryor, on a darkened stage, oozing "earnest" enthusiasm speaks directly to the audience:

> Good evening, ladies and gentlemen. Welcome to *The Richard Pryor Show*. My name is Richard Pryor and I'm so happy to have my own show, I don't

know what to do. I could jump up and down and sing "Yankee Doodle." There's a lot that's been written about me: am I gonna have a show? Am I not gonna have a show? Well, I'm having a show. People say, "How can you have a show? You have to compromise. You have to give up everything." [chuckles] Is that a joke or what? Look at me . . .

The camera pulls back into a medium close-up as Pryor says, "I'm standing here naked—I've given up absolutely nothing." The camera pulls back into a long shot that reveals Pryor in his glory—with all the anatomical correctness of a Ken doll. After the network's decision to cut the sketch, Pryor spoke with both anger and incredulousness: "What it's about is censorship and I can't work under these conditions. The sketch is important because I worked on it, it's about me and I'm the one they hired. If they didn't want Richard Pryor they should have gone out and gotten somebody else."[94] While the implications here are obvious, one wonders how either the network—or Pryor himself—could have thought that the union between the Peacock and the self-proclaimed "crazy nigger" could have ended any other way, particularly given the social and televisual climate.

Yet despite its woefully brief run and the prolonged tussle with Standards and Practices, when one watches *The Richard Pryor Show*, one can discern how the comic's persona was in conversation with the era.[95] The series premiered in September of 1977: a year after Jimmy Carter had beaten Gerald Ford in a presidential election that failed to meaningfully engage the postindustrial realities of the urban poor, the same year that *Roots* became A Novel for Television and sociocultural sensation by depicting an unseen chapter of African American history. On the network front the Tandem years of social sitcoms were coming to a close. With *Maude*, *All in the Family*, and *Good Times* limping through their last seasons, the brief ghetto sitcom boom was ending as televisual representations of black kids moved from their neighborhood (*What's Happening*, ending in 1978) to that of their white benefactor (*Diff'rent Strokes*, beginning in 1979), and even Sanford (Redd Foxx) had left *Sanford and Son*.[96] The black presence in the Nielsen top twenty in 1977 consisted of Isaac (Ted Lange), the bartender on *The Love Boat*, and Detective Harris (Ron Glass) on *Barney Miller* (unless, of course, you want to include various NFL players on *Monday Night Football*).[97] In terms of prime-time television, in the days before stand-up comedy and the cable boom, there was not a place for Pryor.

Diagnosed with multiple sclerosis in 1986, with the exception of a brief comeback in the early nineties Pryor was unable to perform after the late eighties. Despite declining health, however, Pryor remained until his death one of the most influential American comedians of the late twentieth century, and he is universally regarded as a major comedic influence by the generation of comic actors who followed him and who will be examined later in this volume. His impact is exemplified by the 2003 documentary tribute to the comic, *I Ain't Dead Yet, Motherfucker*, in which a cavalcade of stand-up all-stars (from Whoopi

Goldberg, Robin Williams, and Dave Chappelle to Jon Stewart, Chris Rock, and Margaret Cho) unabashedly sing very specific and personalized praises for the comic's contribution not just to comedy but to *their* comedy. In 1998 Pryor became the first recipient of the Kennedy Center's Mark Twain Prize for Humor.[98] Lawrence J. Wilker, president of the Kennedy Center, praised the comic, saying, "Pryor is an American who has made a significant contribution to humor. He really used humor the same way that Mark Twain did: to show us our foibles and to put us on the right path. He opened up race as a topic to talk about openly, before both black and white audiences perhaps were ready for that."[99] While Wilker's statement speaks to the significance of Pryor's perform-ance in both social and cultural terms, Pryor's comments on being the award's inaugural recipient directly addressed not only the ideological and pedagogical directives in his humor but also the role of humor in life: "It is nice to be regarded on par with a great white man—now that's funny! Seriously, though, [the] two things people, throughout history, have had in common are hatred and humor. I am proud that, like Mark Twain, I have been able to use humor to lessen people's hatred."[100]

Pryor revealed the key element to his comedy in a 2004 interview: "[Be] truthful, always truthful and funny will come." When in its stand-up mode, Pryor's comic persona (even when not completely forthcoming) resounded with humor that *felt* candid and real as it voiced multiple lived experiences and multiple articulations of blackness. His comedic discourse resonated with audi-ences across lines of class and color. Pryor's inability to tone down his comedy to be in step with the slowly changing comedic sensibilities of prime-time net-work television illustrated the wickedly funny and uncompromising nature of his stand-up persona—as well as, one would think, the difficulty (if not impos-sibility) of taking it from stage to *any* screen. Yet that transition did take place. Onstage, the genius of Pryor's comic persona is easily discernible in the wed-ding of dissonant strains of sociopolitical discourse in his voices (his own and those of his myriad characters) at play with and against stereotypical construc-tions of blackness, with and against normative notions of both class and race and with and against delimited notions of "acceptable" topics and content for comic commentary. On the circuitous trek to the big screen and mainstream Holly-wood film comedy, some of his "truth" got lost on the way.

## MOVIN' ON UP? CIVIL RIGHTS ERA
## COMICS AND CINEMATIC CROSSOVER

The stand-up iteration of the comedian's voice is the articulation of the core of his or her comic persona. One must discern, however, the ways in which that voice is mobilized within a variety of media in order to understand the place of the black comic persona in American popular culture. Once the pas-sage onto mainstream stages was secured for these civil rights era comics, the sojourn from stage to small screen followed relatively direct paths. Although the variety show and late-night talk shows provided the entrée to American homes via the electronic hearth (Gregory went from The Playboy Club to Jack Paar, Cosby [and later Wilson] from the Village Gate to *The Tonight Show*, Pryor from The Bitter End to *Kraft Music Hall*), the transition into Hollywood film proved a more arduous endeavor. In solely industrial terms Pryor and Cosby were the most successful of the comics who came of age in the civil rights era, having gained access and success in multiple segments of mainstream media. Ironically, only one of them would actually become a movie star—the comic deemed not ready for prime time, Richard Pryor.

That is not to say that Dick Gregory and Flip Wilson never ventured onto the big screen. There was, however, for Gregory, almost a thirty-year gap between his *dramatic* film roles as Richie "Eagle" Coles, a gifted and self-destructive jazz saxophonist in the independent *Sweet Love, Bitter* (1967), loosely based on the last years of Charlie Parker, and his role as local minister, the Reverend Slocum, in Mario Van Peebles's epic recounting the early years of the black nationalist group, *Panther* (1995). His nearly half a century as comic, activist, and author/cultural critic has, however, validated Gregory's screen presence within the documentary genre—making him an ideal subject for musings on civil rights, comedy, and popular culture in documentaries such as *Eyes on the Prize II* (1990), *Mo' Funny: Black Comedy in America* (1993), and *The N-Word* (2004). His comedic roles, on the big and small screen, are both few and curious: a bit part as minegar, wise, and wary washroom attendant in the 2002 Rob Schneider vehicle *The Hot Chick* (2002), and several spots on Comedy Central's irreverent *COPS* parody, *Reno 911* (2003), as a blind panhandler.[101]

Wilson maintained that television was always his medium of choice and his filmography reflects the preference. His first screen role, a cameo in *Uptown Saturday Night* (1974), allowed the comic to play a role taken directly from his stable of characters (a shady preacher) in a moderately successful black comedy (starring Cosby and with an appearance by Pryor). His two other screen outings—as the beleaguered coach of a struggling basketball team that "turns it around" by using astrology in *The Fish That Saved Pittsburgh* (1979) or in the homage to the wonderful world of roller disco in *Skatetown, USA* (also 1979) as Harvey Ross, the lecherous club owner, who is blackmailed into fixing "the big contest" to keep his wife, Mama (also played by Wilson), from discovering his "skirt-chasing"—did little for Wilson's post–variety show career. Curiously, by the end of the decade Wilson's comic personae, which had been welcomed into American homes so readily in the early seventies, could find no amenable or comfortable fit on either the big screen or small. One might hypothesize that in a different era Wilson's characters (or at least his ability to do multiple characters) might have been utilized on the big screen, thus parlaying his television popularity into a big-screen career in the same way that Martin Lawrence was able to do in *Big Momma's House* or Eddie Murphy in *The Nutty Professor*. As previously stated, neither Wilson's comic persona nor the old Chitlin' Circuit flavor—the (fundamentally) depoliticized cultural specificity and the G-rated (or, at worst, PG-rated) comic content of his comedy—had a place in the eighties, when Cosby was king on television and Eddie Murphy gave new meaning to what it meant when comedy was raw.

Both Pryor and Cosby began making their transition to the big screen in the late sixties and early seventies, a time when cinematic representations of growing black consciousness were still a tough sell in Hollywood, particularly in comedy. In the late sixties, African American comedies still struggled with the conflicting ideologically rooted comedic impulses—one informed by minstrelsy and an *Amos 'n' Andy* brand of humor and the other presenting a more "enlightened" view of black life.[102] In the seventies the same struggles between notions of "ideal" and idealized and stereotypical black comedic representation still existed, which resulted in films that "required black directors and black screenwriters . . . , like the black minstrel performer in blackface, [to] enable [the] naturalization, validation and repetition of minstrelsy in the postmodern age."[103] Despite black directors' and screenwriters' (slightly) increased presence in Hollywood, the tropes of minstrelsy persisted, and the question of where black comedians "belonged" remained uncertain.

Among the most successful humorous black films of the era were action/caper comedies that were situated in fundamentally African American milieus but that did not necessarily confront the realities of black urban life. In the recession years of the seventies, films like *Cotton Comes to Harlem* (Ossie Davis, 1970) (the adventures of two Harlem detectives who uncover a crooked back-to-Africa scheme organized by a black preacher) and *Uptown Saturday Night* (Sidney Poitier, 1974). The latter features Poitier and Cosby as two working guys who go to extraordinary measures to recover their winning lottery ticket stolen during an after-hours nightclub holdup. The film, in which both Pryor and Wilson had small roles (as a shaky paranoid private eye and a cinematic version of the Reverend Leroy, respectively), exemplified a slice of black life without interrogating the sociopolitical contexts in which the narratives were situated. Mark Reid asserts that "the popularity of both *Cotton* and *Uptown* reflects the pastiche quality of hybrid minstrel films insofar as they mimic a dead humor without social or political intent."[104] While clearly these films did not emerge as star vehicles for premier black comics (in terms of crossover success), they did allow black screenwriters and directors to articulate humor in a black urban vernacular that had not previously found its way onto the big screen without certain encoded bias based on class, color, and culture. These films presented neither the stories of the Super Negroes of the sixties nor the Super Niggers of seventies blaxploitation—although in terms of kinship they are closer to the latter than the former. Although black audiences understood and, in many cases, embraced these slice-of-urban-life/caper comedic constructions—within which the struggles of working black everyfolk were shown—the box office success of these films was limited, as were the benefits to their black stars' careers.

It is interesting that Cosby's roles in *Uptown* and its sequel, *Let's Do It Again*, do not mirror the comic persona of "Coz." In "Wardell Franklin," the angling everyman willing to compromise his principles to get his piece of the fiscal pie, Cosby creates an iteration of his comic persona more closely akin to a cynical, working-class Chet Kincaid (*The Bill Cosby Show*) than the likable, Anglo-friendly everyman. Cosby's comic shtick (gestures, facial expressions, intonation) is performed, but his universalist take on life is notably absent. The film represents a milieu rooted in cultural specificity of a black urban working-class world.[105] Onscreen, whether big or small, it would take the better part of two decades for Cosby's comic persona to be seen within a working-class milieu.[106]

For Cosby big-screen success has been as scarce as small-screen success has been plentiful. Films like *Ghost Dad* (1990) and *Leonard, Part 6* (1987) attempted to capitalize on the televisualized Coz persona as an overworked patriarch spirit (a harried widower Cliff Huxtable) and the retired secret agent (who was notably much less capable than Cosby's Alexander Scott) with results that proved to be box office poison.[107] While Cosby's stand-up, his "break-though" television roles, and his work as a humorist—and even his stint as Jell-O pitch-man extraordinaire—have made him a sort of mainstream comedic icon and a recipient of Kennedy Center Honors, the big screen was one of the few communication media that did not wholeheartedly embrace him. Due at least in part to the fact that Bill Cosby enjoys the distinction of being one of the few African American stars to be welcomed into American homes for over four decades, both his humor and his persona are fundamentally televisual phenomena. Thus, by consistently providing variable and yet familiar portraits of "positivity" (from *I-Spy*'s premiere in 1965 to *Cosby*'s series finale in 2000), Cosby attained sovereignty in the color-blind televisual domestic milieu, which, in turn, positioned him as the icon of the electronic hearth, the domestic medium. It seems that a consequence of gaining this high degree of familiarity, intimacy, and prominence in television was that, unless they were going to see him perform live, audiences were unwilling to go out for a dose of Bill Cosby.

The unyielding nature of Pryor's stand-up did not easily transfer onto the big screen either. By the early seventies, Pryor's extratextual activities, as well as his emerging "crazy nigger" persona, had labeled him both "controversial" and "unpredictable"—two qualities that did not necessarily mesh with big-budget Hollywood films. Some of these film and television roles acted as teasers for the characters in Pryor's comedic stable, like the fast-talking hustling sidekick, Slim, in the quintessential "pimp" movie, *The Mack* (1973), and the slick and shady Daddy Rich in *Car Wash* (1976). Others spoke to the bifurcation of Pryor's comic personae (*Silver Streak*, 1976), and still others seem like inane examples of the medium's utilizing vestiges of the comic's persona while ignoring his essential voice. Director Mel Brooks had desperately wanted Pryor to costar with Gene Wilder in the classic western parody *Blazing Saddles* (1975), a film on which Pryor had already worked as a writer. According to Brooks, "every studio in town" passed on the film with Pryor as the lead. One might assume that the role of Black Bart, the black sheriff (which Brooks had written for Pryor), would be a star-making turn, but such was not the case for Cleavon Little, the stage actor who was eventually cast in the role. Little's leading-man good looks and the intellectual (and sexual) prowess built into the construction of Bart produced something that had not been seen onscreen—an African American romantic lead in a mainstream Hollywood comedy (albeit a Mel Brooks comedy).[108] Although Little provided a fine comedic performance as Bart, the mind boggles at the comic possibilities with Pryor in the role. That Pryor was deemed unacceptable for a part that was virtually tailor-made for him reveals how his comic persona was viewed as too volatile, too contentious, and too unruly for the cinematic mainstream without strict narrative limitations to contain his comedic discourse.

Over the course of Pryor's career he appeared in more than thirty films, some of which allowed him to use both his dramatic skills, like his turn as the piano man addict in *Lady Sings the Blues* (1972) and the seriocomic turn as a Vietnam veteran returning home from a prisoner of war camp in *Some Kind of Hero* (1982). Films like *Blue Collar* (1978) and *Bustin' Loose* (1981) incorporated Pryor's comic persona in social comedies that dealt with the actual lived experience of urban blacks, but these had limited audience outside of the black community (and die-hard fans of the comic). However, despite the success of his concert films, *Richard Pryor: Live on the Sunset Strip* (1982) and *Richard Pryor: Here and Now* (1983), and numerous made-for-television stand-up specials like *Richard Pryor: Live and Smokin'* (1985), only his *costarring* comedic roles (those imbued with diluted doses of the Pryor stand-up persona) proved to be crossover friendly and spelled box office success.

Both *Silver Streak* (1976) and *Stir Crazy* (1980) paired Pryor with Gene Wilder and gave birth to the interracial buddy partnerships of the eighties and nineties in the humor-tinged action films exemplified by the *Lethal Weapon* series starring Danny Glover and Mel Gibson. In both these Pryor/Wilder films (as well as in the last two iterations of the pairing that seemed to exhaust the team's comic potential, 1989's *See No Evil, Hear No Evil* and 1991's *Another You*), the stereotypical performances of blackness are utilized less in the service of critique than in a reiteration of minstrelsy. In both films, but particularly in *Silver Streak*, Pryor, as strictly comic counterpoint to Wilder's more romanticized comic lead, gives instruction on performing blackness as a means of disguise. The scene culminates with Gene Wilder in blackface (unconvincingly) strutting and doing "brother-speak." (This same scene is virtually replicated in *Stir Crazy*, where the biracial buddy film goes to prison.) As Ed Guerrero notes, this teaching-blackness sequence "turns out to be a comic interpretation of black

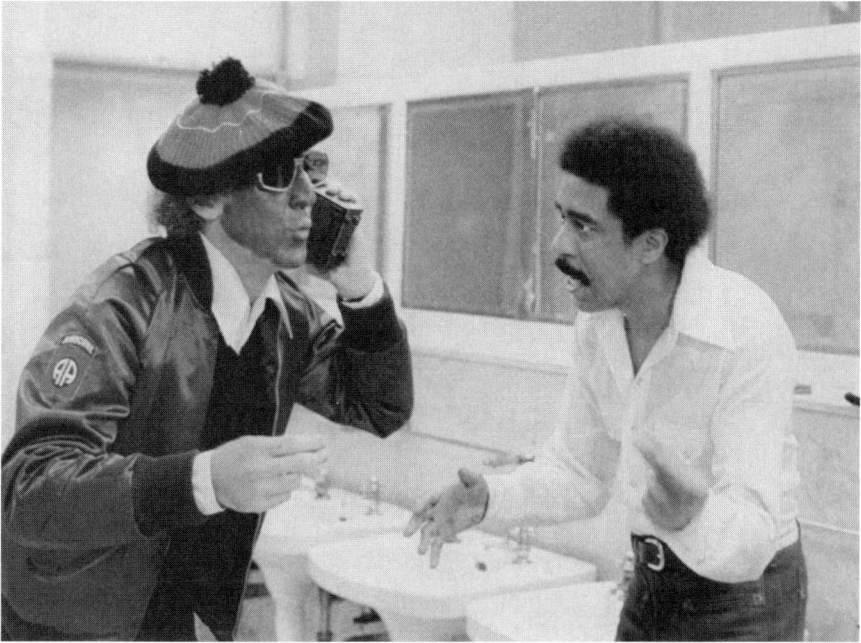

8. Pryor teaches Blackness 101. *Silver Streak* (1976). Directed by Arthur Hiller. Gene Wilder (left, as George Caldwell) and Richard Pryor (as Grover Muldoon). Photo from Photofest. Reproduced with permission from 20th Century Fox.

urban 'cool' and 'toughness'" which would have been deemed offensive if not for the "mediating presence of Pryor."[109] Pryor's persona lends a sense of black-sanctioned credibility to the scene that served to assuage the possible anger of black audiences—over seeing a black man teach a form of urban minstrelsy—and the liberal guilt of white audiences—over laughing at seeing a white man performing this urban minstrelsy . . . badly.

The clear bifurcation of Pryor's comic persona can be seen when one considers that in the same years that he was shining on stage in *Live at the Sunset Strip* and (perhaps a bit less brightly) in *Here and Now*, he was also making films in which his characters came perilously close to "cooning" in both *The Toy* (1982) and *Superman III* (1983).[110] In *The Toy*, a remake of a French film by the same name, aside from the fact that the film depended on broad physical comedy (often with Pryor running and looking scared) and a premise that in and of itself seems offensive (the central element being that a white southerner *buys* a black man as a toy for his child), one can only assume that the opportunity to work with comic star Jackie Gleason and a salary that would continue to support Pryor's self-destructive lifestyle were his motivations. The same could be said of his role as the down-on-his-luck dishwasher turned computer whiz sidekick for the supervillain in *Superman III* (1983). In his autobiography Pryor stated candidly, "It was a piece of shit. But the producers offered me $4 million, more than any black actor had ever been paid. 'For a piece of shit,' I told my agent when I finally read the script, 'it smells sweet.'"[111] While one might argue that Pryor's personal struggles had as much to do with the uneven translation of the comic's persona to the big screen as industrial prohibitions, one must again consider how his attempts to complicate his cinematic construction were received.

Penned by Pryor, along with Paul Mooney and Rocco Urbisci, *Jo Jo Dancer, Your Life Is Calling* (1986) was the biggest project from the comic's Indigo Films production company, part of a $40 million deal with Columbia Pictures.[112] As star, writer, and director, Pryor tells the story of the rise and near demise of Jo Jo Dancer, "a performer raised in a brothel, [who] discovers his own comic style in seedy nightclubs and goes on to achieve Hollywood stardom and comes close to being fatally consumed by his cocaine addiction."[113] At the time of the film's release Pryor maintained that it was only loosely autobiographical, and according to critics it lacked "a satisfactory explanation of how an ambitious, naïve young comic from the Midwest becomes a bitter, paranoid self destructive, drug addict."[114] In the film, a cousin to Bob Fosse's surrealistic autobiographical musical *All That Jazz* (1979), and the fictionalized biography of Lenny Bruce, *Lenny* (1974), the spirit of the horribly burned Pryor/Dancer emerges from his body to search his past for a reason to live and, in the end, chooses life. While the film's moral is life affirming, its harrowing elements—particularly in relationship to the addiction—recount aspects of the public Pryor and are directed, as *New York Times* critic Vincent Canby stated, "with more élan than one has the right to expect of a first time director."[115]

The mantle of the creative tri-hyphenate (writer-producer-star) is often staggering for any artist, and one might assert that the weighty responsibility coupled with the complexity of Pryor's story predestined *Jo Jo Dancer* for accusations of either naiveté or disingenuousness in translating the comic's life to the screen. On one hand, one might agree with *Washington Post* critic Paul Attanasio's contentions: "In *Jo Jo Dancer*, he worships the meekness in himself. . . . There's something lovely about that (that's where his gentle empathy comes from) but there's something dishonest as well. There is, presumably, another side to Pryor—in fact, we've seen it, in the anger behind his early stand-up work."[116] On the other hand, regardless of the deficiencies in either the script or character construction, one may also wonder whether, in this case, it was the strength of the wild, unrelenting, and volatile aspects of his humor that made it impossible for critics—and audiences—to embrace a performance that tried to intertwine the stand-up and cinematic iterations of Pryor's comic persona. The criticism of the film focuses not on problems with Pryor's construction of a comic persona but on his construction of the comic. It seems to speak to some sort of de facto prohibition in terms of what Pryor, as a comic—a black comic—is allowed to do on the big screen and whether allowing the gaps and fissures between the stand-up persona and lived experience can be given cinematic space. If, indeed, the comic persona exists as the performance of the intersection of multiple ideologies and lived experiences, *Jo Jo Dancer* is a significant film for its failures and successes. Whether by default or by design, the wedding of pathos and edgy irreverence, an inherent part of Pryor's stand-up, makes only fleeting appearances in Hollywood comedies.

For both Wilson and Gregory the big screen would never be a vehicle for the dissemination of their comedic discourse, and although Cosby and Pryor both found their way into mainstream comedy, each experiences successes and failures that spoke to the suitability of the black comic persona to American film comedy. The process of making the "crazy nigger" assimilable into mainstream comedy and the difficulty for the fully assimilable Cosby comic persona to transfer from television to film raise significant questions about the place of the African American comedian in screen comedy. One might argue that a dual burden is always placed on the comedian as he transfers from stand-up to screen: he must find a way to retain the essence of his stand-up persona while also conforming to the generic limitations of Hollywood comedy. This quandary is further problematized for the black comedian inasmuch as this process of transition from stand-up to television to film—that is, the negotiation of racial, class, and gender identities, as well as the possible containment of the more unruly (read controversial) aspects of the comic personae—makes a significant contribution to the way that African Americans are viewed at home and abroad. Carrying the burden of his own race, as well as the burden of representing the race, undoubtedly inflects the way the black comedian has been integrated into mainstream Hollywood comedy. Although Gregory, Cosby, Wilson, and Pryor had all established themselves as comedic forces in the stand-up world, to make it in Hollywood film comedy, their performance of black identity and cultural specificity had to be contained and sanitized.

Gregory, whose political activism eventually led him to abandon stand-up's microphone for the lecturer's podium, turned down numerous film opportunities early in his career based on disputes about black representation. Cosby, who has come to personify the image of the universalist African American humorist, has been able to supply a positivist, integrationist image of the "buppie" (black urban professionals) home front, happily consumed in the domestic space and internalized by mainstream audiences as the exception and the rule for the quality of black life in urban/suburban America. Why has Cosby failed on the big screen? Comedy more often than not reaffirms the status quo, so one must consider whether the positivist imaginings of a fully assimilated black man on the small screen provides comfort while the same image on the big screen might be seen as a threat to that status quo. Furthermore, Cosby's attempts to embody a less "Super" construction of blackness have been met with a certain degree of indifference. While finding a niche is essential for the comic/comedic actor's success, the reaction of both the audience and the industry to his or her breaking out of that mold is often as fierce as it is capricious. Wilson's genuine amenability to audiences allowed him, like Cosby, to cross into home spaces with ease, but it did not afford him the ability to grow beyond the comic character types for which he had become beloved. In many ways Pryor's compartmentalization of his stand-up and screen persona may be seen as supplying most directly the template that has been adopted and adapted by comedians like Eddie Murphy, Whoopi Goldberg, and, to a lesser degree, Chris Rock. One cannot dismiss the powerful sway the possibility that iconic status like Cosby's can have over any performer, regardless of race, gender, or pedagogy.

The comedian/comedic actor has to do a dance between the uncompromising (sometimes vulgar) stand-up persona—with all its personal, sociopolitical, and historical baggage—and the screen persona, a construct that is constantly being retooled, reframed, and reenvisioned from multiple industrial sources, as well as from the comedian turned comic actor him- or herself. Pryor was particularly adept at this dance, and, in terms of his stand-up persona, the culturally specific aspects of his humor remained undiluted. The rest of this book is dedicated to interrogating the nature and necessity of the dance in new and variable comic venues (televisual, theatrical, and cinematic) by the next generation of black comedians, exemplified by Eddie Murphy and Chris Rock.

CHAPTER 2

# Murphy and Rock

## FROM THE "BLACK GUY" TO THE "ROCK STAR"

CHRIS ROCK'S BREAKTHROUGH Home Box Office special, *Bring the Pain* (1998), begins by invoking a personal canon of stand-up comedians. "Ladies and Gentlemen, are you ready to bring the pain? Give up the love for Mr. CHRIS ROCK!" The sound of pandemonium accompanies a medium close-up of Rock's black-and-white leather shoes as he swaggers toward the stage. A series of comedy album covers is then superimposed over his strut, including Bill Cosby's *To Russell, My Brother, Whom I Slept With*, Dick Gregory's *In Living Black and White*, Richard Pryor's *Is It Something I Said?*, Steve Martin's *Comedy Isn't Pretty*, and self-titled albums from Woody Allen and Eddie Murphy. The sequence provides both a historical context within which Rock would have the audience view his comedy and a genealogy of comedians who have stepped out from behind the mike to ply their wares as comedic actors. Just as the personae and careers of Gregory, Cosby, Flip Wilson, and Pryor can be seen as emblematic of both the possibilities and pitfalls for black comics who came of age during the civil rights movement, Eddie Murphy and Chris Rock represent the first and second waves of black comedians in the post–civil rights era, respectively.[1] While both the roots of their comedy and the routes of their careers might differ from those of their civil rights era brethren, many of the quandaries remain the same: how to cross over to the mainstream promised land and, if indeed that is possible, how to retain their point of annunciation, voice, and comedic pedagogy on that arduous trek.

## "THE BLACK GUY" NO MORE: THE EMERGENCE OF EDDIE

Historically, the comedians of the pre–civil rights era—the comic forbears of Gregory and Cosby—generally passed through the Chitlin' Circuit before they could access the white comic venues that filtered the "talent" into the entertainment mainstream. By the eighties there were two frequently intersecting roads for stand-ups of all colors into American film comedy—one through *Saturday Night Live* (*SNL*, 1975– ), the other through comedy programming on

HBO. Although the first era of *SNL* can be hailed as cutting-edge television humor, it was not a place for black comics to shine. Over three decades the "black guy" (or girl) on *SNL* has often been an underutilized player whose screen time is minimal and whose characters are ancillary to another player's central role (from Garrett Morris's "Chico Escuela" on Chevy Chase's "Weekend Update" to Tim Meadows's lampooning of Oprah Winfrey). Eddie Murphy was the notable exception to the "black guy syndrome." Before the end of his freshman season (1980–81) on *SNL*, Murphy was a major presence. In fact, Murphy's recurring characters (the grownup Buckwheat as a post–*Little Rascals* celebrity; a Borscht Belt, cigar-chomping version of Gumby; and Mr. Robinson, the Mister Rogers of the 'hood) ended *SNL*'s first comic slump era in the early eighties. By the time Murphy left the series in 1984, he was already a bona fide crossover star on stand-up's main stage—an act captured in *Eddie Murphy Delirious* (1983)—and was well on his way to big-screen superstardom with *48 Hrs* (1982) and *Trading Places* (1983).

Clad in the type of red-and-black leather suit that he would later lampoon as Axel Foley in *Beverly Hills Cop* (1984), Eddie Murphy prowled the stage in *Delirious* with all the swagger of a stand-up virtuoso turned sex symbol. Parading a new sort of audaciousness, Murphy's routines utilized the blue tone of Pryor (particularly in terms of language and sexually explicit content) while excising Pryor's sociopolitical edge. Murphy's stories of family and childhood are jadedly nostalgic but touch on issues of race and class in uncritical terms. Murphy's kid routines are not "cleaned up" idealizations of childhood like Cosby's material, nor are they intended to be points of departure for Pryoresque social commentary on black life. Murphy's ice cream routine begins with the joyous moments a child spends with his freshly scooped cone:

> You don't eat your ice cream for, like, a half-hour, you'd be dancin' around singing, "I have some ice cream, I have some ice cream. And I'm gonna eat it all . . . eat it all" . . . (The joyous song transforms into a musical taunt directed at "that one kid on the side who didn't get no ice cream"). Kids didn't give a fuck, they'd say, "You didn't get no ice cream. You didn't get none . . . you didn't get none. You didn't get none cuz you are on the welfare and can't afford it, you can't afford. You can't afford it" . . . all the other kids are chiming in, "he can't afford it."

While it may not provide an incisive commentary on black urban life, this brief example of kid cruelty touches on stereotypes about the African American community while providing a view of black child life that has almost no relationship to the collectivity of Fat Albert and the Gang. These kid stories lack the "feel-good" payoff of Cosby's work. Instead, the comic tone of Murphy's routines reflect the same ethos as his adult material: insolent, idiosyncratic, and, ultimately, self-interested. While, arguably, Murphy's kid "bits" supply humorous "black-on-black" social commentary, they are not placed within a larger (and more complicated) sociopolitical context for his crossover audiences. Without this contextualization the critical bite of Murphy's routines is lessened, if not lost altogether—as is the possibility that they might threaten white audiences.

The Buckwheat routine exemplifies that when Murphy did engage with representations of African Americans in popular culture, his impressions were encased in routines that only halfheartedly confronted the media mechanisms that perpetuated minstrel archetypes:

> I was standing outside getting ready to come in here and this little Jewish guy came up to me and said, "Hey, Buckwheat." There was some brothers standing next to me and they said, "What did that guy call you, man? Buckwheat?" Then I started thinking about the *Little Rascals*—period. Who the fuck thought up the names on that show? Because I am from a predominantly black family and I have yet to run into a relative named Buckwheat. Go to a cookout and say, "Hi, my name is Ed. What's yours?" "I'm Buckwheat, man. Yeah Buckwheat, that's my name. No, Buckwheat. I ain't got no last name—Buckwheat, that's it. . . . Don't believe me? Ain't that right, Stymie? . . . I want you to meet my brother. Yo, Farina! [pause] Buckwheat and Farina . . . You know how most people are named after their fathers, we was named after our father's favorite breakfasts."

The opening of this bit addresses the absurdity of being identified only with a parody of a pickaninny archetype (Buckwheat), but it soon becomes a riff on the issue of naming in its most simplistic form. Consequently, it stops short of actually questioning the ideological agenda informing the representation of black children in *The Little Rascals*. Like much of Murphy's consciously racialized humor, the routine does not endeavor to deconstruct or debunk either issues of race or racial representation. His pronouncements are rooted more in cynical banter than in social criticism.

The uninhibited bravado of *Raw* (1987), directed by Robert Townsend, makes his earlier onstage persona seem almost self-effacing by comparison. The first ten minutes of *Raw* establish Murphy as rebel and multimedia "rock star."[2] The footage of the multiracial crowd of men and women holding headshots of Murphy, as well as concert posters, programs, and t-shirts emblazoned with his leather clad silhouette, reframes the way the stand-up comic is viewed. Murphy is not the nice, funny guy in the suit (Cosby) or the irreverent young man on the fringes of society (Pryor); he is the young Elvis as stand-up—a comic sex symbol. Murphy's comic persona in *Raw* served the same role for the second wave of post–civil rights era black comics (including Chris Tucker, Martin Lawrence, and Rock) that Richard Pryor's *Live in Concert* (1979) had for Murphy himself: it established a new comic paradigm.

Like Pryor, the irreverence at the core of Murphy's humor seemed to capture the imagination of young audiences across lines of race and class.[3] Whereas Pryor had managed to push the boundaries of good taste while maintaining his status as an "equal-opportunity offender," Murphy revels in taking a particularly adversarial stance toward women, whom he casts as predators looking "to get half of what's mine," and gays, whom he fears may be "taking too long a look" at his physical attributes. His heterosexist attitudes permeate his stand-up (providing some of its most sexually explicit material)—whether in his re-visioning of *The Honeymooner's* Ralph and Norton's sexual preferences in *Delirious*, or his recounting stories in *Raw* of the "24-hour homo-watch" that is on the lookout for him across the country. This analysis of Murphy's stand-up, while only touching on the openly homophobic content in his act (also present in the acts of "shock" comedians like Andrew "Dice" Clay and Sam Kinison), illustrates how the content of even the most controversial stand-up comic responds to popular sensibilities. The blatant heterosexism of Murphy's act, which played easily in that era's contemporary comic mainstream, would not play as well in the post–*Birdcage*, post–*In and Out*, post–*Will and Grace* new millennial comic milieu, which is decidedly more gay friendly. However, perhaps more significantly for the purposes of this study, the vehement antigay sentiments of Murphy's stand-up persona replicate the strains of homophobia in the black community (a notion rooted in the questionable connection between homosexuality and centuries of actual and virtual emasculation, and, a Leviticus-informed antigay dogma for certain segments of Christianity).

One might argue that in order to be considered "daring," the stand-up comic's persona, informed by Lenny Bruce, George Carlin, and, of course, Richard Pryor, must embody a challenge to popular sensibilities (read the status quo). The sexual politics of Murphy's stand-up does challenge the status quo—but it reaffirms it as well by reasserting black masculinity through the degradation of black women (and women, in general) and annunciating the beginnings of a backlash against feminism. In Murphy's 1987 stand-up act depicted in *Raw*, his persona of comic as rock star reduces complex questions of performing black masculinity (why black men have to act like they can fight), gender equity in relationships (how sex is a weapon for men and a commodity for women), and the justification for infidelity (how sexual conquest is male manifest destiny) to a simple catchphrase: "it's a dick thing." This de facto mantra for much of *Raw* treads on that slippery slope between comedic sexism and misogynistic comedy—neither of which is easily justifiable. The phrase also resonates with the assertion made by bell hooks—first in her essay "Reconstructing Black Masculinity" and later in Marlon Riggs's cinematic rumination on identity, *Black Is . . . Black Ain't* (1995): "If the 'black thing' i.e., black liberation struggle, is only a 'dick thing' in disguise, a phallocentric play for black male power, then black people are in serious trouble."[4] One might bemoan the inherent regressiveness of Murphy's articulation of gender identity, in which the black male is judged by a quantifiable measure of sexual power (the figurative and literal measure of the man) and women are referenced in primarily anatomical terms (*pussy* being the favorite); however, what is perhaps more disconcerting is how it seems to respond to other sociopolitical discourse about the place of black women in particular and women in general. There is an unsettling kinship between the infamous assertion made by Stokely Carmichael (Student Non-Violent Coordinating Committee/Black Panthers), that "the place of women in the movement was prone," and Murphy's explanation of why women will put up with bad treatment from men once they have been made to "cum hard." While mobilized differently in these two instances, the notion of black masculine identity rooted in a phallocentric articulation of traditional gender roles—inherent in both Murphy and Carmichael's statements—still holds powerful sway in black popular culture. By being one of the first black comics to directly vocalize this standpoint (without critique or social comment), Murphy's stand-up persona defines an ideological paradigm for comedic discourse about sexual politics—in terms of both gender and sexuality—that has been embraced by the male and female comics of the Def Jam generation.

Given that the articulation of identity is as significant to this study as the black comic's espoused ideologies, one of the most interesting moments in *Raw* provides both: the routine that centers on the battle between Cosby and Pryor for Murphy's comic "soul." Although it begins simply as an opportunity for Murphy to reveal his mimicry skills, this routine transforms into a blanket indictment of Cosby (for his "outmoded" views regarding what a comic can or cannot say) and a quasi-canonization of Pryor (for his "proselytizing" of outrageous curse-laden humor). In the routine Murphy recalls being excited about receiving a call from Bill, but the excitement turns to anger as Cosby chastises him: "[As Cosby] 'You cannot say filth, flarn, flarn, flarn, filth in front of people. . . . I can't use the same language that you do but you know what I mean when I say flarn, flarn, flarn, filth.' [As himself] 'I never said no filth, flarn, filth. I don't know what you're talking about. I'm offended that you called. Fuck You.' . . . That's when I got mad, he thought that was my whole act—that I cursed and left." A stream of obscenities follows, culminating with "Goodnight everybody—suck my dick." Murphy then turns to Pryor for guidance: "Richard says, 'Next time the motherfucker calls tell him I said he can suck my dick. . . . Tell Bill to have a Coke and a smile and shut the fuck up.'" This bit thus serves both to sever and to establish ties with Murphy's black comedic forefathers. The skillfulness of imitations aside, the discourse surrounding "appropriate" black humor plays out in fairly superficial terms. Cosby is cast as a dinosaur, out of touch with the "current" edgy and outrageous humor that Murphy traces back to Pryor.

Yet even as Murphy attempts to position himself as a sort of heir apparent to Pryor, the linkage seems weak because the kinship is based more on style than substance. As Donald Bogle puts it, "It was apparent that Murphy was influenced by Pryor. It was apparent also that he had never understood Pryor's work. For Pryor had gotten inside his winos, junkies or numbers runners, uncovering their vulnerabilities, their troubled histories, and revealing at times their sadness and touching beauty. Murphy, however, seemed to see his various

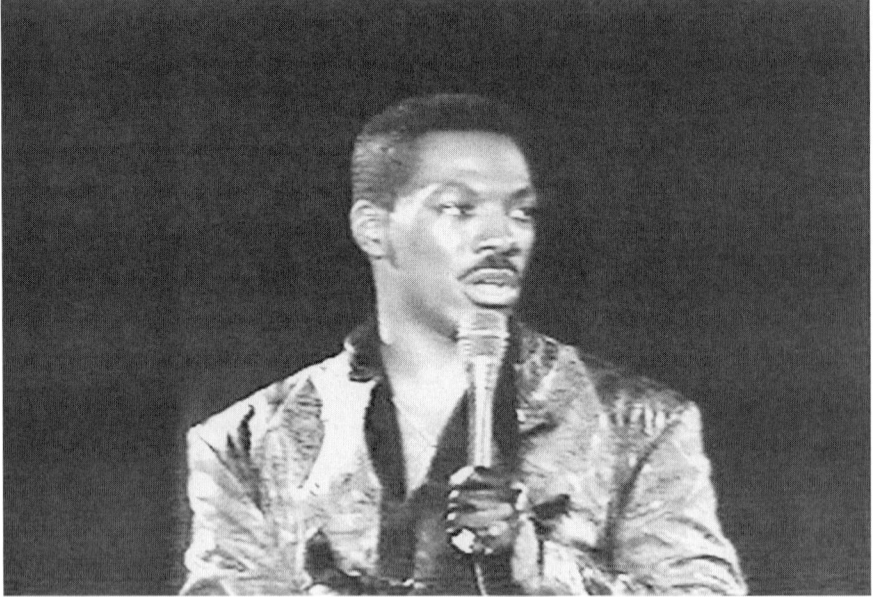

9. Eddie Murphy does his best Cosby in *Eddie Murphy Raw* (1987). Directed by Robert Townsend.

characters as lowlife characters without any innate dignity. . . . And obviously missing from his television skits were the social/political concerns of a Dick Gregory."[5] A sort of "I got mine" ethos informs Murphy's comedy and its apolitical production of black identity. In a *New York Times* article on "bad boy" comedians of the Reagan era (both black and white), Stephen Holden defined Murphy's stand-up—in which he curses, mocks, and rages without any clear sociopolitical or intellectual agenda—as "the perfect symbol of post-hip, survival of the fittest humor."[6]

Although the word *audacious* is an apt description of Murphy's stand-up comedic persona, his televisual iteration, for the most part, lacked the sociopolitical bark and bite of either Pryor or Gregory. From Velvet Jones's guide to pimping to Mr. Robinson's adventures in his whack neighborhood, Murphy's *SNL* characters, while undoubtedly funny, provided caricatures of specific segments of black life without providing sociohistorical contextualization. In other words, his Buckwheat might have been a "player," but, in the end, he was still Buckwheat—a pickaninny with some degree of agency still remains the embodiment of a minstrel trope. Even the character of Tyrone Green, the prison poet, which appeared to be inspired by Pryor's misspeaking black nationalist, was presented in a stylized but uncritical filmed segment, "Prose and Cons." Performed with mock menace by Murphy, the portrayal of Green seemed a missed opportunity for critique; like the character's poem, "C-I-L-L, my Landlord," the sketch ultimately made the incarcerated black male's attempt at self-expression a laughable endeavor. One cannot discount Murphy's comedic brilliance—as a mimic, as a quick-witted observational humorist, as an African American comic who takes control of mediated tropes of race and ethnicity for his own comedic purposes; however, his comic persona on *SNL*, which seemed to be constructed in opposition to positivist constructions of black comedy (like *The Cosby Show*), failed to provide an ideological alternative more complicated than "more power to me."

In a retrospective on the comic for *Salon.com*, Michael Sragow asserted that Murphy "specialized less in rage than in effrontery."[7] Nevertheless, Murphy's very existence, as a very successful, very young black man, who embraced both (seeming) industrial autonomy and international celebrity, provided a new generation with a comic hero who embodied the sociopolitical moment. In many ways, Murphy was the first "successful" post-soul comic. His comic persona was informed as much by the "I'm Black and I'm Proud" style—if not the substance—of the black power movement as the media images of black subjugation (the continued proliferation of minstrel archetypes embodied by Stymie, Buckwheat, and Farina in *The Little Rascals* to those in ghetto sitcoms like J. J. in *Good Times* or Re-Run in *What's Happening*) and black idealization (the Super Negroes of the sixties in *Julia* and *I-Spy*). Murphy presented black humor for media babies—across lines of race, class, and color. Yet one might argue that by failing to engage in direct sociocultural critique, Murphy's comic persona rebelled against one form of containment while engaging in an unproblematized standoff with another. As the unqualified star of the show in his *SNL* days, Murphy brought black humor and sensibility to a series in which it had previously only played an ancillary role. The first African American comic of the post-soul era to gain rock-star status, Murphy inspired a generation of young black comics. Nonetheless, his stardom was a product of the eighties—a time when progressive and regressive representations of blackness were intertwined in the rhetoric of Reagan America. In the days of trickle-down, greed-is-good, aspirations to yuppiedom, truly contentious sociocultural critique did not play well in mainstream popular culture. However, there were moments of rupture that provide gaps and fissures in what might be seen as hegemonic comic sensibility—particularly in relationship to race relations. From a new millennial perspective these moments may seem somewhat innocuous, but their resonance is undeniable. Like the "Word Association" between Chase and Pryor, the ideological work done with Murphy's short film, "White like Me" provided a problematic televisual text that engaged popular conceptions about the experience of blackness by calling into question the experience of whiteness.

The filmed segment, which was arguably Murphy's most overtly political televisual segment on *SNL*, aired December 15, 1984, on an episode hosted by

Murphy a year after he had left the late-night series. The segment begins with Murphy, dressed completely in black (shirt, pants, and leather jacket) walking down what appeared to be the white corridor of the television studio. Speaking directly into the camera, Murphy states: "You know, a lot of people talk about racial prejudice. And some people have gone so far as to say that there are actually two Americas: one black and one white. But talk is cheap. So I decided to look into the problem myself, firsthand. To go underground and actually experience America: as a white man." Murphy enters the studio makeup room and is transformed into "Mr. White" complete with slightly feathered brown wig and mustache, which, Murphy states, is reminiscent of seventies porn star Harry Reems—and, of course, "white face." His "training sequence," which included reading Hallmark cards and watching episodes of *Dynasty*, foreshadows a plethora of "white people be like" jokes; it also confronts (and confirms) long-held assumptions about white privilege. When he emerges, charcoal gray three-piece suit and glasses with briefcase in hand, he seems both the eighties version of the "Organization Man"—an anonymous cog in a corporate wheel—and a cartoon version of whiteness. From the free newspaper at the convenience store to the transit bus that is transformed into a mobile party vehicle (after the last black rider disembarks), the disparities inform Murphy's revelation: in voiceover he intones, "The problem was much more serious than I'd ever imagined."

The final perk of whiteness takes place when a collateral-free "Mr. White" applies for a loan from a black loan officer. Incredulous over White's request, the officer's unequivocal rejection is cut short by the entrance of a white loan officer, who, albeit nicely, takes over handling Mr. White's business.

WHITE LOAN OFFICER: [laughs, then sits] That was a close one, wasn't it?

EDDIE MURPHY: It certainly was.

WHITE LOAN OFFICER: We don't have to bother with these formalities, do we, Mr. White? Huh?

EDDIE MURPHY: What a silly Negro!

WHITE LOAN OFFICER: Just take what you want, Mr. White. Pay us back anytime. Or don't. We don't care.

EDDIE MURPHY: Tell me, do you know of any other banks like this in this area?

The segment concludes with Murphy in the makeup room, again speaking directly to the camera: "So, what did I learn from all of this? Well, I learned that we still have a very long way to go in this country before all men are truly equal. But I'll tell you something." As he walks across the length of the room, the camera pulls back to reveal three black men and one black woman applying white makeup to their faces. "I've got a lot of friends, and we've got a lot of makeup. So, the next time you're huggin' up with some really super, groovy white guy, or you met a really great, super keen white chick, don't be too sure. They might be black." All of the prospective "whites" wave to the camera. While some may assert that this final segment asserts a subversive directive, a way to "work the system," if you will, its resonance is somewhat shallow. In an era when the realities of racial inequity, particularly in relationship to black access to the era's financial bounty, which had not managed to trickle down to those with credit histories that were much more economically viable than Mr. White's, the notion of racial masquerade may have very well seemed like the only option. However, the "solution" in this mockumentary on disparity, while clearly offered with tongue firmly wedged in cheek, is still rooted in individual action and initiative. Even this absurdist answer has traces of the notion that if one only tries "hard enough," then there are ways to "work the system and win" making the de facto "losers" a part of the critique as well as the system. In "White like Me," working the system is still only for a privileged few—in this case, "friends of Eddie." While contradictory ideological impulses are often a part of comedy, this provides a glimpse of how Murphy's comic persona, at its most progressive, is constrained by regressive tendencies in the popular cultural consciousness. Later examination of the successes and the failures of Murphy's film career will reveal how this idiosyncratic approach to the articulation of blackness corresponds to the Reagan era, when black success and black failure were framed within a rugged individualist "up by your own bootstraps" construction of the American Dream.

### ROCK IN THE SECOND WAVE

The nineties would see Murphy forsaking live performance and the small screen for the movies. His meteoric rise to stardom through the eighties proved an inspiration for the second wave of black comedians in both media. Chris Rock clearly demonstrates such an influence, as well as mining the wealth of earlier black humor styles presented by Pryor and Gregory. Like Murphy, Rock began his career as a teenager on the New York club circuit. After seeing the young Rock do fifteen minutes at New York's The Comic Strip in 1987, Murphy secured a place for him on the HBO special *Uptown Comedy Express*. This appearance led to Rock's first screen role, as a parking valet with an attitude at the Playboy mansion in *Beverly Hills Cop II* (1987). After appearing as the kid in search of a single rib (a cameo) in Keenen Ivory Wayans's blaxploitation parody *I'm Gonna Get You Sucka!* and a rare but affecting dramatic role, as a crackhead informer in *New Jack City*, Rock was cast, like Murphy before him, as "the black guy" on *Saturday Night Live*. Despite Rock's insistence that he was "just happy to be here," he was one of a succession of underutilized black cast members to experience minimal screen time and few running characters (the notable exception being Nat X). Rock's association with the series allowed him to branch out as a performer, leading to big-screen supporting roles in such films as *New Jack City* (1991). However, his profile for mainstream audiences was enhanced far more by his post-*SNL* gigs as pitchman: for example his voicing of "Lil' Penny" Hardaway, the Nike puppet or the hostile info guy he did for 1–800-COLLECT.

On his 1992 comedy record Rock raged against the depiction of African Americans in popular culture and the real-life consequences of such mediated assumptions. As the title of the album exclaims, young black men in America today are "born suspect." One begins to see the scathing sociocultural critique in this stand-up set—a discursive set of skills that he also utilizes in *Chris Rock: Big Ass Jokes*, his first HBO special. In the early nineties (and, arguably, even today), the half-hour comedy series often acts as a comic's televisual audition for the big break: the hour-long HBO special. Like many of the markers for the comedian's performance process—moving from opener to headliner in the club, to being invited to the couch by Johnny, Jay, or Dave on late night—making the jump from the half-hour comedy special to the hour-long set was a significant marker in terms of creative "heat" and industrial viability. For Rock, who had never become more than "this year's black guy" on *SNL* (a designation he shared with Tim Meadows during his tenure on the series), this marked a pivotal moment in his career. Ken Tucker, *Entertainment Weekly* critic, articulates what many viewers of the short set on HBO in June of 1994 must have been thinking: "In a crisp 30 minutes, *Chris Rock: Big Ass Jokes* proves just how much of comedian Chris Rock's talent was wasted during his three-season stint on *Saturday Night Live*."[8] Watching the twenty-something Rock strut onstage in Atlanta, to the driving guitar licks that begin Living Color's "Cult of Personality," clad in a flowing blue satin shirt with a very early-nineties red, gold, and black funky paisley, short black vest and modified fade haircut (all of which is a far cry from the all-black, Calvin Klein hipper-than-thou costuming of the stand-up to follow), one can see the comic's intensity. Rock is coming onstage "to kill," to use the comic vernacular—and he does. Despite the comic prowess that the young Rock exhibits, watching *Big Ass Jokes* feels a bit like watching home movies of Michael Jordan play street ball at sixteen: the talent is unquestionably there, but the style has not been refined.

Rock immediately launches into material that is meant to shock the audience by its candor and create an atmosphere for his personal brand of sociocultural critique. His rapport with the audience, their shout-outs and his responses, establishes a conversational tone for the special as he paces back and forth. The rarely stationary Rock uses the entire lip of the stage to engage the crowd—whether in the front row or the "nose bleed" seats. Creating this sense of intimacy, regardless of the venue, is vital for a comic like Rock, whose material will, at some point or another, challenge the sensibilities of the audience: "I cannot complain. I got my special, doing a new movie, got the TV show. [Patting his chest] Successful black man. [The crowd cheers] You know what's next, right? [He pauses, staring straight into the audience with a huge grin] White girl. [Giving a sly throaty chuckle] You cannot be a successful black man without a white girl."

By using his first joke series to interrogate the notion of interracial dating as status symbol, a concept to which he returns many times over the course of the thirty-minute set, Rock plays with, and against, popular opinions on the subject espoused within the black community. By exposing the tensions around interracial dating from an insider's perspective, Rock may well be airing "dirty laundry" in a public venue; however, his critique reveals the discursive complexity of the "white girl or white guy" issue. He covers multiple stances on the issue. By stating that people blame everything that goes wrong in your life on a dating choice—"Chris got hit by a truck." "Fucking around with them white girls . . . that's what he get"—he touches on the anti-interracial sentiments that flourish within the black community—particularly in reference to successful black men—which speaks to larger issues about the fate and the plight of African American males in contemporary America. On the other hand, his response to interracial dating when it is a "white guy" reveals a gender politics that often falls into the regressive camp. Stating incredulously that there are white girls that only go out with black guys and "sisters" who don't date black men, he recounts asking one such woman about her partner choice. The voice he gives her resonates with both belligerence and ignorance:

Girl, why don't you date black men?

[As the black woman] No reason. No reason.

No reason?

So I punched her in the face. [Peals of laughter]

Now she's got a reason. [(The crowd—male and female—howls]

While the violence described for the sake of a punch line is fleeting (and, seemingly, goes unquestioned by the audience), Rock's gendered double standard continues as he bemoans black U.S. figure skater Debbie Thomas's marriage to a white man. Using his usual pattern of phrase repetition, he beseeches Thomas, "Debbie, what do I have to do to get with you?" After conceding that she "probably didn't meet many brothers on the ice," he finishes the bit with a familiar note of condemnation: "Debbie Thomas went to the Olympics and bust her ass. (As he pauses, he smiles slyly) Fucking around with them white boys— that's what she get." While other examples of sexual politics make their way into his act, even at the earliest stages of his stand-up career, Rock's forte was comedic discourse on race. In fact, he clearly states his point of enunciation in this set:

I do a lot of racial humor. You know why? I was bused to school when I was a kid. I had to get up every morning at 6 o'clock in the morning to compete with white kids who didn't have to get up until 8. And that's not fair. Say I get a lower mark on a test, I got a teacher saying, "Chris can't read." I'm like, "No, Chris is fucking tired." You supposed to get bused to school to go to better schools in a better neighborhood. I got bused to school in a poor white neighborhood—a neighborhood worse than the one I lived in.

. . . Beyond white trash, they were like white toxic waste. . . . They hated me. They hated my guts because my family had more money than them. . . . That's when I learned my lesson, boy, there is nothing that a white man with a penny hates more than a nigger with a nickel.

This personalized commentary on intersections between race and class, the vestiges of New Society programs (like busing) and the final adage that sounds like something that, if you're African American, you might have heard from an elder relative, enables Rock to use a thirty-minute set as teaching tool. Thus, this joke series can be seen to function either as an ideological refresher course or as a primer on the African American condition. Although then, as now, Rock maintained that his primary directive is being funny, the subversive power of his sociocultural critique was present in *Big Ass Jokes* (without much of the political edge).

The overtly political spin in Rock's comedy was further honed and achieved wider exposure during his stint as a "correspondent" for the 1996 presidential campaign on Comedy Central's *Politically Incorrect with Bill Maher*. His sardonic reports from the campaign trail provided a forum for Rock to meld his stand-up sensibility with an incisive sociopolitical critique that obliged audiences to laugh even as they squirmed. Rock's commentary on why Colin Powell could not run for office (which was retooled for the "Roll with the New" tour and quoted on his first HBO special) directly confronted white liberal sensibilities—not allowing the audience off the hook.[9] In the conclusion of her book, *Revolution Televised: Prime Time and the Struggle for Black Power*, Christine Acham's discussion of Chris Rock's position on the televisual landscape cites Malcolm X's speech, "A Message to the Grassroots," in which he gives black people the directive to "stop airing our differences in front of the white man."[10] Placing the significance of airing the community's dirty laundry as "a possible means to divide and conquer" into perspective by exposing the social and historical ramifications of making the rifts in the black community visible to the greater American public (namely the division between the civil rights and black power movements often embodied by Martin Luther King Jr. versus Malcolm X), Acham asserts that Rock's *Bring the Pain* was "one of the most significant moments of black popular culture to test the bounds of Malcolm X's philosophy."[11] Rock's choice, to unflinchingly tackle whatever he deems hypocritical or unacceptable—regardless of race, creed, or color— opened up the discussion of issues reserved for what Acham refers to as "black communal sites of the Chitlin' Circuit or the privacy of one's own home" to the "very mainstream venue of U.S. cable television."[12]

In his first HBO special, *Bring the Pain*, Rock's initial verbal assault called into question the politics (and the logic) of the black leadership: "Washington, DC . . . Chocolate City. The home of the Million Man March. Had all the positive black leaders there—Farrakhan, Jesse, Marion Barry. How did he even get a ticket? It was a day of positivity. Marion Barry at the Million Man March. You know what that means? That even in our finest hour, we had a crack-head on stage. [A mixture of laughter and boos] Boo if you want—you know I'm right." Rock's target is not simply Marion Barry, the Mayor of Washington, D.C., who secured another term in office after a drug addiction scandal because he had remained (at least politically) in the bosom of the black community. Rock uses this scenario to critique the kind of unconditional solidarity that seemingly defies the logic of self-preservation. Rock's take on the sensational trial and acquittal of O. J. Simpson is similarly designed to take a shot at everybody, regardless of race: "Black people too happy, white people too mad. Black people saying, 'we won . . . we won.' What the fuck did we win? Everyday I look in the mailbox for my O. J. prize and nothing. [Some folks say,] 'Ooh, it's all about race.' This shit wasn't about race—it was about fame. If O. J. wasn't famous he'd be sitting in jail right now. If O. J. drove a bus, he wouldn't even be O. J., he'd be Orenthal, the bus-driving murderer."

As an equal-opportunity chastiser, Rock directs his comic ire at no single target because he recognizes the complexity of race/power relations and their impact on every aspect of American life. He forces the audience to confront this racial discourse amidst the laughter. In both *Bring the Pain* and his follow-up HBO special, *Bigger and Blacker*, filmed at Harlem's Apollo Theater, Rock directly challenges notions of black identity in ways that few black comics have

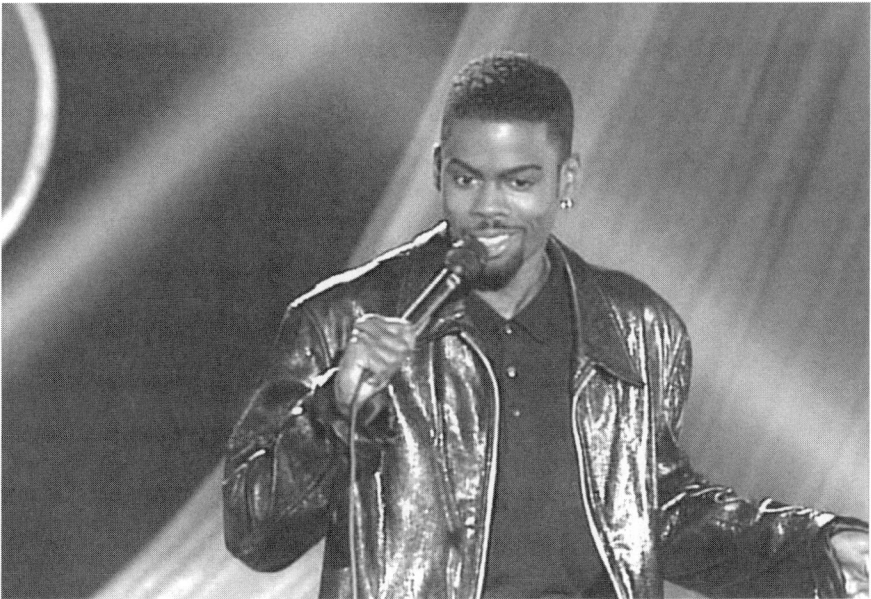

10. Chris Rock as the equal-opportunity offender in his HBO special *Bring the Pain* (1996). Directed by Keith Truesdell.

attempted. Like Pryor he mines the characters and stories of multiple black communities to comment on larger political issues. Like Gregory he unambiguously
states his views regarding the politicized sphere of race relations, whether by
underscoring the way the war on drugs disproportionately affects the African
American community (particularly young black men) or the politically informed
views of the criminal justice system: "Whole damn country is so conservative.
Everybody's saying jails not tough enough . . . jails not tough enough . . . we got
to have the death penalty. Jails are fucked up—don't believe the hype. The problem is jails are overcrowded because life is fucked up, too. People are broke.
People are starving. Life is fucked up. Shit, life is catching up to jail. If you live
in an old project, a new jail is not that bad." His causal analysis of the complex
politics of incarceration, while not comprehensive, emphasizes economic
inequities and forces the audience to recognize how issues of class and race necessarily inflect burgeoning attitudes toward crime and punishment.

Paradoxically, around issues of gender Rock's comic discourse lacks the same
incisiveness. While Rock's act speaks from multiple positions on the political
spectrum, reactionary impulses can be discerned in his ruminations on gender
roles. All of Rock's HBO specials have moments when they dally on the slippery
sexist slope tread by Murphy—as illustrated in Rock's condemnation of domestic violence but his "understanding" the impulse that might drive a man to it, or
the difficult male choice between "commitment and new pussy."[13] By no means
is Rock's act focused on issues of gender, but the sexual politics in his stand-up
comedy—from *Bring the Pain* to *Bigger and Blacker*—becomes progressively more
problematic as the comedic discourse becomes more reductive.

In *Bigger and Blacker* Rock's tirade against the impact for young single
mothers "getting their groove on" when they *should* be "getting their kid on"
acts as a setup for an overly simplistic comic payoff: "If a kid calls his grand-
mamma 'mommy' and his mama 'Pam,' he's going to jail." The statement elicits
nervous laughter from all segments of his audience but fails to interrogate the
sociological implications that inform this particular phenomenon.[14] Furthermore, as Rock off-handedly condemns this particular iteration of the multigenerational matriarchy in the African American community, he espouses and
reaffirms the preferential status of patriarchal gender roles. "If kids can't read . . .
it's Mama's fucking fault [but] if the kid can't read because there are no lights
in the house, that's Daddy's fault" represents a throwback to the days of stay-at-
home moms and single-income families—neither of which is the norm for
contemporary American society in general, and the black community in particular—nor has it ever truly been.[15] It seems that Rock is still, to some extent,
under the sway of a culture that equates black male power with regressive gender roles—even Rock, the Pryor/Gregory heir apparent, is seemingly blind to
the race and class issues generating this attitude.

While Rock's sexual politics adhere to traditional family values in terms of
gender, his views on sexuality, unlike most of his Def Jam brethren, are fairly

progressive: his support of gays in the military ("let 'em fight, cuz I'm not fightin'") and his literal condemnation of homophobia ("don't go in for that ... because whoever you hate is going to end up in your family"), while more practical than radical, reflect more acceptance of gays and lesbians than most black stand-up comedy. The radical impulses that drive Rock's comic persona toward uncompromisingly critical assessment also separate him from Murphy by demonstrating his "ability to set [himself] firmly against the grain, to perceive wrongheaded proscriptions and [to] speak out against them . . . [which] has always been the cornerstone of socially relevant humor."[16] Thus, for better and for worse, Rock's stand-up persona embodies both progressive and regressive forces in cultural criticism—with the ideological bias being entirely dependent on which social issue is up for his comedic dissection.

Arguably, the most controversial material is rooted in intraracial intro-spection: Rock's "Niggas vs. Black People" routine speaks directly to rifts within the black community. "There's some shit going on with black people right now," Rock asserts. "It's like a civil war going on with black people. There's two sides—there's black people and there's niggas. And niggas have got to go. . . . I love black people but I hate niggas." On one hand, the virulent condemnation of "niggas" requires of the audience a self-critical deconstruction of the histor-ically charged term while pressuring them (black and white) to recognize issues of difference (in terms of class and social practices) *within* the black community; on the other, the failure to address the sociohistorical roots of the group that Rock ahistorically defines as the undeserving underclass "niggas" problematizes the "good black/bad black" binary set up in this routine. Indeed, it is often dif-ficult to clearly discern the political intent of Rock's verbal barbs. While scold-ing possible sites of institutional racism (criminal justice, schools, media), he refuses to frame such issues in essentialist terms. In response to the audience titters that follow the "Black People vs. Niggas" routine, Rock immediately responds: "I see some black people looking at me—mad. 'Why do you have to say that, brother? It ain't us, it's the media. The media has distorted our image.' . . . Please . . . when I go to the money machine tonight, I ain't looking over my back for the media—I'm looking for niggas." The direct address to his predom-inantly black audience calls into question any easy assumptions about social problems and issues of representation. On one hand, by casting himself as both a scathing sociopolitical critic and a devil's advocate, Rock offers perspectives on African American life that speak to the conflicted and conflictual aspects of a blackness that is constructed internally as well as externally. Rock provides a comedic riff on a concretized version of what W. E. B. Du Bois asserted a cen-tury ago, that the black experience is informed by an internal division—a "double consciousness": "One ever feels his twoness—an American, a Negro; two souls, two thoughts, two unreconciled strivings, two warring ideals in one dark body whose dogged strength alone keeps it from being torn asunder."[17] Although the term *double consciousness* does not adequately describe the complexity of either identity formation or meaning-making for most people of color, the sensibility embodied in the phrase, and mobilized in the "Niggas vs. Black people" routine, speaks to the ways in which Rock's work resonates for black audiences. On the other hand, the fact that some of Rock's most biting comic critique is focused on the black community might also explain his popularity with white audiences; as the insider who's "telling it like it is" regardless of whom the listeners might be, Rock constantly treads the thin line between humor and heresy. Not surprisingly, while maintaining that he is first and foremost a stand-up comic, Rock has also become progressively more cognizant of the power of his comedy as cultural critique and that, although he is speaking from and to the black community, the numbers of those outside the community, and in his fan base, are legion. In a 2005 interview with Ed Bradley on *Sixty Minutes*, Rock addressed the continued discussion of that 1997 routine: "I think a lot of people were thinking in those terms ['Niggas vs. Black People'] and hadn't been able to say it. By the way, I've never done that joke again, ever, and I probably never will, 'cause some people that were racist thought they had license to say 'nigger.' So, I'm done with that routine."[18] Nonetheless, for better and for worse, Rock's brand of comedic cultural critique played well for multiple audiences, and, by expanding his relationship with HBO to include a late-night series, the comic had the opportunity to both broaden his appeal and hone his style of comedy. While, for the purposes of this study, greater attention—and close textual analysis—is dedicated to his HBO stand-up special as a means of discerning the *televisual* codification of his comic persona, one would be remiss not to note how his HBO late-night series further facilitated his movement into the entertainment mainstream and A-list. It was the success of the comic's stand-up persona that afforded him the opportunity to stretch the boundaries of the late-night talk genre.

The Emmy-winning *The Chris Rock Show* (1997–2000) emerged as a genuine alternative—an idiosyncratic condensation of the techniques used on mainstream network (and netlet) programming like *The Tonight Show with Jay Leno*, *Late Night with David Letterman*, and *The Arsenio Hall Show*—not surprisingly, on the same premium cable outlet that aired both his breakout specials and, in the first part of the decade, *Russell Simmons' Def Comedy Jam*, one of the first high-profile televisual showcases for black comedians.[19] More than simply an attempt to jump on the counterprogramming train, Rock's show, with Grandmaster Flash of the legendary hip hop group Grandmaster Flash and the Furious Five as the series' musical director/DJ, reflected *his* vision of late-night talk, which provided a prime example of African American cultural production. The series sampled a range of contemporary black music—including the Artist Formerly Known as Prince in his first show, and Ice-T in his last, Snoop Dogg and Dr. Dre, DeAngelo, and Jill Scott in between—providing a space for these acts in the years when hip-hop was just beginning to find its way onto the network late-night stages.

Furthermore, Rock, acutely attuned to the rapid flow of both mainstream and black popular culture, asserted that the show had a "youthful slant," speaking to and about people who had not been the target of Leno or Letterman's monologues: "We're joking about people never joked about before. They are almost happy that their name is in the monologue. It's a new thing 'cause no one ever did [the late Wu Tang Clan Member and trouble magnet] Ol' Dirty Bastard jokes before me. And Letterman is doing it now. . . . No one ever put on a suit and did a monologue and talked about these people."[20]

Rock's statement speaks to the larger significance in terms of providing a black perspective on current events through the entertainment medium. In the same way that Johnny Carson's monologue functioned for decades as a means of commentary (albeit usually pedestrian), Rock's monologue, cutting a swath across politics, culture, and the arts, gave a broad, cable audience *his* view of the American condition. The Carson comparison is problematic, however, in that, during the era before the Leno versus Letterman late-night-taste culture split, Johnny's voice was that of late night on network television. In the postnetwork era, there was no single voice, in much the same way as there was no single audience, but rather multiple niches (some more attractive—read lucrative—to media outlets than others). Rock, like his equally irreverent (and even more difficult to ideologically pin) HBO late-night slot mate, Dennis Miller, spoke to a younger and more culturally and politically savvy audience—both a desirable and diverse demographic.[21] Unlike most late-night fare, each episode ran a fast thirty commercial-free minutes, was filmed live to tape, and consisted of a monologue, sketches, and a single interview segment; the guests appeared not because they were hawking new movies, books, or compact discs on the talk-show circuit but rather because they were figures that the series' ethos deemed *relevant*. Tangentially associated with Arsenio Hall's showcasing of highly accessible aspects of black cultural coding (slang, gesture, etc.) in the realm of late night talk (minus Arsenio's semisycophantic coddling of guests and plus Rock's much edgier comedic awareness), the series reflected the imbrication of Rock's multiple ideologies in much the same way that his act does, both of which are informed by the inherent refusal to be easily pinned, culturally or politically.[22] The show became an entertainment-based forum for all corners of the black public sphere, from cultural critic Cornell West, black female empowerment guru and inspirational speaker Iyanla Vanzant, and director Spike Lee to figures who had been targets of Rock's comic ire, including the Reverend Al Sharpton, University of California regent Ward Connerly, and Marion Barry.

The recurring characters included Wanda Sykes, playing an angry political "insider" who provides her commonsensical commentaries on the state of the union from her post in the White House mailroom, and the enigmatic "Super-celebrity" "Pootie Tang" (Lance Crouthers), whose construction (think "ghetto fabulousness meets blaxploitation") lampooned multiple mediated and colloquial archetypes of black masculinity. Thus, the sometimes hostile nature of sketches is a logical extension of Rock's stand-up ethos in the sketch comedy format. Rock's "man-on-the-street" interviews posed purposefully provocative questions in often unlikely settings: whether interviewing white and black South Carolina public and private citizens about the controversy over the Confederate flag flying over the State House or the residents of Howard Beach about renaming a main thoroughfare for a slain black man. The latter segment exemplifies the same layered form of comedic discourse discernible in Rock's stand-up; what begins as musing about why there are no streets named after slain black men in white areas evolves into a sketch with a critical subtext that conflates two killings that deeply resonate in black popular consciousness: those of Tupac Shakur and Michael Griffith, the young black victim of the 1986 Howard Beach incident.[23] No reminder of historical context is given during Rock's trek around Howard Beach as he asks residents to sign a petition to change the name of Cross Bay Boulevard to Tupac Shakur Boulevard, a request that yielded a full spectrum of responses from chuckling incredulousness to downright hostility; however, the sounds of the in-house audience for that evening's taping provides both the groans and laughter that acknowledge the significance of Rock's site choice. Furthermore, as Acham observes, "Rock does get several white residents to sign the petition but the images of the resentful whites of Howard Beach at the turn of the last century cannot be ignored."[24]

The sketches, the man-on-the-street interviews, and, of course, the monologue took conventional late-night comedy shtick and clearly transformed it by providing Rock's particular black sensibility, inflected by hip-hop culture, and African American social history. Like Rock's stand-up, the source of the praise and the criticism during the series run was his persona as the equal-opportunity offender. After the industrial success of *Bring the Pain* and *Bigger and Blacker*, and the clout that accompanied it, Rock's HBO series exemplified the ways in which the black comic persona could flourish on the small screen—in an amenable televisual space. Rock succeeded on late-night television where other black comics' attempts (like those of Keenen Ivory Wayans and Sinbad) had failed. Rock's comic persona permeated the series, informing both the style and the content. Because it was HBO, where edginess is seen as bankable, there was genuinely a space for contemporary iterations of blackness—at least where comedy is concerned.

The reception of "edgy," however, was (and is) dependent on both the sociocultural and industrial conditions, as well as spectatorial and critical taste. During the run of *The Chris Rock Show*, Eddie Murphy also returned to television—or at least his voice did. *The PJs*, Eddie Murphy's Claymation series (think "California Raisins"), depicted life in the projects. The first volley against *The PJs* came from Spike Lee, who called the series "incredibly demeaning. . . . I kind of scratch my head why Eddie Murphy's doing this. . . . I'm not saying that we're above being made fun of and stuff but it's really hateful, I think, towards Black people, plain and simple."[25] Lee was not alone. *The PJs* was the hot-button series for debates about black-on-black representations even before its premiere. Lee's comments fueled the controversy, as did negative press from black journalists like Denene Millner's cutting remarks about the *PJs*' claim of "keeping it real" in the *New York Daily News*: "Murphy's a Long Island boy from a stable, middle-class, two-parent household, who has never lived in the projects so far as we know. And Lord knows that today, as a multi-millionaire with a worldwide following, he's about as far removed from 'ghetto life' as a Southern Republican."[26] In response to the criticism of the series, *LA Times* critic Howard Rosenberg states that *The PJs* is as much of a "slap in the face against blacks as *The Simpsons* is against whites. . . . In the matter of *The PJs* are some Black skins really that thin?"[27] Larry Wilmore, the cocreator and executive producer, expressed exasperation at the criticism of the series, particularly since this sort of parody, he maintained, was "nothing new"—given that African American urban underclass characters have been staples in black comedy from Richard Pryor's stand-up to *In Living Color*. "I thought we would have gotten to the point now that we can make fun of ourselves," Wilmore asserted, "but people say the images are so offensive they don't even want to hear the point you're trying to make."[28]

Proving that, to some extent, even bad publicity is good publicity, *The PJs* scored the network's second most watched series premiere, with almost twenty-two million viewers, and found a temporary home at Fox. In the series Thurgood Stubbs, voiced by Murphy, is master of his domain as the super of the Hilton Jacobs project; a mixture of Fred Sanford and Kingfish, he is also perpetually seeking shortcuts and schemes to enhance or solidify his position.[29] Life with "Supa" makes poverty perversely pastoral. There are roaches, "forties" of malt liquor, gunshots played for laughs in ambient sound. In other words, *The PJs* makes *Good Times* look like a documentary on housing project life, but, apparently, realism wasn't really the point. As Mark Anthony Neal contends, "As 'supa's' name—a surreal conflation of the late Supreme Court justice Thurgood Marshall and the lead singer of the Four Tops, Levi Stubbs—suggests, he is at once an antiquated reminder of a fictive black community where black folks struggled together amid detrimental and demeaning circumstances and a vivid caricature of a generation of black men who remain hopelessly sexist and vulgar, but who regularly redeem themselves in the name of community."[30]

While Larry Wilmore, *The PJs*' coexecutive producer, has been the public defender of the series, Murphy, for his part as executive producer, did not publicly comment.[31] By the end of the following season, *The PJs*, which had been moved, preempted, and put on hiatus by Fox several times over the course of the 2000 season, was cancelled and promptly relocated to the WB as an unsuccessful midseason replacement (spring 2001). One has to wonder whether the reception of *The PJs* was determined as much by the industrial and sociopolitical climate (namely the network "brownout" threatened by a coalition of minority political groups including the NAACP) as the problematic nature of

the series' "hypercaricature" of the black underclass of the projects. Nevertheless, one wonders whether *The PJs* would have fared better in the age of *South
Park* and, of course, *Chappelle's Show*.

In the five years between *Bigger and Blacker* (1999) and his fourth HBO
special, *Never Scared* (2004), Rock became a presence on both the big and small
screen. After leaving his critically and popularly acclaimed HBO series at the
end of 2001 and experiencing mixed success in his big-screen endeavors, like
*Down to Earth* (2001) and *Head of State* (2003), one might contend that his
return to stand-up took on the dual role of homecoming and de facto comeback show—either way, Rock's status as the era's ultimate stand-up seemed at
stake. Rock's much touted return to stand-up revealed a more mature but no
less irreverent comedic figure. Like the Bone Crusher's hip-hop anthem "I Ain't
Never Scared," from which the special's title seems inspired, Rock's fourth
HBO special resounded with self-assurance and defiance—which was exactly
what the audience expected. While one might contend that *Never Scared* does
not provide the level of biting critique that was present in *Bring the Pain* (the
opening comic assault on Marion Barry) or the intentionally outrageous
dualisms of *Bigger and Blacker* (his post-Columbine confession of "being afraid
of young white males"), it is the skillfully constructed set of a veteran comic.
Like the comics whose albums were superimposed over Rock's initial stroll to
the stage in *Bring the Pain* (as well as others like Moms Mabley, Buddy Hackett,
Carl Reiner, and Mel Brooks, whose acts are on rotation in his I-Pod), his ability to both read and work his audience has been carefully honed by study and
practice.

As Josh Wolk notes, Rock tackles issues that many of his peers only touch
on for shock value—"abortion, affirmative action, racism"—with "brutal,
relentless, honesty."[32] In an *Entertainment Weekly* article proclaiming him "the
funniest man in America," Rock's discussion of the care with which his pedantic joke-attacks are structured seems to resonate with Dick Gregory's musing on
comedy's "friendly relation" and the careful balancing act required of the black
comic:"I never stop the show to get a point across, I get it in there, but it's jokes,
jokes, jokes. You do some weird abortion joke, that thing's gotta be worded just
. . . right. . . . You're literally dealing with nitroglycerine. One drop and the whole
place goes up."[33] The construction of Rock as "comic as truth-teller" is far from
a naturalistic process. The forcefully stated assertions, made as if they are
commonsense pronouncements in Rock's act, are the product of a comic
who obsessively rewrites his jokes with the knowledge of both where and to
whom he speaks. This consciousness of his multiple audiences—and the
"nitroglycerine-like" quality of comedic social discourse—guides Rock's work
as both a comic craftsman and a black stand-up comic. Always cognizant of the
experience of "speak[ing] two languages . . . and perform[ing] for people who
don't look anything like you," Rock states, "nobody else has to do that: Lenny
Bruce, Seinfeld, anybody. . . . I pride myself on being the guy who can do *Def*

*Comedy Jam* and *Charlie Rose*. And do well on both."[34] However, the consciousness and care do not necessarily act as inhibitors for Rock's critique: they simply underscore the fact that his comic "truths" are pointed and purposeful. The content of Rock's act, with his tirades against cultural and institutional practices, facilitates what Michael Eric Dyson refers to as "the seepage of his discourse beyond boundaries of ethnic and racial communities."[35] His cross-cultural appeal seems to extend beyond the simple industrial notion of crossover—because, the careful construction of his act does not involve a homogenizing process. Rather, Rock's discursive game is riskier. Again, as Dyson notes: "We can't pretend that we don't live in a political context in which white Americans say, 'See, what we told you about those black folks must be true since there's a black man on television saying the same thing.' I think we have to run that risk to get the 'truth' as we see it, as we're willing to argue for its existence in given cultural and social contexts."[36] Thus, Rock's persona, comic as truth teller, which draws audiences of myriad different positions on the American sociopolitical spectrum, is granted permission to speak from multiple positions. While the Rock of 1996 caught audiences by surprise with his quasi-caustic candor, the Rock of 2004 is not kinder and gentler—he simply has a more fluid ideological and sociopolitical agenda.

Before Rock comes onstage, the HBO broadcast touts the comic's stand-up prowess by including snippets of interviews with the preshow audience as they enter. In one of the three adulation-drenched clips, a thirty-something African American woman states, "Like he says, there are niggers and there are black people. Chris Rock is a progressive black man." This statement, which ties together a reference to arguably his most famous bit from *Bring the Pain* and the marker of "progressive" on his brand of humor, is significant. Her label of "progressive black man" may speak more to Rock's position in the entertainment world than it necessarily does to the content of his entire stand-up act. While it is difficult to discern whether the woman's complimentary remarks spoke to Rock as a comic who speaks "truth to power," as in the nuanced "realities" of a diverse African American community (as in "Niggers and Black People"), or as an African American entertainer who possesses neither an act nor a comic persona that traffics in minstrelesque buffoonery, one might argue that the construction of his comic persona is progressive—though not always positive.[37] As noted in the earlier discussion of Rock's stand-up, one might argue that the gender politics fall within the realm of the regressive, at worst, and the traditional, at best. Even his discussions of race can be seen to engage class in some essentializing ways. The truth of the matter is that most humor—particularly most African American humor—is inflected by progressive and regressive impulses: and few comics embrace both with the same ferocity as Rock.

By the premiere of *Never Scared* in April of 2004, the thirty-nine-year-old Rock was considered a stand-up virtuoso, and, as such, aspects of his comic discourse have become common knowledge in American popular culture. Unlike

Murphy's stand-up triumphs, *Delirious* and *Raw*, which were the products of a very young and very talented comic superstar, whose audacious observational humor was rooted in problematic sexual politics and popular culture savvy, *Never Scared*, and, indeed, all of Rock's stand-up is sociocultural comedic discourse embedded in an elaborate structure of jokes and jokes and jokes. Murphy was the charming bad boy; Rock, then and now, is part comic and part preacher. Rock has even admitted as much—at least stylistically speaking. His rhetorical strategy of repeating phrases multiple times in the course of a joke series, has become a trademark, a technique that, he states, "I probably got from preachers."[38] Yet for Rock, as an African American comic dealing with formidable social issues, the motivation for utilizing the repetition is rooted in guiding the audience through his particular comic object lesson: "If I gloss over the setup, it could be combustible especially when I get into racial dynamics. If you've got the nerve to be a rich nigger onstage, complaining about the plight of your people, everybody is like 'fuck you. You're doing good.' Like I shouldn't care about my people because I can buy 10 pairs of sneakers."[39]

When actor/comic/rapper Doug E. Fresh announces Rock with the exclamation, "D.C. Are You Ready?" the crowd's frenzy can barely be contained. Rock comes onstage in a tailored deep burgundy suit with subtle black pinstripe, black shirt and black handkerchief, diamonds in his ears and a ten-thousand-watt grin. For this most recent iteration of Rock's comic persona the constant movement across the stage was neither the hyped up pacing of *Big Ass Jokes* nor the cocky strutting of either *Bring the Pain* or *Bigger and Blacker*. His entrance reminded me of watching Ali walk into the ring in the "Rumble in the Jungle": every step, little dance move, and even putting his hand to his ear, signaling them to pump up the volume of their cheers, seemed designed for one purpose: Rock was there to win. While one might argue that the parallels between boxing and stand-up may seem tenuous, Rock refers to his stand-up performances on the 2004 *Black Ambition* tour as being in training for the performance filmed at Constitution Hall in Washington, D.C.[40]

In *Never Scared* Rock's combination (joke) series are also reminiscent of Ali's "rope a dope" in discursive terms. With the original "rope-a-dope" Ali allowed Foreman to believe that he knew the direction that the fight was taking (and to pummel him with body blows on the ropes) until literally, he, who was "the greatest," reverses that direction with a left-right combo. Rock also plays with audience expectations—rather than coming in pounding the audience with scathing critique (his technique in *Bring the Pain*), Rock toys with them with initial material that provides the insight without the critical bite (and, thus allowing them to believe that they can anticipate the parameters of his comedy skills set) before moving into a comedic discourse designed to facilitate more complicated cultural introspection. This particular form of audience play also reveals the ideological swings in Rock's material. His "realization" that, as a new father, his only job in life is to keep his daughter "off the pole" and his further theories on strip club folklore (from, she's stripping her way through college, to the lunch buffet is the real draw for daytime patrons) provide easy commentary on modern morality. His establishment of a traditional paternal paradigm as an ideal, and its causal relationship for women's behavior, while humorous, corresponds with the quasi-judgmental tone (bordering on sexism) that Rock often employs when discussing women's foibles. The sexual politics of the first joke series is simultaneously ambivalent and conservative: by citing the need for someone to fulfill the fantasies of the married man (implying that there are things a "good" woman won't do) and detailing a "wife's" vehement refusal to a "nasty" request (to don part of the stripper's new uniform—clear heels), critiques both the madonna and the whore constructions of womanhood, while still clearly privileging the former.

While Rock's style is unrelenting, moving from one fast-paced joke series to the next, like the repeated phrases within the joke series itself, thematic repetition takes place throughout the eighty-minute act. His gender critique reappears as a sideline in a bit relating to broader cultural commentary that engages both personal and cultural history: his love of rap and his difficulties with defending the recent examples of the genre. Here Rock's persona can be characterized as the "truth-teller" meets the preacher. In this bit, and various times during the set, Rock is giving a comedic sermon that belies both discursive urgency and ideological certainty.

> I'm 39 years old and I still love Rap Music. I love it. I'm that age when I've been loving rap music forever. . . . I love rap music but I'm tired of defending it. . . . And in the old days, it was easy to defend rap music. It was easy to defend it on an intellectual level (raises hand as if to indicate high level at which rap formerly functioned). To break it down intellectually why Grandmaster Flash was art. Why Run DMC was art. Why Houdini was art and music, you could break it down. I love all the rappers today but it's hard to defend this shit. It's hard. It's hard to defend "I Got Ho's in Different area codes."

Rock further lures the audience into his discourse by citing a particular song that is "impossible to defend" and that "we should all be ashamed . . . for liking." At the mention of Lil' Jon, the godfather of the Dirty South "crunk" sound, the audience goes wild and raps with him: "From the window, to the walls, till the sweat drips from my balls, till the sweat drips from my balls, skeet, skeet, skeet." Rock goes through the chorus again simulating a female's crunked up little dance to this extremely popular club anthem—hand waving in the air, low stepping semigrind. Given the clearly sexual nature of the song and its widespread popularity, Rock's quotation is not surprising; the critique of this subgenre of rap takes a very gendered angle. His sly chuckle becomes a throaty guffaw as he relays the fact that women who like rap are not phased by the accusations of misogyny thrown at the genre—"if the beat's alright, she'll dance all night." Using progressively more sexually explicit language, he creates an impromptu crunked up song; Rock, imitating the female rap fan, repeats the low stepping semigrind to a rap that begins with "Smack 'em with the dick, smack 'em with the dick." His reflection upon the rap fan's lack of offense at these lyrics is stated with faux incredulousness: "You know what's funny? If you mention to a woman that the song is disgusting and misogynistic, they all give you the same answer—'He ain't talking about me.'" However, what seems more telling, in terms of his gendered view of rap fandom comes when he conflates questions of virtue and taste: "I pity the guys that got to pick a wife out of this bunch. (In childlike voice) 'Daddy, where did you meet Mommy?' (In a nostalgia-tinged adult voice) 'Oh, she was singing about balls at a club. Skeet, skeet, skeet.'" While Rock's feigned incredulousness, his impromptu sing-a-long, and his dancing imitation take the edge off of his mitigated condemnation, the fact remains that although we should all be "ashamed" of singing along with Lil' Jon, only women bare the brunt of actual shame in relationship to the song's oft-repeated catchphrase: "Skeet."[41] While the gendered commentary on this par-ticular aspect of hip-hop-taste culture certainly possesses markers of regressive sexual politics, the sentiments do not appear to challenge the audience's sensi-bilities—rather, it seems to speak to, and of, a sort of shared cultural knowledge about the pleasures and content of contemporary rap. In other words, the audi-ence is still with him. In annunciating this insider perspective, Rock maintains an affinity with the audience even while introducing commentary that requires some degree of personal introspection—albeit uncritical at this point.

Rock's repeated assertion of his love for rap music, and his exhaustion at being compelled to defend it, also speaks to a generational divide that under-scores the ideological differences between old-school-conscious rap like Grandmaster Flash's "The Message" and the crazy drunk ("crunk") partying songs of Lil' Jon.[42] While condemning neither strains of rap in these passing references, Rock historicizes the cultural significance of rap as a genre rooted in, and associated with, a particular black urban experience—as well as the pos-sible motivations for institutional aversion to the music, its practitioners, and the experience of black life that it can and has chronicled. The notion that "rap killings" are investigated and prosecuted in less aggressive ways ("if you want to get away with murder, shoot somebody and then stick a demo tape in his pocket") has become a staple in the sets of many black comics since the late nineties, and, as Rock aptly notes, since the very public and still unsolved mur-ders of Tupac Shakur, Biggie Smalls, and Jam Master Jay. Thus, Rock draws attention to another sociohistorical legacy that resonates within the African American community—that of a legal system that is far from color blind. As if to pound the point home, Rock chooses an intentionally eclectic collection of classic rockers to underscore the politics of differentiation at play—maintain-ing that if Billy Joel, David Bowie, and Elton John had been murder victims, Bruce Springsteen's house would be encircled by police. Within the rubric of a discussion about rap Rock has moved between discourse on intra- and inter-cultural practices and segues from taste cultures to questionable institutional practices and, quite literally, the lack of equal protection.

Yet attention to the discursive misdirection that Rock employs in *Never Scared*—the mixture of comic combinations that play into the audience's per-ceptions and challenge its (moral/cultural) sensibilities and its intellectual acu-ity—does not negate the moments of direct comic confrontation that followed somewhat predictable targets. His material on the legal problems experienced by highly visible black celebrities yielded big laughs from the crowd. Stating that Michael Jackson is "crazy" and that the "King of Pop's" recurring legal woes seem like "groundhog's day,"[43] or questioning Kobe Bryant's decision not to hire Johnny Cochran because it would make him "look guilty" (stating the merit of being yet another black man protesting his innocence from his jail cell versus "looking guilty at the mall"), is hardly the edgiest material in Rock's comic arsenal. However, the appraisals of the per-ils of high-profile black celebrity are designed to segue into a narrative that speaks to his audience in what are, arguably, racially coded terms. Although in each of these instances, the celebrity's travails are known to mainstream audi-ences, for black audiences it is likely that the discussion of these struggles have also been part of casual conversation (and argument) in communal and home spaces. On one hand, one might say that this practice of "airing dirty laundry" has become an expected part of Rock's act; on the other, the intraracial celebrity commentary in this passage is mobilized as part of a rant that has a universalizing effect in service to a particular purpose: the fact that "we" have all been lied to: "Don't let all this celebrity news fool you. [His meter slows to punctuate the importance of the statement.] It is just a trick to get your mind OFF THE WAR. Trick to get your mind off the war. I think Bush sent that girl to Kobe's room. [The crowd laughs] Bush sent that girl to Kobe's room. Sent that boy to Michael Jackson's house. Bush killed Laci Peterson. Bush was fucking Paris Hilton in that video—all to get your mind OFF THE WAR. Bush lied to me."

This joke passage illustrates yet another instance of Rock speaking across cultural boundaries—not simply because in making intentionally outrageous, conspiracy theory–inflected assertions he deals with black and white victims/defendants/celebrities but rather because he calls attention to the fact that these alleged governmental deceptions are neither race specific or isolated instances. The implied "we" of this passage is the American public—although, I would argue, the ideological wakeup call for the African American community is a bit more pointed. Rock frames his antiwar commentary in the context of one who "loves this country"; however, as he speaks of love of country—prac-tices that take place in the name of patriotism—Rock reminds his audience (black and white) how easily "Patriotism turn[s] into hatriotism," and the mean-ing that should have for the African American community.

There was a lot of accepted racism. "I'm American, man. I'm American, man, fuck the foreigners." And that was cool. "I'm American, man. I'm American, man, Fuck the French." And that was cool. "I'm American, man. I'm American, man, Fuck the Arabs," and [with a dismissive wave of the hand], that was cool. And then they went to "I'm American, man. I'm American, man, fuck all these illegal aliens," and then I started listening cuz I know Niggers and Jews is next. [The crowd howls with laughter and applauds this "logical" progression] Any day now (raising his arm to look at his watch), that train's never late.

His throaty guffaw acts the exclamation mark for the passage. By acknowledging the regressive components of patriotism, Rock once again brings the issue of race to the discursive table. Referencing the Oklahoma City bombing (Timothy McVeigh associated with the white supremacist Michigan militia) and the brutal slaying of James Byrd (random racial violence in Jasper, Texas), the comic makes clear that there are far greater "terrorist" dangers to the African American community. With eyes blazing, staring right at the audience and at the camera, Rock's pronouncement, inflected by race-coded common sense, conveys a declarative intensity and ideological certainty: "I'm from Brooklyn, I don't give a shit about Al-Qaeda. . . . I ain't scared of Al-Qaeda—I'm scared of Al-Cracker. You have to look out for cracker Al. He's a dangerous motherfucker."

The joke series has segued into a sociopolitical comedic sermon with Rock, as heavyweight truth-teller, utilizing the rhetorical strategy of repetition, comic misdirection, and first-person observation to bring the point (and the punch line) home. As a self proclaimed student of comedy and current events, Rock contends that "anyone who makes up their fucking mind before they hear the issue is a fucking fool, okay." In so doing, he defies being posited within any ideological or political camp—and encourages others to do the same in a comic passage that serves as a commonsense civics lesson. Equating performing political affinity to membership in a gang, Rock makes a call for ideological, political, and social individuality: "Be a fucking person! LISTEN! No normal decent person is one thing—I got some stuff I'm conservative about. . . . Crime: I'm conservative, prostitution: I'm liberal." While the directive itself speaks to a certain rugged individualist ethos that is (sociohistorically speaking) very American, Rock here, and throughout his act, annunciates an array of ideologies inflected by lived experience and by national, racial, and cultural identities. The articulation of Rock's stand-up persona is informed by a comic style and discursive strategies that, for all of its irreverent consistency, is inherently fluid, defies being fixed in terms of a specific point on the political spectrum, and underscores the imperative that people listen in order make up their minds for themselves.

Like the "Rumble in the Jungle" did for Ali, Rock's fourth HBO comedy special reaffirms the comic's stand-up prowess; Rock, at the height of his comedic powers—older, wiser, and wilier—demands that audiences examine the world in which they live. Embedded in the act are numerous instances in which Rock, who has created a sense of affinity with the audience (casting himself as a part of the many implied *we*'s of the joke series) contests popularly held notions—whether about patriotism, celebrity, or individual responsibility. His willingness to voice his position—taking into consideration audience and venue but never allowing that to dilute the discursive force of his comedy—makes Rock the poster boy for comedy as sociopolitical discourse. Whether or not one agrees with Rock's multiple ideological agenda, one cannot help but be struck by the degrees of fearlessness in his stand-up. Thus, *Never Scared* serves a dual purpose for Rock, and for African American comedic discourse in the new millennium, as both a description and declaration of blackness, and its primacy in understanding both American popular culture and the American condition.

While *Never Scared* reaffirmed Rock's stand-up sovereignty, neither the critical acclaim nor the industrial hype for his long-awaited stand-up special came close to the media frenzy around his semiautobiographical sitcom, *Everybody Hates Chris*. Like Murphy's return to television with *The PJs*, Rock's considerable industrial and popular cultural cachet focused attention on the series long before its premiere. Unlike the considerable critique of Murphy's controversial Claymation outing, neither the authenticity nor the sensitivity of Rock's sitcom, in comic as well as cultural terms, were called into question. *Everybody Hates Chris* is loosely based on Rock's experience of growing up in the Bedford-Stuyvesant neighborhood in Brooklyn and being bused to an all-white school.

*Everybody Hates Chris* was the most anticipated comedy of the 2005–6 season, which caused even more entertainment media frenzy because of its network (or, more aptly, netlet) home, United Paramount Network (UPN). Before deciding to base the series on the comic's life, Rock and cocreator Ali LeRoi originally pitched the series as a black urban *Wonder Years* (the early-nineties nostalgia dramedy). When Fox, who had the first option on the pilot, ultimately passed, citing concerns over the expense of yet another single-camera sitcom[44] and over whether Rock's involvement after the pilot might be limited, UPN president Dawn Ostroff did not hesitate to make *Everybody Hates Chris* the centerpiece of the netlet's lineup.[45]

"Rock has said *Everybody Hates Chris* is not a literal version of his childhood, but it is a pretty literal version of his comedy."[46] The voice of the series is undoubtedly Rock's, both in comic sensibility and in actuality: the comic supplies the voiceover as the adult version of his teenaged alter ego (newcomer Tyler James Williams). As is true in the comic's stand-up, the sitcom refuses to elide issues of race and class. As LeRoi states, "We're dealing with class issues much more so than race issues. It's not black folks don't get along with white folks. It's which black folks don't get along with which white folks and why. It's broke people trying to do the best they can and we're not going to make a speech about it. We're just going to show them doing it."[47] This nuclear family is neither the Huxtables nor the Evanses (*Good Times*). *Everybody Hates Chris* directly engages class and race within a domestic comedy context where neither the family nor its living conditions are idealized. Given that Rock's comedy and lived experiences inform the series, it also avoids the kind of excessive sentimentality often associated with nostalgia sitcoms.

The setting establishes a clear connection with a post-soul urban experience. The first episode begins with the parents, Julius (Terry Crews) and Rochelle (Tichina Arnold), and their children, Chris, Drew (Tequan Richmond), and Tonya (Imani Hakim), moving from the projects into an apartment in what was assumed to be a better neighborhood. Both the move and his mother's insistence that Chris be bused to the all-white middle school were motivated by the desire for safety and opportunity. Rochelle's fierce protectiveness of her family, her firm but loving discipline (with explicit threat of physical reinforcement: "I'll slap your name out of the phone book and call Ma Bell and tell her I did it"), and her fiscal sensibilities (running the family finances "like the government—on a deficit") embody the continued striving for an iteration of the American Dream that promises that the next generation will have it better than the previous one did. Yet the well-intentioned, pragmatic actions of his civil rights era parents did not always yield the expected results, as Rock's omniscient narration intones, reflecting on the family's 1982 move to Bed-Sty: "Had we known that Bed-Sty was going to be the center of the crack epidemic, I guess we would have moved somewhere else."

Just as the first episode of *The Cosby Show* narrativized aspects of *Bill Cosby: Himself*, the pilot of *Everybody Hates Chris* sampled the comic's autobiographical material—from *Big Ass Jokes* to *Never Scared*. The choice of samples, however, further underscores the post-soul aesthetic in the series. The subtext of the televisualized version of Rock's "school as hell" routine (which recounts being called "nigger" and "getting beaten up just about every day") questions the efficacy of the civil rights era–informed goals of integration for young black teens in 1980s urban America. When Chris attempts to use his purported street cred (being from "Bed-Sty: Do Or Die") to "out black" the quintessential bully, Joey Caruso, the bravado and verbal vivisection prove to be futile: he is only saved by running for the bus out of Brooklyn Beach (the televisual stand-in for Bensonhurst). The altercation with hostile white middle-schoolers, led by Caruso, and the indifference of white authority figures (the school principal, a police officer, and the bus driver) reveal a racial climate that is less than ideal but also less than 1950s Little Rock or 1970s Boston. It also alludes to the post-soul baby, dealing with how far we haven't come.

That is not to say that the series discounts the civil rights struggle. In the final scene of the episode, when Julius checks in on his family, as he does every night "between his night job and his late night job," he asks Chris about school. As the voiceover states, "I didn't tell him about the fight. My dad went to school during the civil rights era. After hoses, tanks, and dogs biting your ass, somehow Joey Caruso didn't compare." Archival footage depicting those trials (as well as a black and white image of the bully, Caruso, just prior to Chris's beating) are juxtaposed with the images of the father sitting on the edge of the son's bed. The son's respect for the father's struggle, in the past and present, is unquestionable. The same scene, a softened reiteration of the critique in "Niggers vs. Black People" dealing with the desire to be lauded for things "you're supposed to do" ("I take care of my kids"), forwards a construction of black fatherhood that acknowledges the father's era as well as the son's. After the notoriously frugal Julius slips a couple of extra dollars to his son, he moves toward the door and says, "I'll see you in the morning." In voiceover, Rock remarks, "He was one of four fathers on the block. 'I'll see you in the morning' meant he was coming home. Coming home was his way of saying 'I love you.'" On one hand, in this scene, as in his stand-up, a traditional familial (arguably, paternal) paradigm is privileged. One might argue that it simultaneously speaks to the inordinate numbers of fatherless black children in the post-soul era and fails to address the sociopolitical reasons for the black male absence. On the other hand, the scene, like the series, might be seen as a comedic discursive attempt to create kinship and bridge the gap between a civil rights era ethos and the lived experiences of post-soul babies.

Murphy and Rock represent two strains of black humor that converge stylistically but diverge significantly in terms of ideological content and their performance of blackness. As Rock himself notes, his humor bears a closer kinship to the socially relevant comics of a previous generation (Gregory, George Carlin, and Pryor) than it does to Murphy and his Def Jam progeny.[48] Interestingly, Murphy embodies in many ways Dick Gregory's prescription for crossover success: he is a black funny man, not a funny black man. However, this semantic difference is problematized within the context of Murphy's stand-up act, where his particular enunciation of blackness does not inform the content in either a critical or an especially progressive manner. One might even argue that Eddie's stand-up is fundamentally about Eddie—his celebrity, his sexuality, his experience of media. On one hand, this is reflective of the idiosyncratic aspect of comedy that allows for the creation of a unique comic persona—a fresh voice. On the other, the post-*SNL* comic persona of Murphy, while being a significant comic annunciation of black masculinity and machismo, arguably, speaks not to the black experience in broader sociocultural terms but rather to the black superstar experience—with a certain brand of observational humor that is descriptive rather than prescriptive.

By contrast, Rock's comic persona is built around sociopolitically informed articulations of blackness and serves as the post-soul era's logical reconstruction of Gregory's comedic discourse—in a slightly less transparent ideological frame. While Rock's kinship with Gregory is clear, so is his nostalgic affinity and semireverence for the position Cosby occupies in the pantheon of American

comedy: "I'd love to be Cosby . . . [and] have a whole new hour and a half of
material at 66. But Cosby is a storyteller. Cosby is from jazz. He loves jazz, worships jazz, and his style is pretty Dizzy Gillespie. Me, I'm from hip-hop. I'm
doing LL Cool J. I'm doing Run [DMC]. The rhythm is of old-school hip-
hop."[49] Unlike Murphy, who plays out the struggle with his comic predecessors
in the Cosby versus Pryor bit in *Raw* and repeatedly states his affinity with
Pryor (and, later, Redd Foxx) in word and action but captures only style not
substance, Rock's musical analogy makes a more nuanced comment on his relationship with the civil rights era–bred Cosby. While both jazz and hip-hop are
clearly associated with black cultural production, it is telling that the former,
positioned clearly with an earlier age, speaks to a more narrow swath of the contemporary audience—regardless of color—than the latter. That is not to say that
there is not an acknowledgment and even reverence for jazz greats from Dizzy
Gillespie to Charlie Parker to Miles Davis and John Coltrane; however, one
might argue that there is the recognition that the music, while oft sampled (in
both senses of the word) and savored, does not necessarily speak directly to contemporary notions of black cultural production.

I tease out this analogy because I believe it also speaks to Rock's relationship to Cosby, as the "personal responsibility" and "airing dirty laundry" aspects
of his comic discourse resonate, in some significant ways, with his forebear's controversial statements about the ills of the black underclass. While I would not
assert that Rock's intraracial commentary embraces a kind of black middle-class
vilification of "those other blacks" that, at least, informed Cosby's now famous
rant, some of the sentiments do express discourse previously reserved for black
communal spaces—not every media outlet imaginable. How could one not see
a connection between his now abandoned "Black People vs. Niggas" routine and
the tone, if not the exact content, of Cosby's orations on "lower class blacks."

Like Rock (and Murphy, for that matter), I am a "tweener," a product of the
waning years of the Baby Boom and just prior to the emergence of Gen X,
which means that we were the first generation of black America to come of age
in the post–civil rights era. Rock's espoused "old-school" affiliation positions
him with the first crop of post-soul babies. As such, his comedic discourse reflects
an understanding of civil rights era sociopolitical directives while also questioning their complete applicability to the contemporary African American condition. It also speaks to the mixture of apathy and anger (and often undirected
desire for action) born and bred in response to the socioeconomic disparities and
political disaffection gifted by Reaganism, the thwarted promises of the Clinton
era, and the growing class and culture rifts of one nation under Bush. Once transferred to the big screen, the convergences and divergences between the comic
personae of Murphy and Rock come into sharper focus, as do the color adjustments required—and endeavored—to achieve crossover success.

# CHAPTER 3

# Post-Soul Comedy Goes to the Movies

## CINEMATIC ADJUSTMENTS AND [POP] CULTURAL CURRENCY

THE TRANSITION FROM stand-up to screen has been markedly easier for Eddie Murphy and Chris Rock than for the previous generations of black comedians. Nonetheless, the creation of their cinematic personae has required the negotiation of comedic identities, as well as industrial and generic conventions and constraints. Thus, for the purposes of this study, their film roles will be examined in relationship to three unique subgenres: the "fish-out-of-water" film, the comedy of color-coded color blindness, and cultural comedies with creative control. To varying degrees these subgenres simultaneously recognize and elide race and correspond to roles played by Murphy—and, to a lesser extent, Rock—during different points in their big-screen careers.

### THE FISH-OUT-OF-WATER COMEDIES

The outsider's struggle to survive and thrive in a foreign, possibly hostile, world has always provided grist for the film comedy mill—from Buster Keaton's city-bred Canfield heir returning to claim the rural family estate in *Our Hospitality* (1923) to Martin Lawrence's thief turning detective to recover stashed loot in *Blue Streak* (1999). This comic staple functions differently, however, when a black comic is placed at the center of the insider/outsider paradigm. In such cases black stars are situated in cinematic milieus cut off from other representations of blackness, or even from other black characters, thereby placing them in the dubious position of representing the race. Ed Guerrero suggests, "One reason for the contextual isolation of the black star (or co-star) is not too hard to discern simply because many of these vehicles were originally written for white stars."[1] For example, the role that catapulted Murphy into superstardom, Axel Foley in *Beverly Hills Cop* (1984), was written for Sylvester Stallone.

Both Axel Foley and Reggie Hammond (*48 Hrs*, 1982) are roles that allowed Murphy to incorporate his stand-up persona within a big-screen role. Although *48 Hrs* "literalizes the metaphor of the black image being in the protective custody of white authority," Hammond acts as the embodiment of street sensibility and stand-up swagger.[2] The film operates within the interracial buddy film paradigm by focusing on the temporary alliance forged between surly, experienced cop Jack Cates (Nick Nolte) and small-time criminal Hammond (the "good" bad guy) in order to catch the latter's former partner. Murphy's character is introduced as a disembodied voice that wafts through the cellblock singing along to The Police's "Roxanne," his fondness for the mainstream pop group signaling a likable and unthreatening Anglo-friendliness. Playing off young/old, black/white, criminal/cop dichotomies, the uneasy but amiable alliance of Hammond and Cates acts as a sort of race relations fable that insists we can all just get along.

Reggie Hammond displays the signature black machismo of Murphy's comic persona as well as the verbal acuity of his stand-up (particularly when he tells barroom rednecks that "I'm your worst fucking nightmare—a nigger with a badge"). Hammond's "quest for flesh," a running subplot, gives Murphy an opportunity to dip into the sexual dynamo shtick he honed in *Delirious*. By film's end Hammond is both a hero and a stud: by refusing to grab the money and run, he wins the respect of Nolte's character and returns to jail transformed, if not reformed, by his interaction with Nolte's embodiment of the fair side of the white justice system. In turn, the cop allows the criminal to get laid as a reward for "doing the right thing."

In *Beverly Hills Cop* and *Beverly Hills Cop II* (1987) Axel Foley mocks, but ultimately serves, the needs of a white populace. The murder of his white running buddy brings him to Beverly Hills in the original, while the sequel motivates Foley's actions by means of his inflated sense of loyalty to BHPD's Captain Bogamil (Ronny Cox). Foley's methods and his savvy prove to be superior to those of his white cohorts, Rosewood (Judge Reinhold) and Taggart (John Ashton), but his performance of a hard-boiled Detroit cop converts much of the casework into comic antics. Murphy's skill at slipping into multiple characters is utilized repeatedly, from his angry black man rant at the Beverly Wilshire to his turn as the egregiously fey "special friend" of the film's villain. His unorthodox methods are eventually lauded because of the fact that, once the case is solved, he will be returned to offscreen (black) space. By utilizing the humor in Foley's cameo of blackness in fundamentally white worlds, Murphy's interloper is constructed as an idealized *and* temporary Other.

Furthermore, perhaps because it was not originally intended for a black actor, *Beverly Hills Cop* occasionally elides and reworks blackness in almost nonsensical ways. As Donald Bogle notes: "Coming from the streets of Detroit (the very city whose ghettoes had gone up in flames during the race riots of the 60s), the character's friends logically would have been black. But Eddie Murphy is plopped into a white environment in order that a mass white audience can better identify with him. . . . It's an unrealistic plot maneuver that reveals Hollywood's cynicism about the major black star and his audience."[3] Both of Foley's closest childhood friends in *Beverly Hills Cop* (Mikey and Jenny) are white. Moreover, although there are fleeting hints of a romance between Foley and

Jenny (Lisa Eilbacher), he is more or less sexually neutralized, despite the swaggering machismo of his step and speech. After all, seeing Murphy woo a white actress would have made the film decidedly less friendly to a mainstream (read white) audience. Ed Guerrero points out that "the source of energy and tension in all of Murphy's movies is race, and to a lesser degree, class, deriving from Murphy's blackness as a challenge to white exclusion (but not privilege or domination) . . . and while Murphy gets the upper-hand in almost all situations, the ultimate result of such a challenge is integration and acceptance on white terms in the film's resolution."[4] Hammond and Foley both clearly exemplify the repackaging of the black stand-up persona for mass consumption, with Murphy's quick-witted wisecracking and street kid charisma informing the iteration of his screen persona as black comic action star.[5]

Although Murphy appeared to have exhausted this generic type by the nineties, it is interesting that his black fish-out-of-water roles garnered the most critical and commercial success. Ultimately, just as Foley acts as the "exception" that can be celebrated within a white milieu on a temporary basis, Murphy can be embraced as black comic action hero so long as he does not transgress other mainstream Hollywood boundaries—such as his construction as a romantic leading man.

In *Bad Company* (2002) Rock had his first opportunity to play in a fish-out-of-water action-comedy.[6] Rock plays "street-smart" hustler Jake Hayes, the long lost twin of "Super African American" CIA operative Kevin Pope, who is pressed into service to impersonate the brother he never knew. Interestingly, the "fish-out-of-water" characterization seems applicable on both textual and extratextual levels. In the cinematic text stereotypical constructions of blackness are mobilized in Hayes's attempt to impersonate Pope (the Alexander Scott for

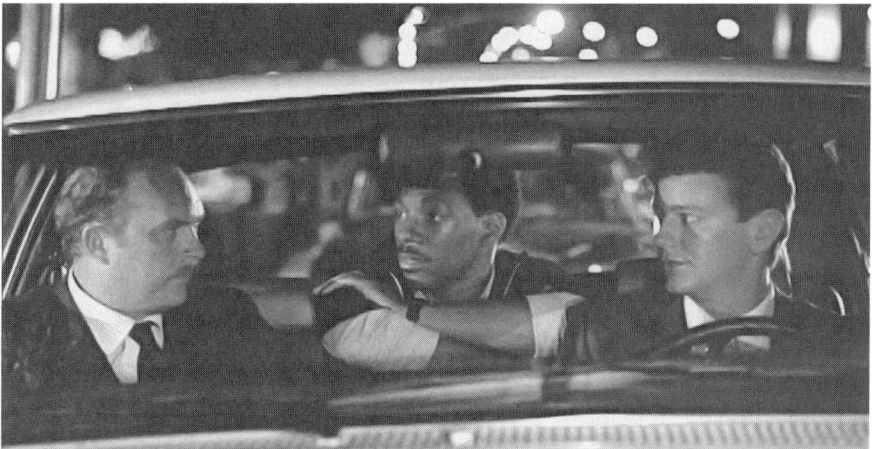

11. Eddie Murphy, as a very savvy fish out of water, does buddy bonding with John Ashton (left) and Judge Reinhold in *Beverly Hills Cop* (1984). Directed by Martin Brest.

the new millennium) and in his transformation from "urban" to "urbane" black-ness—exemplified by scenes in which Hayes changes the music in Pope's apart-ment from classical to hip-hop and when he is "taught" to function in high society during an etiquette boot camp given by the CIA. Extratextually, one can hardly believe that Rock, the usually self-aware cultural critic, is playing Hayes, a sort of urban bumpkin, who spends "much of [the film] being jittery, dys-functional and perpetually frightened in the manner of Mantan Moreland's Birmingham Brown roles in dozens of 1940s Charlie Chan movies."[7] Despite the sprinkling of controversy-free comic bits from Rock's act (as Hayes playing Pope, he renounces the latter's antimeat stance: "Hell, I'll eat a pig's ass if you cook it right"), the cynicism, social, and political savvy, and the razor-sharp wit—the qualities that made him desirable as a costar in this high profile, big-budget Jerry Bruckheimer project—are diluted beyond recognition in a narra-tive where Jake's intellectual promise is signified more by his ability to play chess and scalp tickets simultaneously than in his (questionably successful) masquer-ade as his buttoned-down Ivy League secret-operative twin. As one review simply stated: "This is the kind of movie that Chris Rock the comedian would make fun of."[8]

While the fish-out-of-water film may seem to problematize the black comedian's efforts to interject both his comic persona and some degree of cul-tural specificity into his screen roles, this is not always the case. In Kevin Smith's independent film *Dogma* (1999), Chris Rock plays a fish-out-of-water among fish-out-of-water as Rufus, the thirteenth apostle. Without the expectation of the vast audience pool of a blockbuster, there is more room for Rock to incor-porate his comic persona into the role.

Rock plays a supporting role to renegade angels (Matt Damon and Ben Affleck) who attempt to use a loophole in church dogma to reenter heaven. Operating as the film's philosophical center in a tone very much akin to the comic's stand-up rants, Rock's Rufus tells people what they *need* to know. Rufus agrees to join the holy crusade to save the world, of course, but also to set the record straight—Jesus was black. When fellow holy crusaders scoff at this reve-lation, Rufus puts the error into a sociohistorical context: "Between the time when He established the faith and the Church started to officially organize, the powers that be decided that, while the message of Christ was integral, the fact that he was black was a detriment. So, all renderings were ordered to be Euro-centric, even though the brother was blacker than Jesse." Rufus allows Rock's comic voice to resonate in the character's lines. As the black martyr in this multicultural motley crew, Rock's impeccable comedic timing is well matched by the profane language and scatological moralizing of Smith's film.[9] In this case the black comedian's stage and screen persona are integrated into film comedy without being diluted beyond recognition. One wonders whether the black comic's ability to continue to engage issues of race (and cultural specificity) as directly on film as he does in stand-up routine is dependent upon his remaining outside of the big-budget studio mother lode of crossover success or, as will be discussed later in this chapter, in cinematic vehicles over which he (or she), as a result of industrial clout or individual initiative, has a significant degree of creative control.

### COMEDIES OF COLOR-CODED COLOR BLINDNESS

By the mid-nineties, in the wake of the backlash against multiculturalism, a new subgenre emerges: the comedies of color-coded color blindness. These are not aspirational integrationist tales (the stories of "movin' on up"); rather, they are cinematic versions of *The Cosby Show*: stories of those people who were already living the American Dream. Into this subgenre enter the kinder, gentler (and "bad box office" tamed) Eddie Murphy. Even though *The Nutty Professor* (1996) and its sequel, *The Nutty Professor 2: The Klumps* (2000) heralded Murphy's return to box office prominence, *Dr. Doolittle* (1998) is most emblematic of his transformation into this new "mature" iteration of Eddie. This film not only supplies the most extreme sublimation of the controversial aspects of the black comic persona into an unproblematic integrationist fantasy but also marks Murphy's entry into the family comedy genre. Furthermore, the way that race is incorporated or erased in this film demonstrates the marketability of color-coded color blindness. Two principal changes are made in remaking the 1967 film—it is nonmusical and a black actor plays the title role. Despite the casting of Murphy, the context of the narrative does not engage black culture or identity in any direct or significant manner. Doolittle's "gift" of talking to the animals not only becomes a mark of difference but also operates as a signifier for identity. The lost "gift" that Doolittle had "unlearned" as a result of his father's desire for him to "fit in" reemerges at the point when both his autonomy and his identity are being challenged. A huge corporate Health Maintenance Organization is seeking to buy out Doolittle's practice at the same time that he is striving to teach his daughter to "fit in." After Doolittle nearly runs over a dog, Lucky (voiced by Norm MacDonald), his senses are restored. Once again he is able to talk to the animals and to express his own "individuality."

Race is both inherent in and absent from the film, with Doolittle's extended family (including wife, two daughters, and father) supplying the only black faces in major roles. While actors of color are among the star-studded cavalcade of celebrity voices (most notably Chris Rock, as his daughter's pet guinea pig, Rodney), the story is set in a predominantly white liberal world in San Francisco. The notion of a white liberal setting is central to the film's elision of race. While one might argue that race motivates Doolittle's father (Ossie Davis) to prescribe conformity as a means of gaining access to the American Dream, it is never explicitly mentioned. Within the context of a cautionary tale that warns against homogeneity (figured as the corporate entity or enforced conformity), racial identity and questions of difference are translated into the "special gift" of hearing animals speak. Questions about race are thus displaced

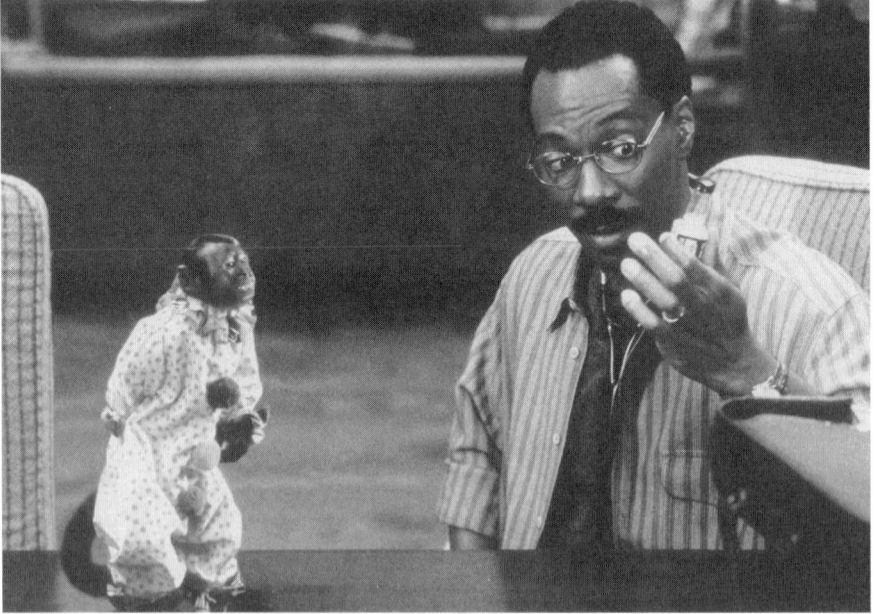

12. Murphy consults with a monkey in *Dr. Doolittle* (1998). Directed by Betty Thomas. Photo from Photofest. Reproduced with permission from 20th Century Fox.

onto issues of the "uniqueness" of individual identity and the struggle between the individual (small-business owner) and the corporation. Doolittle's gift, which *could* mark him as Other, is constructed not as an obstacle to achievement or assimilation but rather as a type of uniqueness (read both rugged individualism and suburban conformity) that has consistently been part of the mythology of the identifiable American Dream. In this way racial identity, coded as uniqueness, slides past Otherness into the realm of a mythic, idealized middle-classness. The clear villain of this film is the corporation, personified by the HMO president (Peter Boyle), an embodiment of soul-less homogeneity and mediocrity. The film's plot may reward the return of the individual's uniqueness (Doolittle opens a dual practice for animals and humans, which will undoubtedly be a lucrative one), but it is also in the business of smoothing out individual difference. On one hand, one might argue that it is especially ironic that a tale that professes to celebrate the expression of individual gifts requires Murphy to dilute his stand-up persona almost beyond recognition. On the other, the family-friendly persona that Murphy employs might be seen as the logical extension of an older comic actor—one far removed from the edginess and energy of stand-up performance—and the father of five children.

Indeed, Murphy's stand-up comic persona plays only an ancillary role in many of his most recent films: as the voice of the puny dragon with codependence issues in Disney's animated feature *Mulan* (1998), which he reincarnates in donkey form for the not-so-subtle Disney-bashing DreamWorks product, *Shrek* (2001) and *Shrek II* (2004); as the mild-mannered Sherman Klump, his megalomaniacal alter ego Buddy Love, and the entire Klump clan in *The Nutty Professor* films; and, as action star Kit Ramsey and his geeky brother Jiff in *Bowfinger* (1999). Interestingly, some of these characters seem to quote different impersonations from Murphy's old act: the Klumps, for example, appear to be refugees from his family cookout material. Yet only the "posse"-laden Ramsey and the hypersexualized Buddy conflate the onstage and offstage public personae of the young Murphy and feed directly from the attitude (if not the content) of the *Raw* years—and these figures are played as parody. Even in Murphy's recent attempts to recapture the "edgier" side of action comic fare—with the egomaniacal Kelly Robinson, the boxing champ and temporary secret agent of *I-Spy* (2002), and the constantly posturing, aspiring actor/television detective, Trey Sellars, of *Showtime* (2002)—his performances seem to be self-conscious impersonations of his former, more fully articulated, comedic incarnations. As *New York Times* critic Elvis Mitchell bemoans in his review of *I-Spy*, "Mr. Murphy is still doing the all-id hostility of Buddy Love, the swampy-depths alter ego of 'The Nutty Professor.'"[10] Murphy's performance of black identity through machismo appears to have been thoroughly domesticated.[11] Nonetheless, one must question whether Murphy's new comedic persona is a kinder, softer iteration and his audience is primed not for the swaggering audaciousness of *Delirious* but for the delightful safety of *Shrek*'s "Donkey" and "Doolittle." In *Daddy Day Care* (2003) his character, Charlie Hinton, the beleaguered "every dad" who ultimately embraces the role of professional "Mr. Mom," serves to codify the preferred (read bankable) Murphy persona for the new millennium. In Murphy's Hinton the profane and culturally specific aspects of his stand-up are replaced by a postracial fantasy in which race is not a problem at all. As Tom Sherak, a partner in Revolution Studios, which produced *Daddy Day Care* for Sony, so clearly articulates: "Eddie Murphy is Bill Cosby. . . . People who grew up with the edgy Eddie Murphy, they're older now and parents, but they still want to see him. He's not the urban kid anymore, he's a grown-up, a good father and family man, and he makes these movies that appeal to families."[12] In these films, as far as his big-screen persona is concerned, the "urban" has been traded for the urbane: in the struggle for the comic soul of the new family-friendly Murphy, Cosby, rather than Pryor, is the victor. Furthermore, the new Murphy is, in some ways, the antithesis of the stand-up/cinematic personae of Pryor, who, whatever the absurd premise of the film, keeps more than a passing aura of Pryorness in his work.

While, on some level, Murphy's G-rated (or PG-rated) film comedies revisit the domestic comedy for the big screen, the absence of race recognition in the narratives is striking—particularly when one takes into consideration other big-screen black family comedies that, while not foregrounding race, still endeavor to deal with issues of cultural specificity. This new spate of "urban suburban" comedies (from *Barbershop* to *Johnson Family Vacation*) presents narratives that are neither integrationist nor separatist—and features actors associated with niched black cultural production (like Ice Cube and Cedric the Entertainer).[13] In Murphy's family films the rich cultural coding that often shades the black comic persona has been thinned out (or redistributed) in ways that allow them to be easily folded into a mainstream cinematic milieu.

In several films over the course of his career, Murphy has channeled aspects of his personae (from his smack talking, smirking form of machismo to his carefully crafted comic mimicry) into a variety of characters. This fragmentation can be seen in *Bowfinger*, as well as in *The Nutty Professor* and *The Nutty Professor II: The Klumps*. While the latter offered an "elephantine showcase for Murphy's virtuosity" and a "Murphy, Murphy, Murphy world," the comic actor first dabbled in fragmentation almost a decade earlier. It was in *Coming to America* (1988), the comic's last big box office success before his 1996 cinematic "comeback," that Murphy first revealed his ability to subsume his comic personae in service to a very conventional comedic paradigm. Although exploring convergences between the Murphy of *The Nutty Professor* series and the original kinder, gentler iteration in *Coming to America* might enable us to trace the trajectory of Murphy's shifting comic personae, there is greater significance to the earlier cinematic constructions—and their relationship to Hollywood comedy. *Coming to America* affords an interesting case study in that it demonstrates how each subgenre supplies a different point of entry for the black comic into mainstream comedy and varying degrees of control over the ways in which his or her comic persona is mobilized as a representational default for blackness. In fact, one might even argue that the 1988 romantic comedy can be seen as a conflation of the fish-out-of-water comedies, those of color-coded color blindness, and the cultural comedies with creative control. As a big-budget romantic comedy—with director Jon Landis at the helm, whose early films, *Animal House* (1978), *The Blues Brothers* (1980), and *Trading Places* (1983) were star turns for Murphy as well as for *SNL* veterans John Belushi and Dan Ackroyd, and with a story penned by the film's black star, *Coming to America*—and Murphy's new star power—were anomalous for the eighties. In all likelihood the film could not have been made without Murphy's industrial status, which in turn yielded him a modicum of creative control. The shift from being a star who has his pick of projects to star who gets his projects made represents a significant movement up the industrial food chain. On one hand, Murphy's choice to throw his new industrial clout into a film that is fundamentally an updated 1930s romantic comedy—a PG-13 version of the runaway heiress tale within a black context with a runaway heir—could be seen as a risky endeavor. The story centers on the quest of Prince Akeem, the future ruler of Zamunda (a country that embodies a storybook notion of the continent of Africa as idyllic, exotic, and resplendent) who takes the forty days allowed him to sow his wild oats before returning to an arranged marriage, to find true love (and intellectual compatibility) in Queens, New York.[14] As will be discussed in greater detail later in this chapter, one of the hallmarks of creative control in the cultural comedies is the reframing of a classical Hollywood genre narrative in an African American context.

One might assert that the story of a Nubian prince in Queens, which also fits squarely within the fish-out-of-water genre, represented an industrial slam-dunk—given Murphy's prior successes with the subgenre. However, as film critic David Ansen noted, the film is perhaps "more interesting as a career move than as a movie."[15] In reality Murphy, who was at the top of the comedy's A-list, with a string of hit films including the record-shattering concert film *Raw* (1987), took only a mitigated risk. Humble, innocent, and sweetly earnest, the prince marked a significant departure for Murphy, and, as the romantic center of the film, Akeem is imminently likable but not a memorable, comic character. While the prince was not Axel, the traces of Murphy's comic personae (from *SNL*, stand-up, and the *BHC* series)—metered out amongst brief supporting roles—were present to showcase his prowess as comic character actor and, arguably, to satiate (and reindoctrinate) his fan base. The search for sociopolitical content in contemporary romantic comedy may yield ambiguous results; however, the analysis of this particular vehicle as the nexus of the transformation of Murphy's comic personae speaks to the sociocultural and industrial moments, as well as their relationship to the film itself and its subgenres. As a comedy of color-coded color blindness, *Coming to America*'s elision of race is intriguing. The cinematic milieu of *Coming to America* is fundamentally black—and, as such, the actual discussion of race is displaced by the unproblematic engagement of class and nation. Although the cultural differences between the mythical Zamundans and African Americans are depicted—primarily through the opulence to which Akeem and his aristocratic companion, Semmi (Arsenio Hall), were accustomed in Zamunda—the film's diversity is rooted in class. The class delineations are represented by three male characters: the middle class by the local fast-food king, Akeem's boss, and father to his love interest, Lisa (Shari Headley), played by John Amos as a self-aggrandizing social climber; the nouveau riche by Eriq LaSalle, the narcissistic heir-apparent to the Soul-Glo [read Jheri-Kurl] fortune, and Akeem's rival; and, the aristocracy by the king of Zamunda, portrayed by James Earl Jones, as both supreme potentate and concerned dad. The foibles of each of these characters (and their social class ilk) are portrayed in broad strokes. This is neither the vehicle nor the genre for genuine social critique; rather, the film functions as a dual celebration of the black presence (read actors working) in a big-budget comedy and the cinematic creation of a mythical African/African American milieu of prosperity, safety, and promise.

The film, and Murphy's creative input, does represent the potential and the promise for a more forceful black presence in Hollywood. Moreover, *Coming to America*, along with Robert Townsend's scathingly funny tale of racism and the

plight of the contemporary black actor in *Hollywood Shuffle* (1987), and Keenen
Ivory Wayans's star-studded blaxploitation parody *I'm Gonna Git You, Sucka!*
(1988), mark the emergence of the Black Pack in Hollywood. In this industrial
moment—a year before Spike Lee became a sociopolitical cinematic force with
*Do the Right Thing* (1989) and three before John Singleton's *Boyz n the Hood*
(1991) would start the stream of ghetto/gangsta melodrama/morality plays—
writer, director, actors like Townsend, Wayans, and Murphy used film comedy as
social discourse on black culture and the African American condition.

Unlike the majority of Murphy's work in the eighties, Townsend and
Wayans employ multiple culturally coded satirical moments in their films—like
classically trained black actors demonstrating the process of "blacking it up" for
their coveted "junkie" roles in *Hollywood Shuffle*. The virtual roll call of blaxploitation stars (including Bernie Casey and Jim Brown) as middle-aged urban
heroes in a literal fight against the (white) Man, Mr. Big, the crime boss of the
ghetto in *I'm Gonna Get You, Sucka!* provides additional spectatorial pleasure for
those "down" enough to recognize the stars' cultural cachet. These moments
depend on some degree of cultural differentiation—an audience with black
popular cultural savvy—and, in so doing, act as comedic social discourse at a
moment when the black audience is being (re)discovered, on the cusp of the
niche marketing and narrowcasting of the netlet era and the explosion of hip-
hop into the popular culture mainstream. While, arguably, the ideological work
being done in these films has a greater critical bite than Murphy's genre films,
the significance of the latter's ability to "go wide" cannot be underestimated in
terms of the industry's willingness to make black-oriented film. Nonetheless,
these films, penned by, helmed by, and starring black comic actors, established a
creative community working in concert and afforded models for the next wave
of comics turned cinematic creators.[16]

In each of the aforementioned texts race, genre, and history (social, political, and industrial) are at play in a new wave of cultural comedies with creative
control. Over the next two decades the presence of these comedies continued
to make sporadic appearances in the cinematic mainstream. During the early
nineties, while black-oriented dramatic films depicted the gritty (and gang
inflected) experiences of black urban life, the cultural comedies of creative control acted as their middle-class (and upper-middle-class) comedic counterparts.
These comedies that emerged early in the decade, as well as those that have
appeared in the new millennium, played with genre to capture the desired rein-
scription of the black experience in contemporary film comedy. Moreover, by
carving out spaces for both their comic personae and their selected black cultural milieu within the context of previously established genres, Rock and
Murphy became significant players in this particular genre game. Additionally,
the examination of the passage of their comic personae into these films reveals
the convergences and divergences between the intent and content of their distinct reimaginings of contemporary and classical Hollywood comedy.

### Cultural Comedies with Creative Control

Undeniably, having creative control over one's films allows any actor greater mobility in molding the way that his or her cinematic persona is conceived. On one hand, the promise of creative control in the film work of a black comic turned "hyphenate" signifies the opportunity for black self-representation within a genre where, historically, socioculturally regressive and essentialized African American images have abounded—from the direct reincarnations of minstrelsy like Mantan Moreland's eye-popping, body-quaking "I'se afraid" performances in the already problematic Charlie Chan films to the "token" presence of "the black guy" in the teen comedies of the eighties sprinkled throughout John Hughes's oeuvre. On the other hand, the comic's persona, whether onstage or onscreen, must possess some degree of idiosyncrasy, thus problematizing the notion that he or she can be seen as representative of the race—which he or she undoubtedly will be. When black comics, like Murphy or Rock, attain the degree of status required to set their own creative agenda, expectations (and the stakes) are high. Often the discussion of the black comic persona being diluted in the movement from stand-up to screen is rooted in the fact that they do not have actual creative control over their vehicles—making the notion of "for us, by us" in filmmaking highly desirable. After all, the transformation to a "hyphenate" (like "writer-director") is not necessarily a stretch for the comic: he or she has been fundamentally a writer-performer throughout his or her career. Long before Murphy and Rock made their presence known cinematically, they were writing material for either stand-up or sketch performances. That's the good part.

Given that neither a sketch nor a set is a screenplay, and that sustaining the "funny" onscreen is an arduous endeavor, Rock and Murphy are faced with a significant challenge—particularly when there is an additional representational burden placed on the work—as both film and black cultural production. Thus, regardless of whether or not these films go down in history as "classic comedies," Murphy's and Rock's comedies with creative control reveal the desire to expand the niche of the black comic presence in American film comedy—in terms of the stories of blackness that can and have been told. Yet creative control is not a panacea for either the loss of comic edge or the dearth of progressive representations of blackness.

By examining film comedies that were written and/or directed by their star, Murphy and Rock, respectively, one can begin to see how the translation of the black comic persona onto the big screen can be just as problematic, even when the creative team behind the camera is African American. Both Murphy's creative trifecta (writer-director-star) and Rock's first venture as writer-star exemplify a desire to capture a distinct black sociocultural moment: *Harlem Nights* (1989), the former's Harlem heyday gangster comedy, and *CB4* (1993), the latter's parodic shout-out to the explosion of gangsta rap (and, by extension, hip-hop) in the early nineties. Regardless of whether one might question either

the aspects of the era that the comic-writer-filmmaker has chosen to foreground or the genre through which they have chosen to explore the moment,
both of these films act as cinematic valentines to richly textured moments of
black culture. In some ways these particular comedies can be seen as For Us By
Us films: although the genre may be familiar to the cinematic mainstream, the
cultural content is purposefully niched for audiences attuned to black culture.

Murphy's desire to do a period piece was, arguably, motivated by the types
of black historical fictions that had come out of Hollywood in the recent past;
from *Sounder* to *The Color Purple*, film tales of black survival and spiritual growth
were not the stuff of which comedy is made—nor did they tell stories of black
success coded in classical Hollywood generic conventions. *Harlem Nights* functions as multiple homage to the gangster genre, to Harlem, and, perhaps most
significant, to two of Murphy's comic inspirations, Richard Pryor and Redd
Foxx. In his article on the "three generations of comedy" in *Harlem Nights*,
Walter Leavy states that Murphy made clear that if he had not made this film,
no one else would have brought these comics together: "Hollywood wasn't trying to hook us up. But I think it's historic that I get to work with these brothers. The privilege of working with Richard and Redd has been the greatest
reward of my career."[17] The film, with its "dream cast," was clearly a big-budget
labor of love for Murphy. The story seems a familiar permutation of the genre:
Quick (Murphy) and his older wiser mentor, Sugar Ray (Richard Pryor) must
outsmart the evil mob boss with an elaborate con in order to save themselves
and their friends. One might even describe it as *The Sting* inflected by blaxploitation machismo. What is striking about the film is the way in which the
performance of a genre archetype, the young "hot head," rarely affords Murphy
any spaces for humor. In fact, neither Murphy's Quick nor Pryor's Sugar Ray
carry the comedy in this film. *Harlem Nights* boasts three generations of black
comedy; however, only one generation—the oldest—lives up to that promise.
Channeling a touch of "Sanfordesque" spirit, Redd Foxx's cantankerous sight-
impaired croupier, Benne, along with Della Reese's Vera, the no-nonsense
madam who's in charge of "the girls" working out of Sugar's, supply some of
the film's funniest moments with their constant, albeit loving, banter.[18]

The choice to keep "Pryorness" out of the construction of Sugar Ray may
have been designed to supply the comic with one of his most suave film roles
(a distinct departure from his most recent screen time, the broad, buddy comedy *See No Evil, Hear No Evil* with Gene Wilder) but left Pryor playing the wise,
old, virtual straight man. The moments when Murphy's comic persona actually
makes cameo appearances are among the film's most misogynistic. An argument
over money with Reese's Vera is punctuated by his signature laugh, before verbal sparring becomes physical—it culminates with Quick shooting her in the
foot, with the rationale that he told her to "shut up." Replete with missed
opportunities to engage the personae of these black comedy heavyweights,
*Harlem Nights* maintains numerous paradigmatic allegiances—to gangster/caper

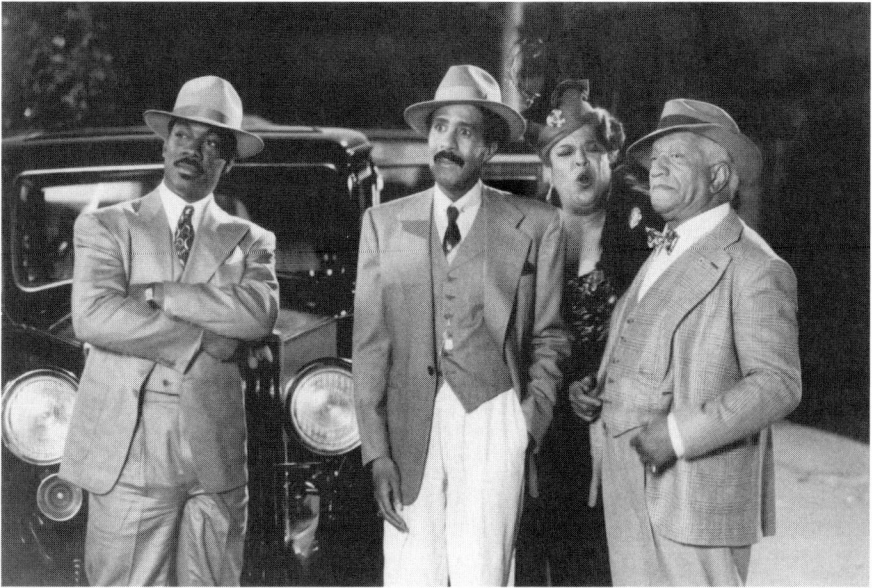

13. Three generations of black comedy in *Harlem Nights* (1989). Directed by Eddie Murphy. Left to right: Eddie Murphy (as Quick), Richard Pryor (as Sugar Ray), Della Reese (as Vera), Redd Foxx (as Bennie Wilson). Photo from Photofest. Reproduced with permission from Paramount Pictures.

comedies like *The Sting*, to the spirit of blaxploitation films (where the black man can actually beat the odds and get one over on "the Man"), and to, albeit elliptically, the historical aura of 1930s Harlem.

From the meticulously costumed integrated assemble of patrons at Club Sugar Ray, the speakeasy, which acts as the film's visual and narrative centerpiece, to the soundtrack featuring vintage Duke Ellington, the mise-en-scène of Murphy's gangster comedy creates an idealized vision of lush uptown nightlife, which, like *Coming to America*'s African kingdom, makes for a nostalgic vision of the way that, on some level, things never were. The film engages the era's racial politics in fairly simplistic ways: blacks and whites frequent the popular night spot, but the harassment of corrupt police (Danny Aiello's Phil Cantone) and the strong-arm tactics of the white mob boss Bugsy Calhoune (Michael Lerner) are reserved for the African American entrepreneurs. In this world, where all the heroes are black, more intellectually adept, and, regardless of their vices, morally superior to their foes, and the villains are corrupt, easily manipulated, and all white, the audience is provided with a black world recentered within a classical Hollywood framework. Moreover, the creation of a world where black savvy and style are privileged—and historically rooted—might even allow the film to be viewed as a progressive representational text—if not for the film's gender politics. The previously mentioned sequence between Quick and Vera, as well as the former's bedding and then killing of the film's Creole femme fatale (and Calhoune's mistress) played by Jasmine Guy, exemplify how the film equates all women with some form of sexual servitude, which can hardly be seen as liberatory construction.

*Harlem Nights* was not a big box office success: grossing roughly $61 million, it was Murphy's least successful film comedy up to that point in his career (even *The Golden Child* outgrossed it). The film was dismissed by reviewers like *Washington Post* film critic Hal Hinson as "Murphy's folly . . . a vanity production if ever there was one, launched on behalf of a star with vast amounts of vanity to soothe. And it's hard to imagine a more wrong-headed, aggressively off-putting exercise in star ego."[19] Nonetheless, through the examination of this film, and its classification as a cultural comedy with its star's creative control, one must ask—by shying away from familiar iterations of both Pryor's and Murphy's comic personae and by constructing a film that conflates related but racially differentiated genres—whether the goal of "going wide" was ever genuinely a motivating force in this project or whether Murphy's vision to make a film with the setting of 1930s Harlem as a character rather than a backdrop was designed to be For Us By Us.

It was industrial clout that got *Harlem Nights* made, and, in actuality, it was Murphy's influence that allowed Rock to make his first For Us By Us film. Murphy, who had given Rock his first break on television (*Uptown Comedy Express*) and in film (*Beverly Hills Cop II*), approached Brian Grazer, the head of Imagine Films and producer of *Boomerang*, about the project at the same time that Nelson George, music journalist extraordinaire and cowriter of *CB4*, was contacting his friend, producer Sean Daniel. In the end it was the combined effort of Grazer and Daniel that was integral to getting *CB4* made. "Brian and I decided to join forces to support Chris and Nelson at Universal. The movie deserved to get made. The material was original and raw and worth fighting for."[20]

Emblazoned on the cover of Nelson George's insightful sociohistorical analysis of the burgeoning musical movement, *Hip Hop America* (1998), there is a quote from Chris Rock that begins, "I love hip hop more than I love my mother." Rock's love of hip-hop, which is present in his later stand-up, television, and film work, can clearly be seen in *CB4*, a film that does for gangsta rap what Rob Reiner's *This Is Spinal Tap* did for metal. Rock and George created a narrative that *required* not only knowledge of hip-hop but a love for it. *CB4's* film within a film is a "rapumentary" by A. White (Chris Elliot) chronicling the rise of the "world's most dangerous band," the gangsta rap trio of MC Gusto aka Albert Brown (Rock), Dead Mike aka Euripides Smalls (Allen Payne), and Stab Master Arson aka Otis O. Otis (Deezer D). The story, which begins with a series of testimonials from hip-hop glitterati, including gangsta rap royalty, Ice-T, Ice-Cube, and Easy E, attesting to or questioning the group's "hardcore" pedigree, shifts gears after an attempted drive-by from the real gangsta from whom Brown had "borrowed" both his name and persona (played with testosterone-fueled comic menace by Charlie Murphy) after he escapes from the actual Cell Block 4. Through the process of revealing the middle-class roots of *CB4*—Albert Brown, as good and obedient son, Otis O. Otis, as the harried de facto head of household for his numerous sisters and genial mother, and Euripides Smalls, as the only genuinely struggling young brother in search of spirituality and black consciousness—Rock and George's story begs the question, "How gangsta are the gangstas?" The hip-hop cultural savvy required to understand the significance of this question squarely posits *CB4* as a For Us By Us film.[21]

In George's and Rock's script the translation of the "big and wild" elements of the rap world takes place through the transformation of the film's central trio from middle-class kids to gangsta rappers. Depicted as a fashion and rhetoric makeover, the "evolution" of the band speaks to the stereotypes of "gangsta-ness." The physical image is changed with a weave, a Jheri-Kurl and prison work shirts, t-shirts, and jeans (procured at the fence of a correctional facility). The trio sits in character: Otis/Stab Master Arson, in backwards baseball hat, swigs out of a 40 in a paper bag; Albert/Gusto, now gold-toothed, gold-chained, adjusts his dark shades and black-knit cap; and Euripedes/Dead Mike (the only non-Jheri-Kurled member of the trio) in dark bandana, arms crossed, doing his best black-militant-inspired glare. However, it was Trustus Jones, the rap record mogul, not the members of CB4, who articulates the band's new rhetoric. Before signing the group, Jones, who knows that CB4 has a gangsta veneer rather than hardcore cred, does a sort of gangsta checklist, communicating what he expects that they will be:

TRUSTUS: I love the image. . . . I have a few questions. Do you cuss?
GUSTO: Fuck, yea.
TRUSTUS: Do you defile women with your lyrics?
CB4 [all nodding with enthusiastic assent]: Mmm-hmm.
TRUSTUS [in a faux whisper]: Do you fondle your genitalia onstage?
GUSTO: Whenever possible.
TRUSTUS: Do you glorify violence and advocate the use of gu . . . [His question is cut short by the sound of guns being readied as each CB4 member prepares his "piece" of choice]
TRUSTUS: Okay, okay. Final question: do you guys respect anything?
CB4 [in unison]: Not a damn thing.
TRUSTUS: You've got a deal. Welcome to the family.

While there are numerous instances that flaunt the popular conceptions of rap, the comedy often resembles a series of thematically connected gag-driven (rather than character-driven) sketches with a not-always-crystalline critical agenda. The fact that the broadness of the comedy, its inherent raunchiness, and its celebration of a certain degree of political incorrectness are deemed necessary to parody a genre that, to some extent, also does all of those things supplies contradictory ideological messages. For example, the film's gender politics are inconsistently regressive. While the objectification of women in rap videos is explored through the conversation of two dancers who boast about the screen time their body parts received (an "ass right behind MC Hammer's head in 'Can't Touch This'" and a "left breast prominently featured in Eric B.'s last video"), the women's industrial complicity seems to elide the issue. Like many other contemporary film parodies—from *Blazing Saddles* to *Soul Plane*—*CB4* is informed by masculine zeitgeist. The two (most) central female characters—Sissy (Khandi Alexander), the entrepreneurial rap groupie who differentiates herself from the "hip hop ho's" due to her prized possession (an album of polaroids of former rapper-lovers just before they begin engaging in oral sex), which yields ongoing profits; and Daliha (Rachel True), the squeaky clean, quasi-virginal embodiment of black middle-classness, whose sole role seems to be *not being Sissy*—are constructed as madonna and whore. While neither could be considered a leading role, Daliha receives significantly less screen time than Sissy, which, arguably, is consistent with the genre being parodied.[22]

Nevertheless, for those not well-versed in hip-hop culture, the film's sporadic moments of biting critique, as well as most of the self-referential humor, is lost. Neither Stoney Jackson's Wacky-D send-up of M. C. Hammer's mainstream hit "Can't Touch This," shown as a video that, much to Brown's dismay, is loved by his family and his girl, nor CB4's performance of their theme song, "Straight Outta Locash," clearly a parody of N. W. A.'s "Straight Outta Compton" (which actually manages to be more profane than the original), will have any resonance for an audience unaware of the source texts. As one review noted: "Like those forms of parodic tribute, it assumes . . . a certain level of hipness. In other words, if you don't know rap, forget about it, you'd do just as well taking an SAT prepared by extra-terrestrials."[23] While *CB4* takes great pains to deal with the foibles of rap culture, it also lampoons the mainstream reaction to the music, style, and content of hip-hop—as illustrated by the unabashed liberal gushing of the documentary filmmaker, A. White (Chris Elliot), and the vitriolic attacks from Congressman Virgil Robinson (Phil Hartman), whose actions are motivated less by the rabid fandom of his adolescent son (J. D. Daniels) than by the political mileage that could be gained by a PMRC-like crusade.[24] As a result of Robinson's campaign, the band is threatened with jail if they perform their hit, "Sweat from My Balls"—which, of course, they do.[25]

The performance sequence provides an interesting mixture of parody and tribute: after CB4, in prison garb and shackles, enter into the elaborate set with a prison motif (complete with searchlights, barbed wire, white guards with guns, and black prisoners inside cells), un-gold-chained Gusto and shirtless Dead Mike kneel in their shackles; with lights swirling as though there has been a jailbreak, an authoritative voice resounds over the booming bass of the beats that Stab Master Arson is spinning: "MC Gusto, Dead Mike and Stab Master Arson, you have all been sentenced by the government of the United States of America to a life of poverty, ignorance and imprisonment in CELL BLOCK 4." What ever poignancy and resonance supplied by this operatic staging and the visual image of a shackled, shirtless black man (in terms of the obvious relationship to multiple forms of slavery) is quickly undermined when instead of launching into a conscious rap credo, Dead Mike and MC Gusto, throw off their shackles, singing "jump, jump" as the lead-in to "Sweat from My Balls." The redirection, or arguably, misdirection, that takes place in this sequence deliberately confronts ideological inconsistencies of CB4's politics by the juxtaposition of one image of oppression (the justice/penal system) against another (blatant misogyny). Perhaps, not surprisingly, in the scenes around the abortive performance sequence, one sees flashes of Rock's witty and irreverent voice and also his fluid ideological positioning in statements made in passing. In one instance, Albert responds to both Euripides' and Otis's questioning of the song's controversial content, for its questionable political agenda and its lack of family friendliness, by critiquing not the legitimacy of their claims but rather the ways in which they had been culturally manipulated to even ask the question: "One brother wants to be Malcolm X, the other one wants to be Richie Cunningham." In another, after being arrested for singing the verboten song, Rock as Albert, sitting in the paddy wagon, can be heard railing against the racialized double standard at play in their arrest: "answer me this, how come a rock group can bite the head off of pigeons, nothing happens, but I'm getting ready to go to jail for doing a song about the

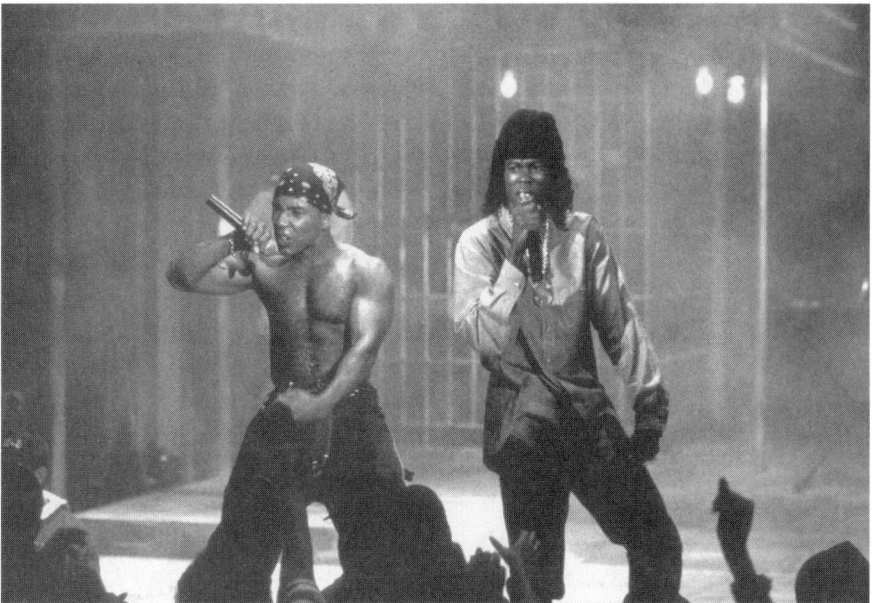

14. *CB4* (1993). *This Is Spinal Tap* for gangsta rap. Directed by Tamra Davis. Allen Payne (left) and Chris Rock. Photo from Photofest. Reproduced with permission from Universal.

sweat from my balls." For the majority of the film, however, neither Albert Brown nor his gangsta alter ego, MC Gusto provides strong articulations of Rock's comic persona.

One might argue that the diminishing of the comic persona was dictated by the "mocumentary" format. Nearly a decade earlier, in the source text for faux "rocumentary" *This Is Spinal Tap* (1984), one of the parody's greatest successes was the translation of metal's iconic personae into the fading metal band; conflating myriad rockers from Black Sabbath's Ozzie Osbourne to Led Zeppelin's Robert Plant, Harry Shearer's Derek Smalls, Michael McKean's David St Hubbins, and Christopher Guest's Nigel Tufnel provided the comic embodiments of the musical genre. While some might argue the parody of *CB4* has not gained the cult status of the 1984 film, it did extend the notion of genre, driving the construction of personae in concrete ways: after all, Rock's trio were performing a performance of gansta-ness. Often, the construction of their "hard" personae, utilized to legitimize their position in the rap world, was in confrontational dialogue with the people who the rappers were "in real life."

Amidst the movement, back and forth, between the earnestness of Albert Brown and the overblown insolence of MC Gusto, the narrative did not leave space for the witty and acerbic rants of comic Rock's persona. Moreover, at this point in his career Rock's comic voice—the scathing sociocultural critique, the unrelenting rants against hypocrisy (inside and outside of the black community), and even the throaty guffaw and devilish grin that punctuate his most biting jokes series—was not yet established.[26] Nonetheless, Rock and George had made clear choices in *CB4*: rather than centering the film on Rock's burgeoning comic persona, their script utilized insider (cultural) humor to parody a genre for which the writers had great affection. In so doing, they created a culturally niched text that explored rap's adolescence, grounded in the cultural and genre conventions of hip-hop. Like *Harlem Nights*, *CB4* was a studio product, coded for a particular culturally savvy audience, whose star's persona was subsumed by his character's genre-driven imperatives. In considering the shortcomings of these two For Us By Us films, one must consider whether it was the cultural and/or racial specificity of the comedies' milieu or the absence of Murphy and Rock's comic personae that was a greater impediment to box office (and crossover) success.

Enamored with different conventions of gangster and gangsta genre, in film and music respectively, *Harlem Nights* and *CB4* were films that, while endeavoring to create culturally specific comedic texts, gave only passing attention to the comic personae of their stars. Furthermore, in absenting the power of those personae, the creative control of the stars was wasted on vehicles that lacked the comedic legs to stand up as genre films (gangster and mockumentary) in their own right. Arguably, Murphy's and Rock's ventures into classical Hollywood comedy presented different problems and possibilities than *Harlem Nights* and *CB4*: both succeeded in placing their comic personae, as well as contemporary constructions of black culture, at the center of the narrative, while achieving varying degrees of popular and critical acclaim. In Reginald Hudlin's *Boomerang* Murphy provided the story for an eighties hypersexualized reenvisioning of the notoriously chaste sixties comedies. Murphy's entry into romantic comedy hinged on a cross-racial audience's willingness to accept the conversion of his action comedy film persona into the idyllic milieu common to the genre, a gamble given the historical exclusion of black actors as romantic leads in the "boy-meets-girl" stories of mainstream American cinema.

"This is the story of a famous dog . . ." are the first words heard in *Boomerang*, and when Murphy's Marcus Graham emerges from the elevator in the swanky eighties chic office building, it is clear who will be playing the dog. As Murphy moves through the office building, we see Marcus as the man that every man wants to be and every woman wants to do: every woman's greeting drips with desire, and every man is trying to gain charisma points, if only by being near him. Marcus's direction to his secretary to send a single rose to a list of women with the "usual message," "thinking only of you," solidifies his construction as a "player." His heroic "dog" status is further underscored by his lunchtime conversation with his two best friends, Tyler and Gerard, played by Martin Lawrence and David Allen Grier.[27]

TYLER: There's a whole world out there we don't know about. Like the letters in *Penthouse Forum*? Stuff like that never happen to me.
GERARD: Stuff like that never happens to anyone—except Marcus.
MARCUS: The only reason stuff like that happens to me is because I pay attention to women. Y'all don't pay attention.

For Marcus, "paying attention" means knowing your prey. His mode of seduction (his self-proclaimed "art form") is simply a means for sexual conquest. With Marcus ensconced in the position of sexual sensei, his buddies function as part commentary of black masculinity and part rearticulation of traditional roles of the supporting male in a romantic comedy; while Tyler and Gerard may engage in banter akin to "playing the dozens" with each other, Marcus is "above" this verbal volleying; in fact, they are constantly singing Marcus's praises.[28]

Marcus Graham is the eighties equivalent of Hudson's Jerry Webster in *Lover Come Back* (1961), the playboy ad man who wins the love (and virtue) of his virginal competitor, Doris Day's Carol Templeton, through duplicitous means but then, in order to win her back, must actually become the virtuous man he pretended to be. Although the details of the two ad-themed romantic comedies differ, both are stories of the "dog's" comeuppance. The love triangle that develops between Marcus; his boss, Jacqueline Broyer (Robin Givens), who acts as the female version of a "player"; and Angela Lewis (Halle Berry), his subordinate, the mildly Afrocentric "good girl," who becomes Marcus's moral compass, plays within the parameters of the romantic comedy formula. For this particular "dog," Marcus, a cross between the old-school construction of the "ladies' man" and the contemporary construction of an upscale "player," his comeuppance is both personal and professional.

Marcus's infatuation with his female counterpart grows, even as Jacqueline treats him in the duplicitous (and objectifying) manner that he had treated countless other women; as Marcus gets in touch with his feminine side (being cast as the "wronged woman"), his ability to retain his swaggering machismo disappears, as exemplified by the ending of the first liaison with his boss/lover. Marcus awakens to see Jacqueline making one of his patented exits (the half-hearted excuse of an early meeting and a quick noncommittal kiss good-bye), and in an act of uncharacteristic modesty, he pulls the covers to his chest and softly intones, "Call me." Not surprisingly, the emasculated Marcus becomes progressively less able to perform in the world of work. In this triangulated boy-meets-girl(s) story, Marcus finds redemption in his friendship-turned-relation-ship with Angela, with whom he finds renewed creative focus and belief in his abilities, and whom he rejects (for an abortive return to Jacqueline) only to pur-sue again for the requisite happy ending.

The construction of both women in *Boomerang* could easily provide signif-icant fodder for the analysis of black women's representations in contemporary African American film. Jacqueline Broyer's treatment of Marcus reflects a certain moral relativism regarding sex and success—which gains resonance given audi-ences' extratextual knowledge of Robin Givens's alleged man-eater status after her much-discussed, short-lived marriage to Mike Tyson. In addition, the lumi-nously lovely Halle Berry is cast as Angela, the "every sistah," who, despite moments of actual agency (when she becomes a professional force in her own right after her breakup with Marcus), ultimately exists to be acted on by Marcus. However, *Boomerang* is Murphy's movie—he is the famous dog, and it's his story, not that of a couple.

*Boomerang* is by no means an ideal romantic comedy, nor is it the worst example of the genre produced in the early nineties. One might fault Murphy's story or Hudlin's direction for the fact that *Boomerang* did not give the mam-moth box office numbers that many of the comic's previous films had gener-ated.[29] One must also consider that in 1992 the portrayal of a thriving black upper-middle-class milieu, which was viewed by a majority of Americans on Thursday nights in *The Cosby Show* (the centerpiece of Must See TV for much of the previous decade), was not commonplace in American cinema. Released during a period when films dealing with black men were predominantly films from the hood (for example, *Boyz n the Hood* [1991], *Juice* [1992], and *Menace II Society* [1993]), *Boomerang* preceded the spate of black-women-centered middle-class melodramedies later in the decade like *Waiting to Exhale* (1995) and *Soul Food* (1997). Earl Calloway of the *New Philadelphia Courier* described *Boomerang* as "a romantic comedy that has style and offers a great contrast to most of the African-American oriented films that have been produced in the last decade."[30]

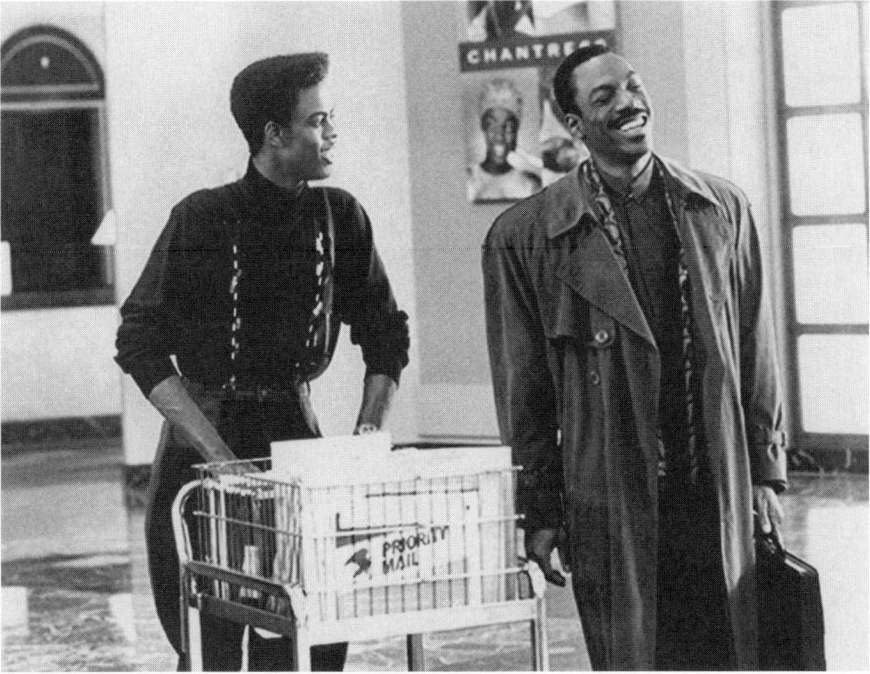

15. The "pup" and the "dog": Chris Rock (left, as Bony T) and Eddie Murphy (as Marcus Graham) in *Boomerang* (1992). Directed by Reginald Hudlin. Photo from Photofest. Reproduced with permission from Paramount Pictures.

Given this industrial reality and, arguably, the ways that varying audiences were "ready" to see Eddie on the big screen, the critique of Murphy's romantic leading man role in the colorized and updated sixties romantic comedy also speaks to the de facto prohibition for a black comic (or any black actor for that matter) to be the boy who gets the girl in a mainstream romantic comedy. As previously stated, in both the fish-out-of-water and color-coded color blindness comedies, Murphy enjoyed enormous crossover success. When constructed as an anomalous figure in a sociocultural milieu only tangentially connected to reality—a Detroit cop in Beverly Hills, an African prince in Queens, or a former executive running a rainbow coalition day care center—Murphy is consistently embraced by the mainstream. Indeed, it seems as though the black comic actor is only afforded a space in comedies with romance when a broad comic premise is foregrounded: whether it is Murphy in a fat suit (and multiple other disguises) in *The Nutty Professor* films or Martin Lawrence in drag for a majority of *Big Momma's House*. However, drastic departures from those formulae—namely the attempts to construct Murphy as a conventional leading man (regardless of genre) have yielded inconsistent results as illustrated by the strikingly disparate reactions to Murphy's first genuine attempt at a romantic comedy. Although it would be reductive to say that the black entertainment media praised *Boomerang* and the mainstream press panned it, the most unforgiving negative reviews came from the critics belonging to the latter group. Some of it was fairly mild: Janet Maslin's disappointment in the fact that "the person to disrupt the status quo in an Eddie Murphy Movie was Eddie Murphy. But in this new role Mr. Murphy becomes part of the establishment he once made fun of."[31] In contrast, Calloway, the film critic for a black paper, asserts that this construction of Murphy as part of "the establishment" is what is so significant about the film: "he is an African American executive and has everything he wants . . . something one hardly sees in movies"; and Calloway lauded the comic actor's concern "that the character, while maintaining professionalism, should reflect [an actual] African American."[32]

While one might argue whether Marcus should be lauded for sleeping with an aging diva (played by Eartha Kitt) in order to (unsuccessfully) secure his promotion and position at the agency, Murphy provides a black male professional who is both hypersexualized and hypercapable. The "hypersexual" nature of Murphy's persona inspires reviewer Peter Travers's ire. Travers begins his vitriolic review by attacking the notion that *Boomerang* was Murphy's attempt to "make amends for the relentless misogyny of his recent films" and ends with a critique of the PG-13-ness of its cinematic depiction of sex: "for all the sex talk . . . there is very little nudity. The only thing naked is Murphy's vanity. . . . What Murphy is doing isn't acting, it's masturbation."[33] The vehemence of Travers's barbs stands in opposition to several critics (in both the black and mainstream press) who viewed *Boomerang* as marking the emergence of "a new maturity for Murphy, which leaves the loudmouth behind and introduces an actor willing to play on a level playing field with his peers."[34] While one can argue the merits of each of these positions on *Boomerang*, and the multiple subjectivities involved in the processes of reviewing African American films, the one thing that is indisputable is the fact that, until recently, no African American actor has emerged as a romantic comedy leading man in a mainstream American comedy. (An arguable exception to the rule, Will Smith's *Hitch* [2005] was given a lukewarm box office reception.) Given Murphy's crossover success, one might think he was the black man to do it. That was not the case. After *Boomerang* Murphy's leading man roles were few and fundamentally unsuccessful (remember *The Adventures of Pluto Nash*). Murphy had to return to the role of the anomaly in the mainstream comedy in order to receive the full mainstream embrace—or he had to become Cosby.

While Murphy's foray into romantic comedy proved problematic for aesthetic and sociocultural, as well as industrial, reasons, Rock's *Down to Earth* and *Head of State*, acting as literal and figurative remakes, sought to posit revered populist Hollywood comedic narratives in an African American context. While Rock had become a screen presence in supporting roles, 2001 provided his first opportunity to "open" a film: Paramount's *Down to Earth*. Arguably, the comic potential was great, with Rock doing double duty as writer and star in a film directed by Chris and Paul Weitz, the white boy-wonders responsible for the *American Pie* films (1999, 2001, 2003). This remake of Warren Beatty's *Heaven Can Wait* (1978)—itself a remake of *Here Comes Mister Jordan* (1941)—features Rock as Lance Barton, a stand-up comedian who dies before he can "kill" at Harlem's Apollo Theater and is then reincarnated in the body of a murdered fifty-something white millionaire, Charles Wellington. The question of whether or not the uncompromising stand-up persona of Rock would translate into a PG-13 Hollywood vehicle was answered within the first twenty minutes of the film: the answer was yes *and* no. Despite Rock's characterization of the film's humor as "race neutral," cultural specificity inflects the film throughout—particularly in terms of Lance/Wellington's relationship to popular culture and, of course, stand-up. Soon after his reincarnation as Wellington, Lance requests a television in the mansion that has BET (Black Entertainment Television). Later, the film presents alternating images of Lance (tall, skinny, black man) and Wellington (short, pudgy, white) as he rides in the Rolls, jamming to Snoop Doggy Dogg's "Gin and Juice" while flashing the three fingered sign for "Westside."

Rock's stand-up persona is omnipresent, with his act metered out over the course of the film. Lance/Wellington's first stand-up gig directly lifts the "black mall vs. white mall" routine from *Roll with the New* ("there's not shit in a black mall except sneakers and baby clothes") with the comic twist that such material is now voiced by an elderly white man—to a stunned reaction from the club's black audience. Coming from Rock, this routine serves as a critique of corporate America's perception of the black community as a collection of pregnant women and wannabe athletes. When it is delivered by Wellington, a privileged white male, the material is compromised—and the critique's bite is entirely negated. Rock's act also informs the social conscience that Wellington develops as he determines to save Brooklyn Community Hospital for the community, inspired by the urgings of the activist (and love interest) Sontee (Regina King). His answer to the hospital board of directors regarding uninsured patients is a tirade straight out of *Bring the Pain*: "Insurance . . . Insurance ain't enough for people. I don't even know why they call it insurance. They should just call it 'in-case-shit-happens.' I give a company money in case shit happen. Now if nothing happens, shouldn't I get my money back?"

With an opening-weekend take of $18 million and a finish in the number two slot in domestic box office, *Down to Earth* promised to deliver crossover success for Rock—but at a cost.[35] As one critic noted, "Like many of Pryor's movies (*Brewster's Millions*, *The Toy*), *Down to Earth* takes pains to soften and bland out its star's more scabrous characteristics."[36] Another reviewer simply states that if "Mr. Rock's fans . . . are going to want a movie with the same acidulous funkiness that he brings to his standup, they are not going to get that."[37] Or, as a fellow moviegoer commented on the film's opening night in Ann Arbor, Michigan: "It was a'ight but . . . it wasn't funny like I thought it'd be."[38] In the process of mainstreaming Rock's stand-up humor for a studio film, the race issues that motored his biting social critique now provide the setup for a string of running gags. There is little difference in the type of laughter elicited when Lance celebrates his inability to hail a cab—"I surely am a black man again"—and the punch Lance/Wellington receives after his impromptu duet with DMX's "Ruff Riders" from one of the "homeys." By streamlining Rock's abrasive and edgy performance within a mainstream Hollywood narrative, *Down to Earth* delivers humor that could be described as race neutralized rather than race neutral. Although racial difference is interwoven throughout its narrative, the film deals with race relations as evasively as the integrationist fairy tale of *Dr. Doolittle*. The literal color coding of these films supplies mainstream audiences with comforting but empty signifiers for race in America, wrapped up by happy endings that celebrate inclusion and acceptance. "Funny is funny," they seem to say, "regardless of race, creed, or color."

As previously discussed, Rock's political discourse in his HBO oeuvre exemplified his facility for unflinching and incisive sociopolitical commentary. Despite the "blanding" that had informed the critique in *Down to Earth*, as the story of a black presidential candidate, *Head of State* (2003) had the potential to be the film where Rock's stand-up and screen persona could be joined seamlessly—particularly given the fact that Rock scored a creative triple crown with the film, acting as star, writer, and director. Instead, in the sociopolitical climate of the cinematic milieu, as well as the construction of Rock's presidential candidate, Mays Gilliam, and the other major players including a Condoleezza Rice clone and Bernie Mac playing . . . well, Bernie Mac, multiple ideologies seem to be smashing into each other.

Although *Head of State*'s political critique itself is not new for die-hard Rock fans, seeing a cinematically realized version of what would happen to a black man who ran for president (candidate Rock as the virtual center of a bull's eye), or the reaction of white "quasi liberals" to the actual possibility of a black president (swarms of suburbanites pouring out of the Orange County subdivisions to the polls), is not a common sight in a mainstream Hollywood film. As Manohla Dargis notes, *Head of State* speaks to a deceptively benign and, thus, particularly duplicitous social moment: "America loves hip hop culture and Colin Powell but for Rock what's more instructive—and grist for his comic mill—is that divide between white love of Black culture and white fear of a Black planet."[39] In this light Rock's film arguably serves a dual purpose. It is a Hollywood film that addresses the convergences and divergences between trends in popular culture and forces in public policy in the ways that both race and class are articulated and contained. More significant, it is an intervention in American screen comedy that attempts to appropriate a classical Hollywood narrative and reframe it within an African American/multicultural context. After all, the film could just as easily have been called "Mr. Gilliam Goes to Washington," with the politics voiced by Rock's politico everyman informed by almost Capra-esque populist sentiments: "The politician's style (and Rock's delivery) is 'Showtime at the Apollo' brash but the politics could be straight out of Barbara Ehrenreich's bestseller 'Nickel and Dimed.' If this were the 1930s, and Mr. Gilliam were, like Jimmy Stewart's Mr. Smith, mounting a filibuster from the Senate floor, the rhetoric would sound less radical. In the current climate, Gilliam's unfashionable insistence on poverty as a deeply American issue is more than just startling—it's downright heretical."[40]

Dargis's assessment of the film's inherent "radicalism" might easily be contested: the populism-tinged reframing of a postracial "us" in Gilliam's presidential bid—regardless of the hip-hopification of the campaign—creates a narrative where cultural and racial specificity is less about ideology and pedagogy than about preference and style. The Nate Dogg–led version of a Greek chorus provides commentary on both Gilliam's rediscovery of self and his trek on the campaign trail; however, their presence seems more like an additional spice progressively hip-hopified cinematic roux than the genuine tool for self-reflexivity that it might have been.

On the other hand, it is easy to argue that the PG-13 version of comic social commentary that emerges in *Head of State* often recirculates and sanitizes quotations from the "black president" material from Rock's act. Furthermore, Rock and Ali LeRoi, his writing partner, play with stereotypical constructions of blackness: the ghetto fabulousness of Gilliam's retooled campaign—complete with candidate clad in Kangol cap and Sean John sweats—and campaign ads that look strangely like Snoop videos, the haphazard insertion of Tracy Morgan's hilarious, if almost minstrelesque, street hustling "meat man" as well as Robin Givens playing . . . Robin Givens. Unfortunately, these events are played with minimal self-reflexivity. Even in the "House Party" fund-raiser sequence, which was the preferred ad clip for the film, the electric sliding White Gilliam supporters supply one long sight gag punctuated with the literal frenzy over the old-school chant "the roof . . . the roof . . . the roof is on fire." This "look at the silly white folks" moment seems like the cinematic incarnation of a BET *Comic View* "white people be like . . ." joke. Less satire than shtick, it underscores the somewhat puzzling choices made in *Head of State.*

In the *New York Times* review of the film, A. O. Scott notes that the "satiric possibilities" of the film are often squandered: "The result is a political comedy that refuses to address a single political topic. It is all well and good to poke fun at the empty, platitudinous dishonesty of political oratory, but the mockery is blunted when the opposing view is just the same boilerplate in more vivid language. What does Mays stand for? Better schools, better-paying jobs, public transportation. Just imagine a politician brave enough to stand up and call for such things."[41] One might argue that, as a new millennial political comedy, *Head of State*—with the populist paradigms seemingly formed outside of concrete contemporary issues of race, class, gender, and sexuality—may seem fairly pedestrian politically. However, some might also argue that there was some modicum of sociopolitical critique embedded in the cartoonish construction of the opposition, the incumbent vice president, Brian Lewis, whose spouting off about family values (and family fame) barely mask megalomania and multiple levels of entitlement.[42]

One might theorize that *Head of State*'s lack of commercial success was caused by either its dearth of or its inculcation with political content. Regardless, the film has established Rock's ability to have access and control over all aspects of his film work. As an A-list black comedic actor, one of a handful of African Americans who is deemed able to open a film, one might assume that Rock's ability to articulate his comic persona within the context of his film roles would become less problematic—although that clearly has not been the case. The notion of artistic autonomy is always difficult for the African American actor to attain—and it is no different for the black comic/comedic actor. It is no accident that the best moment of *Head of State* finds Rock in the familiar position behind the mike, his speech and demeanor transformed by his older brother (Mac): "When are *you* going to start talking?" In his "That Ain't Right" speech the voice of the cultural critic can definitely be heard and Chris Rock is on the campaign trail—not necessarily Mays Gilliam. For that moment there is, albeit fleetingly, the sense that this could indeed be *social* comedy. The indignant tone of Rock's delivery is undoubtedly the impetus for this particular reading of this anomalous cinematic moment—when the negotiations of race, class, and comedy play as text rather than subtext in a mainstream movie.

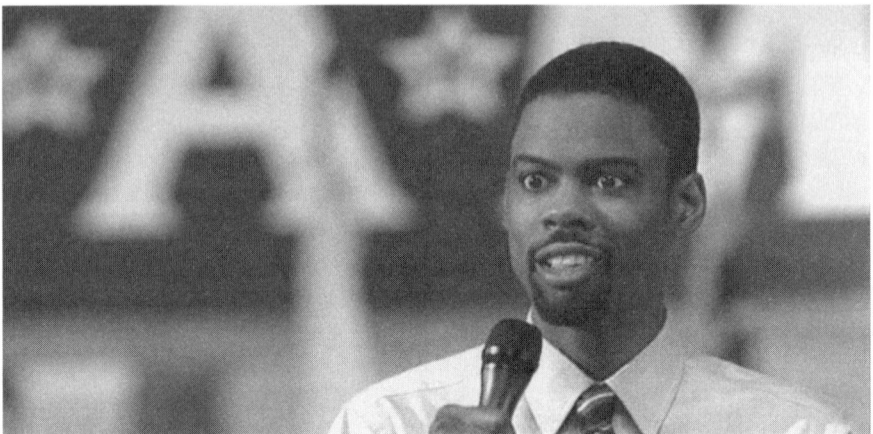

16. The impossible dream: Rock for president in *Head of State* (2003). Directed by Chris Rock.

In his 1997 book, *Rock This*, the comic made clear his desire to have a greater presence in American cinema—with a significant caveat: "I've been in movies. I want to make more movies. But I don't want to be the gimmicky black guy. I'm holding out for something normal. But nothing scares white audiences more than black people being normal. Please, let me be a normal guy! . . . Hollywood keeps looking for another *Trading Places*. They want something that plays with black/white differences."[43] When one looks at the range of Rock's roles, one must ponder what exactly he means by "normal." Is Mays Gilliam, a black new millennial Jefferson Smith, normal? Doesn't Rock's role in *Down to Earth* (and his stand-up, for that matter) play with black/white differences? Doesn't his mainstream role as Caretaker in the remake of prison football film *The Longest Yard* (2005) work within the same rubric as the Murphy/Ackroyd buddy paradigm found in *Trading Places*, with Rock in, what Manohla Dargis refers to as "the humiliating job of playing second banana to a less gifted comedic talent [the more box office bankable Adam Sandler]."[44] I pose these questions not to chide Rock's role selection but to highlight the tenuousness of the black comic actor's position—even after he has made his way onto the industry's A-list. It is not surprising that Rock's earlier jab at the industry's desire for *Trading Places* is countered by his later (2005) assessment of the significance of Murphy's presence onscreen to him—not necessarily as a black comic actor but as a black spectator: "[Murphy] was the first Black guy [on the big screen] that I can remember being cool. I can't remember going to see a movie with Black people before him. I barely remember my parents taking us to see *Sounder* or *Let's Do It Again*."[45]

While the two films Rock barely remembers—the former a historical family drama about pre–civil rights black struggle, the latter one of Cosby's [few] forays into black film comedy in the seventies—hearken back to earlier forms of black cultural production in American cinema, Rock seems to call into question the applicability of those cinematic constructions of blackness to the contemporary African American cultural milieu. Furthermore, by juxtaposing the construction of Murphy's persona as "Shaft with jokes" and the cinematic iteration of Pryor as depicting someone who "was scared in every movie: Oh, my what'm I gon' do?" Rock also speaks to the historical constructions of black masculinity onscreen (either Shaft or Sambo) and the disparity between the stand-up comic persona (as you may recall, Pryor is evoked in the roll call of comic influences in *Bring the Pain*) and how it is retooled for mainstream cinematic consumption. Undeniably, Murphy acts as the not-so-much-older brother of Rock (and the Def Jam generation), and his first wave of post-soul black comedy marks a departure from those who came before by allowing for a degree of black masculine agency and sexuality to be incorporated in the stage and screen incarnations of his persona(e). But, it is not a linear progression for either Murphy or Rock.

The quest for "normalcy"—for a space to survive and thrive in films with the black comic actor's name above the title in a multiplicity of comic roles—has not been completed in the film careers of either of the first- or second-wave comics—despite their crossover popularity, their attempts to reframe classical Hollywood genre in African America contexts, and their integration into mainstream film. Neither Murphy nor Rock is consistently relegated to playing the "black guy," the token presence of color on the big or small screen; however, one sees the dualities of their positions still exist—which comes most sharply into focus in relationship to the cinematic iterations of their personae. The evolution of their comic personae is always in conversation with the black cultural past as articulated within and outside of American popular culture and the mainstream industrial present, which allows space for (minimal) black comedic stardom, within certain narrow and all-too-familiar constrictions.

Whether Rock can open a film again or Murphy's career path veers from the cinematic iteration of the new millennial Cosby (*Daddy Day Camp*) toward the multiple character comedies like his original "comeback" film, *The Nutty Professor* (or the untitled Brett Ratner project with Rock), or back into an action-based comedy form (Quentin Tarantino's remake of *Dirty Dozen*–like WWII film *Inglorious Bastards*), both men's comic personae continue to inform notions of what a black comic can be and can do in contemporary American film. Furthermore, the significance of their comic persona to the mediated cultural production of blackness should not be underestimated. Having said that, it is necessary to view the persona (and career paths) of either Murphy or Rock not as emblematic of new millennial black comedy but rather as possible models for those who will follow in terms of the style, content, and ideological directives of their brands of African American humor. These first- and second-wave post-soul comics are in culturally powerful positions. With increasing industrial and popular cultural cachet, their voices are endowed with depth and resonance: they can often be heard more clearly and more widely than the black politico.

### ROCK IN THE MAINSTREAM: THE OSCARS

In 2005 the Academy of Motion Picture Arts and Sciences' choice of Chris Rock to host the 2005 telecast was designed to draw a younger audience—a self-conscious attempt to hold on to as much of the lucrative eighteen-to-forty-nine demographic as possible in a year when televised award fetes were being tuned-out in droves.[46] Far more interesting than either Rock's actual performance as host was the fact that Rock's *persona* became the lead story of a rather lackluster Oscars' season.[47] Rock, acting both as an agent of the Academy PR machine and as a protector of his particular comic brand, was everywhere—from the pages of multiple magazines and newspapers to the talk show/news magazine circuit. In this instance the industrial market value of the terms, "edgy," as it related to a black comic, had risen significantly. As noted by Bruce

Davis, executive director of the Academy, "edgy is the word that keeps coming up. I like to hear that people are nervous, because that means you're likely to watch."[48] The frequent mobilization of Rock's cutting-edge comedic brand was constant—like an extended period of duplicitous foreplay with the audience, or at least the desired audience.

The "controversial" statements made in the comic's February interviews (particularly those published in *Entertainment Weekly* and the *New York Times*) included his assertion that "no straight black man watches the Oscars" and his admitting that he hasn't watched the Oscars because "they don't recognize comedy and you don't see a lot of black people nominated, so why should I watch it?" He also hailed comic turned dramatic actor Jamie Foxx (*Ray*, 2004): "Foxx is not going to walk out of that place without an Oscar." While the remarks seemed part of Rock's candid and offhanded rap, they also possessed more than a whiff of calculation. The reaction of longtime Oscar producer Gil Cates to the controversy—"poor Chris, in the sense that he's a comedian, he's supposed to make people laugh. And he gets bombarded for doing that"—seems to reverberate with the idea that there is no such thing as bad press.[49] Furthermore, the particular type of irreverence (about the "stuffiness" of the ceremony, emotional reactions to nominations, gender, and sexuality-coded fandom) speaks to a problematic kind of populism that Rock exhibits in these interviews, which Nelson George addressed in his comments about the comic's impending Oscar gig: "The reasons the Oscars have him there hosting is not to make Warren Beatty laugh, they have him there to make Joe Six-Pack laugh."[50] George contrasts the Hollywood politico and a color-blind, but decidedly blue-collar, construction of the everyman in the television audience, thus recognizing both Rock's mainstream status in American popular culture and the movable ideological feast encompassed in his humor.

Given the host network, ABC's renewed commitment to "family friendliness," Rock's "edginess" was the award show's hot commodity—particularly in the wake of the Jackson–Timberlake "wardrobe malfunction" and the Sheridan–Owens towel dropping controversy.[51] In fact, The "threat" of something "unexpected" happening with Rock at the helm was so appealing that ABC directly made the connection between these controversial events and the new poster boy for edginess (Rock) explicit in an Oscar show promo spot. During the *Desperate Housewives* timeslot Rock was shown "fondling" the "naked" Oscar statuette and declaring, "You won't believe the halftime show." As *New York Times* columnist Frank Rich noted: "Mr. Rock, as skilled at PR as he is at comedy, ran around giving cheeky interviews making the 'outrageous' charge that the Oscars might have a gay following. Matt Drudge took the bait and assailed the comedian for indecency. Mr. Rock was soiling the 'classiest night in Hollywood' he said on Fox News, by taking 'a lewd route . . . to the gutter.'"[52] Conservative blogosphere pundit Matt Drudge's assault on Rock (and the Academy's choice of the comic) proved the assertion that there is no such thing as bad press: it solidified Drudge's position as champion of "traditional values" and Rock's as an "edgy" and "dangerous" comic force.[53] In the end the media frenzy around Rock's hosting duties became an exercise in smart marketing.

Given that the "dangerousness" and "edginess" of the comic's persona were the centerpieces of the Academy's advertising onslaught and the fact that the show, even with a much-touted seven-second delay, was appearing on prime-time network television, Rock was placed in the unenviable position of being able to meet the expectations of neither his fans nor his detractors. As the comic promised in his *60 Minutes* interview, he did not abandon his comic persona; Rock did not sing, "there [was] no soft shoe [and] there [was] no tapping"— the performance he gave, although muted, was still Rock.

Interestingly, it was not his political humor—exemplified by his assertion that Bush must be a genius to "reapply for his job" and get it the same year that "there's a movie in every theater in the country that shows how much you suck" (*Fahrenheit 9/11*)—but rather his industry digs—his statement that "there are only four real stars, and the rest are just popular people." Despite the fact that there was self-deprecation built into the jokes series where he stated, "If you want Tom Cruise and can only get Jude Law—wait" (expanding a bit on the British actor's overexposure) before drawing the same conclusion about himself as an inadequate replacement for Denzel Washington, some actors (most publicly, Sean Penn) took umbrage to the remark.[54] In an evening of comedy that could be easily characterized as "Rock Lite," the most memorable moment was the-man-on-the-street segment filmed at the Magic Johnson Theaters in Los Angeles, asking black patrons to list their movie of the year. As Paul Brownfield recounted, "one guy said, '*The Chronicles of Riddick*' [a Vin Diesel sci-fi/action vehicle]. Several others said *White Chicks*, which became a running joke."[55] The coda to the segment was the statement of the only white "patron," erudite comic actor and director Albert Brooks, proclaiming that *White Chicks* was the best movie and that "Wayans, you were robbed." The segment spoke, not simply to differences in taste culture based on race, as well as genre, but also to the notion that, as Brownfield declared, "Applaud yourself all you want, Hollywood, but your business is built on the opening take of 'White Chicks' at the mall in the predominantly Black neighborhood. You could feel the self-congratulatory air back at the Kodak Theater being sucked out of the room, and, for a brief moment, it felt as though Rock had blown the show open."[56] Such moments of comic subversiveness were few, however, and although Rock proved to be a more-than-adequate host, he was hardly dangerous and barely edgy. As Rock would later state on Oprah Winfrey's post-Oscar special, "It wasn't my show, it's the Oscars. And I was there—I was working for people . . . when I'm working for me, then I'll be a little more dangerous."[57]

While Rock was not the Oscars' first black host, the unpredictability and outspokenness of his African American predecessor, Whoopi Goldberg, was not seen or marketed as the ceremony's greatest (ratings) asset. Although "his open-

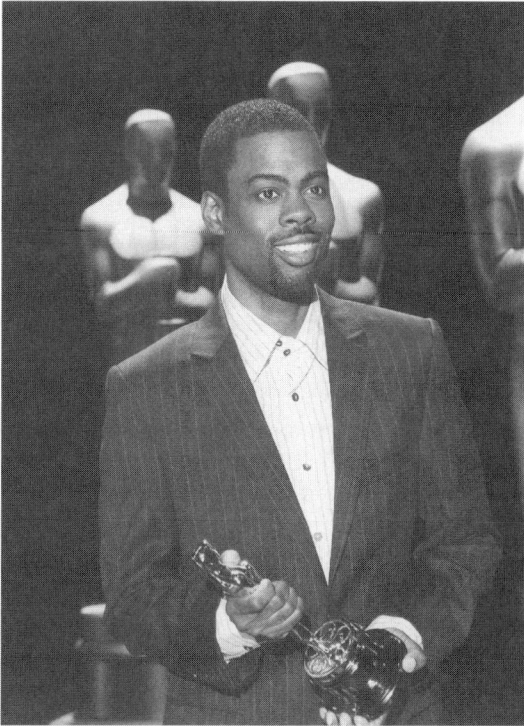

17. The equal-opportunity offender as host of the Oscars. Chris Rock in ABC's Oscars On-Air Promo (2005). Directed by Jon Favreau. Photo by Danny Feld, acquired from Photofest, and reproduced with permission from ABC.

ing monologue and later bit made repeated reference to black performers and black culture as he sought to add his race-based comedic voice to a telecast that nonetheless remained cautious and bland," his centrality at an event that is classically Hollywood makes a statement about the position of his comic persona in American popular culture.[58] At this particular sociocultural moment Rock is absolutely correct when he states, "I hosted the Oscars, how much more mainstream can you get?"[59] However, one must also question whether it signifies another instance of the commodification of black cultural production—in this case, of a persona often seen as emblematic of an unbridled, uncompromising voice in black comedy—or whether the older notions of crossover must be interrogated in a popular cultural milieu where Chris Rock actually is mainstream.

PERSONA POLITICS: MURPHY AND ROCK
IN THE NEW MILLENNIUM

Rooted in an explication of the social conditions of African American life, black humor carries an inherent critique of cultural and racial inequalities. Implicitly or explicitly, such humor explores the conflicting (and conflicted) allegiances of being black and American. The personae of the black comic are always supervised by the history of race relations in America—from what venues he or she can perform in to the assimilationist negotiation of blackness in mainstream media showcases. As in the civil rights era and earlier, issues of race continue to inform daily life in black America—in terms of media representation, social mobility, and political agency. How, then, could they not play a role in its humor?

Indeed, the very qualities that have enabled Chris Rock and Eddie Murphy to attain a significant cross-racial following is the comic tradition of truth telling. Whose truth and to what end becomes a significant question. Even Rock, who whose "transgressive" notion of blackness elicits praise from Michael Eric Dyson, sometimes shifts uncomfortably under the cultural-critic mantle. In a *New York Times* interview the week before the opening of *Down to Earth*, Rock commented on what it meant to be a black comedian: "Being a comedian is like being in a boxing ring but when you add the subject of race, it's like you get to use a bat, too. Few guys can't resist using that bat. But then journalists start analyzing it and talking to me like I'm Kwesi Mfume [the president of the NAACP]. I don't need that gig. All I care about is being funny."[60] Even though Rock's comment reveals a desire for a comic tradition that is "outside of history," it acknowledges the power that black humor offers to the "bat" of social critique. Four years later, Rock, while adhering to the same premise, seems far more circumspect about the burden of responsibility borne by the black comic.

In Rock's 2005 interview on *60 Minutes*, broadcast one week before the Oscar telecast, Ed Bradley read Rock a quotation from a *New Republic* article on Rock by Justin Driver, in which he stated that "Rock is attempting to shuck, jive, grin, shout and bulge his eyes all the way back to the days of minstrelsy. His act often legitimizes white racists' views of the world." Rock appears less taken aback than tiredly exasperated by Driver's comment as he responds: "Comedians are verbal clowns. . . . I don't have the red nose on and floppy shoes . . . but who am I kidding here? . . . The sad thing is, the black comedian has a weird responsibility and a weird line that we have to walk that sometimes offends people like the guy you just quoted."[61]

In much the same way that Rock was in a win/win and lose/lose situation as the host of the Oscars—given that any adjustment of his persona to the venue would create contention and consternation in supporters and detractors alike—Murphy and Rock are placed in untenable positions as the comic emissaries for the post-soul generation. Their personae are always already constituted in relationship to absence—as the fortunate few who are given the ability and responsibility to convey black culture and experience through comic discourse. Whether Rock's *Everybody Hates Chris* becomes the new sitcom gold standard and Peabody-winning darling or Murphy decides to return to the stand-up stage after an almost two-decades absence or to retool his comic persona in the image of another civil rights era comic (Gregory instead of Cosby or Pryor), some will undoubtedly be disappointed in the choices made by these first- and second-wave comics. Whether in terms of stasis or changeability of style, ideologies, or politics; of courting and/or achieving crossover, embracing or rejecting genre, narrowcasting or typecasting, their actions are scrutinized industrially and culturally. With their success (and the burden of representation) comes an additional responsibility—to actually speak to the African American condition in all its myriad forms while contending with the mutability of the aesthetic, cultural, industrial, and historical moment.

One must ask whether it is unfair to expect black comedians to operate within a pedagogy informed as much by cultural criticism as by the need just to "be funny"? Yes, but I would maintain that it is necessary nonetheless. This necessity is illustrated by the color adjustments that take place in the mainstreaming of the black comic persona for Hollywood comedy—and in the miniscule number of black actors or black-themed films that are actually deemed able to "go wide" or television programs deemed to have an appeal beyond the "urban niche." The ability to "go wide" or to "open" a film is, however, a guarantee of neither a consistent box office success nor wholesale acceptance from all segments of the moviegoing populace—black and white—as exemplified in the audience's ever-shifting love affair with the personae of crossover diva Whoopi Goldberg.

CHAPTER 4

# Crossover Diva

## WHOOPI GOLDBERG AND PERSONA POLITICS

SINCE HER LANDMARK one-woman show in 1985 Whoopi Goldberg has been somewhat of an entertainment anomaly: a black comic diva. On stage and screen Goldberg has gained a degree of critical and financial success attained by few African American comics—and industrial clout accorded to even fewer women. With the notable exception of Jackie "Moms" Mabley and Pearl Bailey, whose careers, like Goldberg's, straddle stage and screen, Whoopi has acquired what few black female comic entertainers of either the pre–or post–civil rights era have been able to gain: access to white main stages and the entertainment mainstream. All of these women, with varying degrees of success, knew how to play to their audiences. The differences between the Moms of the Chitlin' Circuit in the forties and fifties (and mainstream clubs of the sixties) and the Moms on *The Ed Sullivan Show* in the late sixties and seventies can be found in nuances of language and delivery rather than substantive content, while Bailey's Pearlie Mae persona, which was center stage in most of her stage work in nightclubs and on Broadway, made only cameo appearances in a majority of her screen roles. Like those of her predecessors, Goldberg's career navigates crossover waters by mobilizing multiple personae—dependent on both intended audience and the limitations of the given medium. However, unlike Mabley and Bailey, the many facets of Whoopi often seem at war with each other—particularly in relationship to her comedic work.

Goldberg, who first came to prominence for her inventive and transgressive comic characters onstage, often seems to flounder in tired genre pieces such as *Eddie* (1996) and *Bogus* (1996) or to be woefully underutilized as the virtual Rhoda of melodramedies—*Moonlight and Valentino* (1995), *Boys on the Side* (1995), and *How Stella Got Her Groove Back* (1998). Furthermore, the roles of the put-upon, disempowered mothers of the African American family dramedies *Kingdom Come* (2001) or *Good Fences* (2003) seem to have a greater kinship to Celie in *The Color Purple* (1985) than to her Oscar-winning role as Oda Mae Brown in *Ghost* (1990), Sister Mary Clarence in the *Sister Act* franchise of the early nineties, or Sarah Matthews in *Made in America* (1993). Goldberg's extratextual presence also frames the popular understanding of her comic persona: the outspoken cultural critic's impromptu remarks have cast her alternately as advocate (her work with and performances on *Comic Relief*) or saboteur (most recently, her anti-Bush remarks endeared her neither to the hipster Kerry faithful nor to Slim-Fast, for whom she had acted as spokesperson, and, possibly, voters in swing states). Goldberg's stature in the industry remains problematic, tenuous, *and* high: the significance of the fact that the Whoops is the only female to host the Academy Awards–and has done so multiple times—should be neither under- nor overestimated.

In exploring Goldberg's comic personae in relationship to those who came before and those who followed her, one begins to discern how race, sexuality, and gender are played with and against by female black comic actors and how the construction of their personae are inextricably tied to tropes of black femininity—for better *and* for worse. In her introduction to *Not Just Race, Not Just Gender*, Valerie Smith mobilizes Kimberlé Crenshaw's concept of *intersectionality* "as a mode of cultural or textual analysis, what it means to read at the intersections of constructions of race, gender, class and sexuality."[1] This concept seems particularly apt for the discussion of the multiple ideological and sociocultural impulses that inform the personae that are Whoopi Goldberg. It is in this intersection that we all exist—our identities and our articulation of them, fluid and never fixed, always already being impacted by our past and present as well as by histories of race, class, gender, and nation. Undoubtedly, the complex process of identity formation for black women in the United States is in conversation with Goldberg's evolving comic personae. As one might expect when dealing with an individual who consistently endeavors to defy both convention and expectation, it is not always a friendly conversation. On one hand, the evolution of her persona and her sometimes contentious relationship with her audiences (black and white) calls to mind Dick Gregory's reflections on the "friendly relation" involved in being a black comic.[2] This "relation" is further problematized for Whoopi by gendered notions of "how to be funny" and those tied to the function of racial and cultural specificity in stand-up comedy, in the theater, and on the big and small screens in the post–civil rights era. Furthermore, as with Gregory's act, the high level of sociopolitical critique that has informed much of Goldberg's stage work has, in the past, complicated the friendly relation—and it continues to do so. While Gregory's political activism would eventually pull him out of the entertainment mainstream, Goldberg, holding fast to her industrial position, continues to speak her mind—in multiple venues and with varying results. On the other hand, as I suggested in my introduction, one could argue that Goldberg *began* crossed-over. Thus, her outspokenness, her unabashed disdain for being "niched," and her idiosyncratic sense of humor and appropriateness have sometimes had the effect of setting her apart from the black community—for which, like it or not, she will always be seen as a representative.

Furthermore, when viewing Goldberg in relationship to other post-soul (and even civil rights era) comics, issues of gender, comic tradition, and trajectory, as well as what one might call her "era," come into play. Goldberg is a contemporary of Eddie Murphy; both came into comic prominence in the 1980s. However, as the elder statesperson of the post–civil rights era comics examined in this volume, Goldberg occupies a position that straddles the civil rights and post-soul era in her life and her comedy. While Whoopi enjoys high visibility in film, theater, and television, to a degree that could be seen as comparable to Flip Wilson in his heyday or even Bill Cosby (pre– and post–*The Cosby Show*), her acceptance by both mainstream and black audiences has always been mitigated by the textual and extratextual construction of both her personal politics and her comic persona. Like Gregory, Pryor, and Chris Rock, onstage her comic discourse is imbricated with sociopolitical discourse. Yet Goldberg is granted "equal-opportunity offender" status begrudgingly—particularly in the black community. After following the trajectory of her career, one might even argue that both her ideological bent and her comic content are informed more by the San Francisco counterculture, vestiges of Oakland radicalism (like Richard Pryor) and theater (in California and on and off-Broadway) than the comic legacy of the Chitlin' Circuit, the treks through comedy clubs, or the Reagan era black urban experience.

I use the phrase "crossover diva" to try to capture the conflicted and conflictual position that Goldberg occupies in American comedy. A slew of adjectives come to mind when one thinks of a diva: *gifted, unique, uncompromising*, and, of course, *prima donna*. The term *diva* is thrown around a lot these days—usually in association with events starring a few pop stars du jour and a couple of one-of-a-kind performers whose body of work has given them venerated status or when referring to someone's unreasonable self-importance or selfish demands. I choose to mobilize the word as a signifier for a unique black female comic presence who occupies a space in the entertainment world that, as much as possible, she defines (or tries to define). Thus, the choice to focus upon persona rather than star, which necessarily forces one to foreground the comic actor's body of work rather than his or her personal life, is further complicated because the diva, one might argue, is always "on." Again, the notion of intersectionality comes into play, not only in the construction of the persona in relationship to race, class, and gender but also in the ways she is perceived at this same intersection. To understand the significance of Goldberg's various personae, one must see how their trajectory was directed by and, in turn, directs other black women's comic personae. While the apolitical "sassiness" of Bailey may have less of a kinship to Goldberg than the raucous sexual candor of Moms or the irreverent brand of lived black feminism expounded by diva-in-training Wanda Sykes, the complexities of Goldberg's choices of comic personae, as annunciated in her stand-up/stage performance and in film comedies, reflect and refract their articulations of African American womanhood in myriad forms: the hypersexualized *and* desexualized, the stereotypical and the anomalous, within "integrated" milieus and homogeneous media texts. One might assume that the multiplicity of variations on the theme of black women's humor would marginalize Goldberg's comic voice.

Surprisingly, in reality Whoopi Goldberg has been afforded a dually—albeit mitigated—privileged space from which to speak for—if not always to—the African American community. Sadly, for audiences whose knowledge of Goldberg is limited to questionable comedic fare like *Bogus* and *Eddie*, the onstage prowess of the actor seems more like an antiquated legend than a popular cultural reality. Just as one might question Pryor's iconic status in American comedy if one had only viewed his Gene Wilder buddy films and not the pinnacle of the comedy performance film, *Richard Pryor: Live in Concert*, those who came to know Whoopi in the late nineties and the first decade of the new millennium have a woefully limited picture of her comedic discourse. While this study focuses on the cinematic constructions of Whoopi, one must recognize the (minimally) bifurcated nature of her comic persona—existing as if the split between the onscreen and onstage personae, between the audacious sociocultural critic and the amiable trickster, is the function of sort of a willed schizophrenia. Like Richard Pryor, the cinematic construction of her comic personae often provides only the vestiges of the scathing sociopolitical critique and expansive notions of the American condition. Yet in order to understand the multiple functions of Goldberg's comic personae, it is necessary to trace its evolution from the beginning—from the moment of Whoopi—and *The Spook Show*.

## CONSTRUCTING THE COMIC WHOOPI:
### *THE SPOOK SHOW* AND BEYOND

From the choice of her stage name—"Whoopi," of cushion fame, and "Goldberg," either a homage to Borscht Belt comics or the name suggested by her mother (depending on which bio one consults—and there are many differing accounts), the former Caryn Johnson was compelled to challenge and defy predetermined conceptions of who she was and what she would be like.[3] After Johnson became Goldberg, her comic personae began to take shape—honing her acting skills at San Diego's Repertory Theatre, then in its infancy, and her comic instincts in the improvisation troupe Spontaneous Combustion. The moment of Whoopi, however, coincides with the creation of *The Spook Show*, written by Goldberg with additional material by David Schien, with whom she also codirected the production. This first iteration of what would later be her Broadway debut was first presented at Berkeley's Hawkeye Studio in 1982, before touring Europe and landing at New York's Dance Theatre Workshop in 1983. The series of monologues in the show attested not only to Goldberg's range as an actor—playing diverse characters from a black male junkie to a teenaged white surfer chick—it revealed her affinity for those on the margins of society. Like her chosen name, the title of the show was designed to play with audience expectations. As Mischa Berson states in "Whoopi in Wonderland," expounding on the creator's intentionality in relationship to the show's title, the word *spook* is a derogatory term used for blacks, (usually within the African American community); "the word is also a synonym for ghost—an invisible presence, just as many of the underclass characters Goldberg portrays remain invisible with mass culture."[4] The off-Broadway performance of *The Spook Show*, which had already provided Goldberg with a cult following on the West Coast, came to the attention of renowned director Mike Nichols. "I've never seen anyone like her," declared the award-winning director of stage and screen, "one part Elaine May, one part Groucho, one part Ruth Draper, one part Richard Pryor and five parts never before seen."[5] By 1984, the self-titled show, *Whoopi Goldberg*, was in production at the Lyceum, and the actor was rapidly becoming a darling of Broadway.

With the unabashed success of *Whoopi Goldberg* the comic actor, who had been doing theater since the mid-seventies, became an overnight phenomenon and went from stalwart actor in the provinces to diva. In Enid Nemy's piece for the *New York Times*, "Whoopi's Ready, but Is Broadway?" Goldberg voiced her insistence on not being bound by so-called "traditional" casting. "I'm going to change all that because I'm good. I can be a dog, a chair, anything, and people are shocked and surprised because they don't see too many actors these days, only personalities."[6] The audaciousness of Goldberg's claims could only be made because of the virtuosity of her performance. Onstage she moved fluidly from satire to pathos, from stand-up comedy to the brink of tragedy. In retrospect, one can see pieces of later iterations of Whoopi's stand-up and cinematic personae in each character's monologue, as well as the sociocultural themes that informed her work for the next two decades.

With characters that continued to resonate with audiences long after they left the theater, the show, which ran from 90 to 120 minutes any given night, allowed Goldberg to truly occupy different personae: "the Surfer Girl," whose singsong, Valley Girl–informed whine intones, in denial-filled casualness, her botched self-abortion; "the Crippled Girl," who, embodied with physical and vocal dexterity by Goldberg, waxes poetic on what living with difference actually means; and the Jamaican nurse, who talks candidly about caring for and, later, loving the old man she refers to as "The Raisin." Two characters that speak most directly to the personae that Goldberg would continue to inhabit were "the Little Girl with Blond Hair" and "the Junkie."

In the "Little Girl with Blond Hair" monologue Goldberg engages the struggle with budding media-induced racial self-hatred as depicted in a little black girl, who wears a white shirt on her head to simulate her "long, luxurious blond hair." With a soft, childlike, semi-shy lilt in her voice, swinging her body back and forth in the gentle rhythm natural to a child speaking to an adult, she confesses her desire to attain a "Breck Girl" existence, in language that is both funny and poignant: "I told my mother I didn't want to be black no more. . . . Man, she say even if you sitting in a vat of Clorox till hell freezes over, you ain't gonna be nothing but black. And she was right too, because I sat in the Clorox and I got burned. And she say I just got to be happy with what I got, but look. See? It don't do nothing. It don't blow in the wind. And it don't casca—cascadadade down my back. It don't." While very directly addressing racialized notions of beauty, Goldberg doesn't offer a simple solution; rather she makes visible experiences that the audience might never otherwise see. Furthermore, with Goldberg as the little girl—dark-skinned, dreadlocks, with features not considered beautiful by Eurocentric standards—this monologue challenges narrow definitions of beauty and testifies to the damage done by them.

Despite the power and the prowess shown in the other monologues of the show, the segment that comes closest to the voice of Whoopi—irreverent, outrageous, and, arguably, outraged—is Fontaine, the junkie, who opens the show. Fontaine's entrance immediately lets the audience know that this is not going to be a night of traditional theater. He is heard—singing—before he is seen:

Around the world, in 80 Motherfucking Days . . .
Da dooby doo,
Da dooby do,
Da dooby do be do be do-waaah.

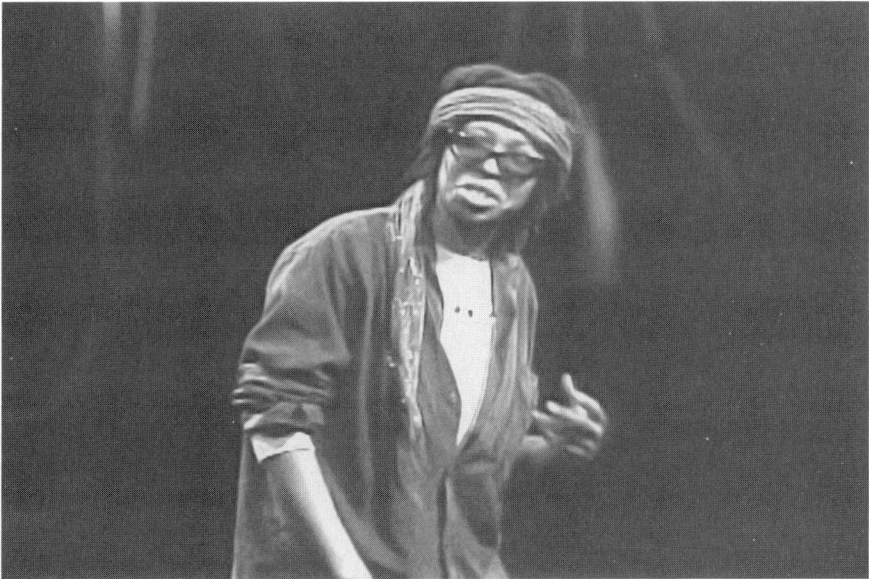

18. Whoopi Goldberg channels Fontaine in her one-woman show, *Whoopi Goldberg: Direct from Broadway* (1985). Directed by Thomas Schlamme.

On the second time through the chorus, the audience sees Goldberg as Fontaine, scarf tied around her head, dark glasses and a slow, hipster strut. Fontaine continues to sing as he moves toward the center of the stage. Like all the characters, Fontaine speaks directly to the audience; unlike the others, he expects them to answer back:

> What's happenin'? [Exasperated] What's happenin'?
>
> Look, I say what's happenin,' you say everything is everything, whatever the fuck you all say. So we're gonna try this shit again.
>
> [Fontaine leaves the stage and begins the show again.]
>
> Around the world, in 80 Motherfucking Days . . .
> Da dooby doo,
> Da dooby do,
> Da dooby do be do be do-waaah.
>
> What's happenin'?
>
> [Audience speaks out with multiple muddled responses]
>
> That wasn't shit.

Although breaking the fourth wall is clearly significant here, as is the choice of song, which connects thematically to the monologue that will follow and begins the disruption of the audience's notions about the breadth of Fontaine's cultural fluency, perhaps more important is the relationship that Fontaine immediately establishes with the audience: he is in a position of authority. Goldberg, speaking in a low growl reminiscent of a blaxploitation movie hustler, endows Fontaine with toughness and just a touch of menace—the kind that might induce the clutching of pocketbooks if the upscale Broadway patrons were to pass him on the street. Fontaine, aware of this possible perception, toys further with the audience: "Lot of people real uptight around me—I don't understand it. I think I'm real friendly. [Pauses, staring over his dark glasses out at the audience] Don't you?"

Fontaine's monologue, which is the longest in the show, takes him from JFK airport to Amsterdam. His description of a visit to the Anne Frank House provides the opportunity for universalizing experiences of hope, loss, and oppression. It also gave Goldberg the opportunity to challenge, yet again, audience expectations—to complicate their conception of the junkie by constructing for him a life that responds to real-world possibilities. His discovering of the room where Anne and her family hid is preceded by a passage that, within the context of the story, makes a statement that calls into question the civil rights era ethos that higher education is the ticket to "a better life": "And, as I was perusing the area, I noticed a small staircase leading up to a big bookcase, and I'm into books, you know, I got a Ph.D. in literature from Columbia. [The audi-

ence's uproarious laughter is met by a cold, incredulous stare] . . . I know you
don't think I was born a junkie. I have an education. I got a Ph.D. I can't do shit
with so I stay high so I don't get mad."

After that moment of sociopolitical critique, made in passing, Fontaine confesses breaking down in the hidden room, "and I'm not a crier, I'd just as soon
cut your throat as look at you." To let the audience share the reality of twenty
hours a day in silence required during the Franks' time in hiding, Fontaine stands
silent for a minute, before stating, "Twenty hours of no movement? I could've
done it." Overwhelmed with emotion, he describes trying to leave "because my
manhood was on the line" when he was filled with righteous indignation at a
quotation posted on the wall: "In spite of everything, I still believe people are
good at heart." Realizing that the words were Anne Frank's, his indignation is
replaced by wonder at a child's ability to "to see the good in the worst situations." The semipoetic rumination on the horror of that historical moment, what
it meant for people who "didn't see it coming," and the contrast between the
violence of the civil rights movement and the experience of the Holocaust create an interesting frame for Fontaine's journey into the hinterland, where "the
only thing black was the forest and me" and where, despite his expectations of
the contrary, he finds the people to be kind. In the end, after a return flight filled
with mechanical difficulties lands him in Bellevue, Fontaine's unconventional
"American Abroad" story becomes a work of philosophical introspection in
regard to how we treat one another and our own forms of intolerance: "I had a
lot of time to think you know, in between freak bouts. 'Cause it turns out, you
know, I'm one of those people, 'if you don't speak English don't come up to me
in the street and ask me where shit is.' Yeah, you're the same way, right? . . . It is
real hard to be that cold once you've been the alien. . . . It don't take nothin' but
a little bit o graciousness, Mon." Yet the possible sentimentality of life's truisms
proffered by a junkie philosopher is cut by Fontaine's awareness of the "real
world" and his place in it: even as he gives the directive to appreciate "that life
is a constant thing, it's constant live and learn," he repositions himself in the
social order, as if to underscore his doubt that they will actually listen to him:
"Never get over that shit, not even a junkie. Not even a junkie."

In Fontaine, Whoopi Goldberg found a comic alter ego that, if not auto-
biographically informed, was certainly inflected by her lived experience. As a
former heroin addict, Goldberg understands that the addict is more than the
addiction, and certainly this understanding is part of what allows Fontaine to
be the most fully realized character in the show. Moreover, Fontaine's irreverently incisive critique and his candid self-assessment provided the truest indication of Goldberg's actual comic voice up to that time. Interestingly, endowing
Fontaine's monologue with the greatest degree of discursive power provided a
masculine voice for Goldberg's persona. Thus, in this instance gender is displaced by race, which informs not only Fontaine's worldview but also the
authority with which he speaks—even if he is speaking from the margins.

In the intervening years between her Broadway debut in 1984 and her second HBO special in 1988, Goldberg continued to gain both acclaim and industrial cachet.[7] Goldberg returned briefly to the Bay Area stage, where she starred in *Moms*, a play she cowrote based on the works of Jackie "Moms" Mabley, whom she states was one of her comic idols. Between 1985 and 1988 Goldberg made an auspicious film debut as Celie in *The Color Purple*—which yielded her first Academy Award nomination and her first taste of controversy within the industry and within the black community.[8] A string of less-than-memorable comedies followed, including 1986's *Jumping Jack Flash*, which was Penny Marshall's directorial debut, and *Clara's Heart* (1988), her first melodramedy, in which she plays the Jamaican caretaker to a pre–*Doogie Howser*, Neil Patrick Harris. Despite inauspicious roles in film comedies not written with Goldberg in mind (*Jumping Jack Flash* was intended for Shelly Long and *Burglar* for Bruce Willis), her comic cachet continued to grow—due at least in part to her work as an activist as well as a comic during the Reagan era.

By the time *Fontaine: Why Am I Straight?* (HBO) aired in August of 1988, Goldberg's reputation for being outspoken in terms of her political beliefs was well established. Whereas the construction of the junkie philosopher in its earlier iteration had been informed less by a political agenda than a common-sense form of humanism, the clean and sober Fontaine of 1988 ripped into the status quo with a vengeance. Whereas Goldberg had previously used Fontaine's reflections on his European experiences as idiosyncratic yet universalizing object lessons—from the emotional catharsis at the Anne Frank House, resulting in the desire to do "better," to the transformative power of his own "alien" experience as a means to encourage tolerance, the new Fontaine was not showing; he was telling. The hour-long special was less a monologue than it was Whoopi doing stand-up *through* Fontaine. Furthermore, there are moments when the line between Goldberg and Fontaine blurs. In one joke series Fontaine castigates Nancy Reagan, whom he dislikes "because she doesn't live in the real world. . . . You cannot live in the real world and tell teenagers, 'Just Say No.'" He then extols the virtues of Lady Bird Johnson, who was "the only First Lady": "Nobody remembers Lady Bird but me. I remember because she *employed* me—she put up theaters. She built the arts." It seems that Goldberg's biography—not the character's—is being referenced.

As Goldberg's political agenda comes, unfiltered, through Fontaine, so, too, does a more direct form of sociopolitical discourse, less concerned with seeking the audience's empathy than with unequivocally stating a point, regardless of how the audience might react to it. This pedagogical shift is demonstrated in Fontaine's unanticipated de facto defense of Jimmy "the Greek" Snyder's statement about blacks' athletic superiority and their deficiencies in terms of being part of team management, by citing that, in the old days, they "bred us" to be athletically superior. The mitigated defense also includes chastising those who jumped on the castigation bandwagon as harboring a double standard. Fontaine states that the "flip side" of Jimmy the Greek, and signal of the fluctuation in the nature of the public's outrage, was the liberals' embrace of Jesse Jackson's 1988 presidential campaign:

> Jessie when he ran the first time talked about a beautiful idea—the rainbow coalition . . . a great utopian vision where everybody was equal except the people in Hymietown. . . . People say to me, why are you fucking with the brother, mon. Because I ain't gonna vote for him 'cause he's black 'cause it didn't work for the white folks. See you can't vote based on this. . . . [Pointing emphatically to his skin] Yes, it good to be the first and the forefront—but you damn well better be the best.[9]

Fontaine's reiteration of the disparaging remark from the 1984 campaign and his condemnation of those who support Jackson based primarily on racial affinity forms a sort of two-tiered attack—on what Goldberg sees as hypocrisy in liberals, who condemn Jimmy the Greek and forgive Jackson, and on African Americans (the target audience for the last comment), whom she constructs as politically naive if they believe that the same race means the same political agenda.

Over the course of the sixty-minute set, the targets of Goldberg/Fontaine's ire are varied and many—and sometimes couched in celebratory language that turns quickly to wry criticism. Such was the case in the discussion of the national frenzy over the welfare of Baby Jessica, who in 1987, at age eighteen months, fell into a well in Midland, Texas, and became the lead story worldwide as rescuers worked feverishly for three days before safely retrieving her. Fontaine applauds the national "concern":

> America, when we get behind stuff, is incredible. We are like a symphony in motion. The American people together is what makes the country great. Baby goddam Jessica . . . Baby Jessica fell in the hole . . . and America went catatonic. . . . Had nothing but CNN everywhere you looked . . . the Baby Jessica report, the Baby Jessica minute, the Baby Jessica second. . . . When they brought her up, it was like the end of a Busby Berkeley musical. . . . That's what's great about the country because everybody was glad. She got dolls, she got candy, bitch got a Toyota truck.

As the emphasis builds in this passage, it is Goldberg's voice, not Fontaine's, that achieves auditory dominance; as the low, slow growl becomes deep and clear, the emphasis on the "patriotic" component of the national concern is undeniable: "She got a telegram from the President of the United States saying that 'as spokesman from the American people, we're glad you're safe.' She couldn't read it but she'll have it to show her children. This is what makes America great."

As with the passage exposing the Jimmy the Greek/Jesse Jackson duality, Goldberg/Fontaine reveals another national double standard. By employing the same sort of comic misdirection, the monologue's celebration of the wealth of concern for "our children" as an American virtue turns into condemnation for the dearth of compassion as a national sin: "The flip side of [the concern for Baby Jessica] is the Ray brothers. The three little boys, who were hemophiliacs, who got AIDS from a transfusion, who got bombed out [of] their own house in [the] neighborhood they grew up in. There was no fervor. There was no 'Oooh, the Ray brothers.' Nothing." Although the intensity builds in this speech, the voice remains Fontaine's, wry, incredulous, and progressively more angry: "There certainly was no telegram from the President saying, 'Look guys, this is un-American behavior, and as your president, I'm going to let the country know that I stand behind you, and I'm going to let the country know because this is not how we handle things here.' Nothing. See, I don't understand that. I don't understand where we were."

Goldberg/Fontaine calls into question the unspoken prejudices, the "acceptable" forms of passive discrimination, implicit in silence and lack of demonstrative concern for the Ray brothers. Fontaine's rhetorical question drips with venom as he acknowledges both the absence of care and of outrage.[10] Goldberg/Fontaine's outrage over there being no "kiss" for these children, or for those adult victims of the AIDS epidemic, from either the general public or the administration, is recontextualized within the character's new sense of clarity and accountability: "See I'm straight now and maybe that's why it's so angering."

As Mel Watkins notes, "In that special, Goldberg proved that she could be as blasphemous as [Eddie] Murphy but her humor spotlighted social and political satire as well as straightout parody."[11] Watkins's comparison of Goldberg to Murphy, while apt on some levels, draws attention to the gendered dimensions of stand-up comedy, in which, the audaciousness of the male's content is viewed differently from that of a female's—with greater license being granted to the former in terms of being as "nasty as you want to be." One might even argue that Goldberg's initial decision to disseminate her scathing critique through the masculine filter of Fontaine speaks to these gendered assumptions. Furthermore, while the audaciousness of Murphy's humor, particularly in *Raw* (1987), was rooted in masculinist discourse on sexual politics, popular culture, and celebrity, Goldberg, who was always overtly political at this point in her career, did not use extended discussions of sexuality as a comic staple.

Goldberg's rise to national prominence in the mid-eighties coincided with an increasingly difficult period for black America. This was an era when the gift of Reaganomics was the ever-expanding gap between rich and poor, and poverty among blacks was at an all-time high. The crack epidemic (another eighties phenomenon) was accompanied by the expansion of violence (gang- and drug-related) and wreaked havoc in urban black America. In the same era when Martin Luther King Jr.'s birthday was established as a national holiday and Jesse Jackson's run for the presidency seemed to act as testaments to how far we had come in the struggle for civil rights, the incarceration of black men rose to record numbers. The eighties marked a period in which African American women writers (from Toni Morrison and Alice Walker to Terry MacMillan), whose work gave voice to a multiplicity of black women's experiences, emerged. At the same time, media images spun new tales of black female archetypes to join the mammy and the jezebel, namely, those of the welfare queen and the black female "buppie" (black urban professional) or the "black lady." Taken in tandem, these emergent tropes of black femininity, like their predecessors, served as yet another means by which black women could be blamed for their own oppression and could be used to offer justification for the cutting of social welfare spending or the limitations sought in relationship to affirmative action. As Wahneema Lubiano notes, "Whether not achieving and passing on bad culture as welfare mothers, or by virtue of having achieved middle-class success . . . black women are responsible for the disadvantaged status of African Americans."[12]

By the mid-eighties the administration's domestic policy had a devastating impact on the underclass—namely, the homeless and the working poor—especially in urban America: from the lost revenue sharing to cities and reduced funding for public service jobs and job training to the elimination of the antipoverty Community Development Block Grant program and the reduction of funds for public transit. One of Goldberg's first public political acts responded to this glaring need in the "greed is good" days in the land of plenty. Goldberg, along with Billy Crystal and Robin Williams, became the public face of Comic Relief, a nonprofit organization created by writer-producer Bob Zmuda in 1986, which used the increased popularity of stand-up to raise funds and awareness to fight homelessness. For Goldberg the telethon stand-up show provided a venue to espouse her strongly held political beliefs with like-minded comic actors. Goldberg became associated with this crusade against homelessness, a cause that cut across boundaries of race, gender, and region and, in so doing, became a high-profile equal opportunity activist.[13] By the early nineties, emboldened by the significant industrial currency from her Academy Award–winning role in *Ghost*, Goldberg became even more insistent on bringing her particular political agenda to the public's attention—regardless of the venue. No longer using characters as vehicles for her discourse, Goldberg's voice, unfiltered, expounded on glaring social and political ills.

Whether pitching a movie on the talk show circuit or hosting an awards show, Goldberg utilized these personal engagements and her high entertainment profile to provide commentary on the current political climate. As the host of a showcase of alternative comedy on HBO, *Chez Whoopi* (1991), held at The Comedy Act, a premiere club for young black talent in South Central Los Angeles, Goldberg's opening monologue focused on the popular conceptions of "the hood" in post–King beating (pre–LA uprising) America:

> Thanks to HBO for being brave, brave white people, thank you. I know how uncomfortable it must be for folks because now that Daryl Gates is gone, I feel a lot better on the streets. [Laughter] No, it's true. And they put

out the Christopher Report and people been saying this shit for two years, have been trying to get the motherfucker out but they said "Mmm, Mmm, [no,] we have to do it the right way." Now, eight motherfuckers [are] saying to get his ass out. Now, if they had read the Goldberg report, they would have known. It had one page said "Fuck him." Bye, bye, Darrel [Gates] . . . good riddance—you can kiss all of our black asses.[14]

Although Goldberg's presence is actually relatively minimal in this special, her monologues acting as the bookends for the show, it clearly illustrates how, by utilizing racially informed politicized observational humor with a clearly articulated agenda, Goldberg used stand-up as a bully pulpit for both her causes and her grievances. While humor was never secondary to her sociopolitical agenda, she was not simply doing a set. Goldberg was giving a lecture, as illustrated in her appearance in *Comic Relief V*, held in Los Angeles in May of 1992, less than a month after the upheaval that, arguably, brought race relations back into the center of American political discourse. This fifth installment, a hip-hop flavored edition, began with Goldberg, Crystal, and Williams's rapping on social ills including homelessness. In so doing, the trio's opening number acted as a concrete recognition of the ways that the understanding of black culture and experience were/are central to dealing with what ails American society—as did their close-up of the Angeleno sociopolitical, economic, and cultural milieu, constructing it as a microcosm of American society rather than as an urban anomaly. Unlike cohost Billy Crystal's monologue, which was delivered as the sexagenarian proprietor of a black-owned business, who had spent his lifetime in the 'hood, which provided an elliptically historicized vision of the post-verdict aftermath in the black community and ended with a vow to rebuild and heal the wounds of the city, Goldberg did not take a reconciliationist tact. "Makes you wonder, 'cause it is hard to justify to young people these days, why the law is there. . . . Now if you break the law, you're supposed to go to jail, right? Right? Oliver North broke the law and now he's out. Bush and Reagan broke the law and they're free. So you're pissed at me for looting?"

By reframing the discussion of the LA uprising in relationship to a different absence of "law and order," Goldberg offers an additional spin on the notion of "equal justice," which was one of the core issues sparking the rebellion. Moreover, by *not* calling for everyone to pull together and, as mayor of Los Angeles Tom Bradley suggested, stay home and watch *The Cosby Show*, Goldberg stood at the beginning of what would be a long line of comics and commentators who contested how the events in April had been televisually constructed and sociopolitically rationalized:

There were a lot of white folks down there. Didn't see them on television. I saw more black folks on TV in the past couple of weeks than I have seen in my entire life. My entire life I have never seen so many black people on TV. I was like, "Hey look, we got households, we got homes and families."

Suddenly, it became interesting for people to know how many folks were out there . . . all because of this. I said to people I don't understand why everyone's surprised, because they knew it was coming. The nation had a nervous breakdown, not just in LA, all over the country.

Goldberg's monologue on *Comic Relief*, like her act on *Chez Whoopi*, gave explicit articulations of the intersections between her blackness and the state of African American community. Given that Goldberg's mediated position within the African American community has been marked by sporadic expressions of ambivalence and antagonism (as will be discussed in greater detail in relation to her film roles), the content of her commentary, its astuteness and insight, is sometimes lost in the impulse to *ignore* the messenger. Whoopi Goldberg—as activist, comic actor, and diva—will not be ignored.

When Goldberg acted as the first African American host of the Academy Awards in 1994, she brought her highly politicized brand of humor to the usually fundamentally apolitical proceedings: speaking directly to supporters and detractors alike, she made her personal political agenda explicit:

I seem to cross so many ethnic and political lines. I'm an equal opportunity offender and to make sure that you don't feel shortchanged on the political soap box department, I'm gonna get it all out of my system right now: save the whales and the spotted owl, gay rights, men's rights, human rights, feed the homeless, more gun control, free the Chinese dissidents, peace in Bosnia, health care reform, choose choice, act up, more AIDS research, less Frank Sinatra finish, Lorena Bobbit please meet Bob Dole, and somebody stop these damn earthquakes. I think I took care of everything . . . including my career.

As self-professed equal-opportunity offender, Goldberg offers a broad swath of critique and establishes her affinity with multiple communities; she also makes clear her unwillingness to being limited by the political agenda of any one of them. While one might argue that Goldberg's construction of her comic personae, onstage (literally and figuratively) was tailor-made for her very personalized politics, the intentionality of the comic in the creation of his or her persona is only half the story; the way in which the personae are seen to mobilize, represent, and speak to varied ideological and cultural impulses in American popular culture is the other half. Clearly, Goldberg's forthright comedic persona posits her in unique and problematic space within the entertainment industry: a sort of A-list star with an asterisk next to her name. The power of that asterisk both signifies her highly politicized public persona and suggests a negative spin on Mike Nichols's early praise—"I have never seen anyone like her." In the film industry, which never seems to know exactly what to do with her, her uniqueness is not necessarily a good thing. This fact becomes progressively and more painfully apparent when examining the body of her comic film work.

In a 2001 interview Goldberg, with characteristic acumen, observed, "I've never been offered a lot of scripts because nobody is sure what to do with me."[15] As a black woman in American film, Goldberg is indeed an anomaly: neither a Hattie McDaniel, known for playing quintessential "mammies," nor a Dorothy Dandridge, whose talent and beauty (in Eurocentric terms) afforded her a wider (although still narrow) field of roles, nor is she a Pam Grier, the blaxploitation queen, who established new parameters of black beauty and female agency during the genre's short reign. Onscreen, Whoopi Goldberg plays with and against these iterations of black womanhood—sometimes subverting and sometimes reifying problematic constructions. While Goldberg's personae offer unique voices for comedic sociopolitical discourse, I would argue that the lineage of their divadom can be traced back to the humor of black women, who—onstage and around the kitchen table—offered their reflections on their American condition. Goldberg is not the only comic presence to play with expectations and to use humor to forward both critique and complacency. Indeed, Jackie "Moms" Mabley and Pearl Bailey are two such black female comic figures who, while not achieving either the industrial success or widespread notoriety of Goldberg, managed to cross over to the mainstream promised land with their divadom intact. If, indeed, as Valerie Smith states, "by reading intersectionally," one might ascertain "the ways racism, misogyny, homophobia, and class discrimination have functioned historically and in the present to subordinate all black people and all women," one might also be able to address the manner in which industrial and cultural practices play out in the movement of mediated images (like comic personae) and the ways in which the images themselves are in conversation with multiple forms of limitation and/or subjugation generated by those aforementioned practices.[16] While the rewards for crossover—in terms of exposure, industrial cachet, and fiscal remuneration—are not insignificant, neither is the price of the ticket, determined by American taste culture as well as the times. Although Bailey, Goldberg, and Mabley thrived in a male-dominated genre, the terms of success, like the times themselves, offered unique struggles and unexpected opportunities.

At first glance, race and humor might be seen as the only qualities that join Pearl Bailey, Moms Mabley, and Whoopi Goldberg. Bailey's Pearlie Mae persona blended lackadaisically saucy sexuality with "down-home" acceptance (and, even celebration) of the sociopolitical status quo. As Dorothy Gilliam noted in her review of Bailey's *Between You and Me: A Heartfelt Memoir on Learning, Loving, and Living*, Bailey "used humor to communicate her view of the world as a joyous, harmonious place that had no great problems or tensions."[17] Mabley adopted the wise, folksy, and risqué "Moms" persona to speak to social and political issues not seen to be within the purview of female comedians during her five decades in show business—from Chitlin' Circuit to Carnegie Hall. "Her ability to move from folksy homilies to ribald double entendre and on to social and political satire was remarkable. Perhaps more than any of the other early

Apollo comics, she foreshadowed the shift to direct social commentary and stand-up techniques that would define humor."[18] Like the multiple and multi-faceted personae of Goldberg, Bailey and Mabley each possessed a distinctive style that captivated audiences across boundaries of class and color, each used humor tied to her respective era to illuminate her worldview, and each was able, within the limits of her chosen medium and personae, to articulate an idio-syncratic, sociopolitically, socioculturally informed brand of comedic discourse. While one might place Goldberg to the left of the political spectrum, Bailey on the right, and Mabley somewhere in the (liberal-leaning) middle, their bodies of work and the working of their bodies (how they were visually constructed) speak to historical constructions of black womanhood. Both Bailey and Mabley have merited studies of their own; however, for the purposes of this study their comic kinship with Goldberg will be examined in relationship to their articu-lations of sexual and political agency and integrationist Americanism, respec-tively, as well as, of course, their shared diva status and the audience and industrial understanding of that construct.

### Remembrances of Divas Past, Part I: Moms Mabley

Elsie A. Williams, in her extensive study *The Humor of Jackie "Moms" Mabley: An African American Comedy Tradition*, captures the comic's status as one who has both mined the history of black humor and sets the trajectory for its future. Mabley made "extensive use of homespun folk imagery, colloquial sayings, stories and jokes commonly known by the African American community—a body of lore which points to the perpetuation of a cultural tradition," while her "womanist stance provided [her] with the strength and character to define her persona and to establish herself as free to say what others of her gender, race and time often had to suppress."[19] Jackie "Moms" Mabley took over five decades to cross over. Mabley's "Moms" persona was born on the vaudeville stages of the Theater Owners' Booking Association (the black venues of the Chitlin' Circuit) while she was still in her twenties and was honed for more than thirty years in performances at the crown jewel of the black theater world, the Apollo Theater in Harlem. By the time Dick Gregory did his famous stint at the Playboy Club in Chicago in 1961, Moms Mabley, using the granny persona as a means to soften her cutting sociocultural critiques (and to lighten the "blue" of some of her more salacious material), also proved to be primed for crossover success— only forty years after she started working on the TOBA circuit. "Her matronly, offbeat appearance and down-home ruminations about politics and the Civil Rights movement, and her fondness for younger men, were perfectly suited to the club's racy image."[20]

In the years that followed this appearance Mabley's crossover success, which had been a long time in coming, was impressive: after her auspicious debut album, *Moms Mabley at the UN*, she made more than twenty recordings on the

Chess label and remains the highest charting comedienne on Billboard.[21] As Williams notes:"With the integrated audiences of the sixties and seventies, the comedian continued to perform, basically, the same kind of folk humor that she had developed on the earlier 'chitlin' circuit,' where the boundary of segregation made the question of boundary practically irrelevant."[22] Through the Moms persona Mabley retained her comic voice in the crossing from TOBA venues to white main stages and beyond—onto the stage of traditional television variety and talk shows (*The Merv Griffin Show*, *The Mike Douglas Show*), as well as those with varying degrees of countercultural hipness (*The Flip Wilson Show*, *Rowan and Martin's Laugh-In*, and *The Smothers Brothers Comedy Hour*). With the exception of lightening the blueness of her "old man" material, Moms remained Moms on the small screen, which solidified her persona and limited her options. Like Goldberg, her black comic diva daughter, Mabley's discursive choices, in terms of the construction of her persona and the content of comedy, played with audience expectations and won popular acclaim. Both comics were also inherently constrained not only by their times but by the multiple and conflicting ideological impulses that inflected the choices in their comedic discourse.

Interestingly, as with Goldberg, there was subversiveness built into Mabley's choices—both of name and of the purposefully desexualized (in Goldberg's case, androgynous) construction of gender. Whereas there was a certain arbitrary (and, arguably, anarchic) component to Goldberg's choice of moniker, Loretta Mary Aiken became Jackie Mabley in response to the actions of two men in her life: a brother, who expressed his embarrassment about his sister's life on the boards, and her first boyfriend, whom she said took so much from her that the least she could do was take his name; the "Moms" nickname was given to her because of the maternal streak that endeared her to fellow performers on the TOBA circuit. Furthermore, after a forced marriage at fifteen to a much older man, who provided the fodder for her myriad "old man" jokes series, Mabley's choice to take the name of her ill-treating beau, not because it was given as a part of wedlock but rather because he "owed" her something, signaled the feminist underpinnings of her persona—as did her choice to construct her appearance. Goldberg's consistent choice of baggy unisex clothing corresponds to Moms' attire, which was, arguably, suggestive of a mammy of sorts (frumpy, oversized housedresses, mismatched colorful clothing, floppy hats, socks with slippers) in that neither had made a fashion choice intended to construct their bodies as objects of desire—rather, they had purposefully covered their bodies in ways that made their female sexuality unobtrusive.

The physicality of their personae seemed intended to contrast directly with the content of their comedy: for the early onstage Goldberg persona her body was a sort of tabula rasa on which she detailed the characters she embodied, with her dark-skinned, dreadlocked androgyny acting as their counterpoint—whether the Surfer Girl or Fontaine. Mabley, on the other hand, modeling "Moms" physically after her own grandmother, constructed a purposefully desexualized persona with touches of both masochism and pathos: the fact that the only thing that "an old man can do for [her] is to deliver a message from a young man" does not negate the frequent waves of self-deprecating and self-denigrating humor. It does not seem an intellectual stretch to hypothesize that the act of taking on the "Moms" persona at such a young age was an extension of Mabley's lived experiences—many of which had robbed Loretta Mary Aiken of both her youth and her innocence.[23] The disparity between the libidinous nature of her monologues (often on the merits of young men and the deficiencies of the old) and her rubbery-faced mugging, gravel-voiced delivery, and desexualized appearance did not diminish the liberatory potential of her comedic discourse, as illustrated in this passage crediting her grandmother for her "hipness":

> I never will forget my granny. . . . You know who hipped me, my great-grandmother. Her name was Harriet Smith; she lived in Brevard, North Carolina. This is the truth! She lived to be 118 years old. And you wonder why Moms is hip today? Granny hipped me. She said, they lied to the rest of them, but I'm not gonna let you be dumb. I'm gonna tell you the truth. In fact when they'd tell me them fairy lies, Granny'd tell me the truth about it. One day she's sitting out on the porch and I said, "Granny, how old does a, does a woman get before she don't want no more boyfriends?" She was around 106 then. She said, "I don't know, honey, you'll have to ask somebody older than me."

By foregrounding both her sexual agency and autonomy from what had to be seen as a highly marginalized position, Mabley forwarded a commonsense feminist agenda "allow[ing] for public discussion of the female's sexual needs and . . . focus[ing] on the inadequacy of the [usually old] male to fulfill such needs, both off-limits as subjects in comedy routines by women until very recently."[24]

Despite the sometimes socially defiant content of her act, Mabley's comedic agenda was varied and, at times, also supported a sociopolitical status quo. In the introduction for one of her song-as-position papers, "Pray, Little Children, Pray," on *Moms the Word*, which was fundamentally a musical indictment of the 1962 Supreme Court's decision banning state mandated prayer,[25] Mabley made clear her willingness to speak her mind regardless of whether her particular stance was particularly popular with her audience: "They did wrong when they gave Moms freedom of speech 'cause I'm gonna tell the truth about it. Although they might put Moms in jail for what I'm gonna say—but by God, I'm gonna say it anyway." Furthermore, in the Cold Warrior years of the mid-sixties (and later on the aforementioned album) Mabley's persona gained a new dimension, constructed as doing "government business . . . lyin' and spyin', you dig. Got Khruschev and the Chinaman [Mao Tse-tung] fussin'," she annunciated a clearly anticommunist sentiment and reified African American ties to the Democratic Party, in general, and, perhaps less enthusiastically, to Lyndon Baines

Johnson.[26] In her commentaries on civil rights Mabley's adherence to the revolutionary directives of the movement was unequivocal. Her observations about both racial violence and the struggles of black activists were encased in vaudevillian-styled joke series, which provided pointed critique within the guise of old-fashioned entertainment, as exemplified on her album *Moms at the White House*:

> Colored fellow down home died. Pulled up to the gate. St. Peter look at him, say, "What do you want?" "Hey man, you know me. Hey, Jack, you know me. I'm old Sam Jones. Old Sam Jones, man, you know me. Used to be with the NAACP, you know, CORE and all that stuff, man, marches, remember me? Oh, man, you know me." He just broke down there, "You know me." He looked in his book. "Sam Jones," he say, "no, no you ain't here, no Sam Jones." He said, "Oh, man, yes, I am; look there. You know me. I'm the cat that married that white girl on the Capitol steps of Jackson, Mississippi." He said, "How long ago has that been?" He said, "About five minutes ago."

While the light blueness of her humor and the barely disguised socio-political commentary may seem mild by contemporary standards, Moms Mabley was an innovative force in American comedy. As a veteran of both the Chitlin' Circuit and the overt discrimination and racism its performers experienced, Mabley created a comic persona informed by the sensibility of the trickster, common in African and African American folklore, and by utilizing verbal sleight of hand, she simultaneously employed and critiqued those archetypal constructions for her own purposes. In other words, her persona still operated within a stone's throw of the mammy, thus supplying some degree of comfort to audiences to whom the minstrel archetypes still appealed, but the content of her comedy was inflected by a mitigated sense of rebellion. She constructed a comic persona that subverted long-held social predispositions as the desexualized, alternately cantankerous and kindly sort of revisionist mammy, who uses comedic strategies associated with masculine forms of black humor (playing "the dozens" and "signifying"). Through this construction she positioned herself not simply within the black comic traditions of the past, in which the critique of mainstream America had to be coded and hidden, but also, in the spirit of the civil rights era, within a new form of direct comedic sociopolitical discourse, in which the voices of marginalized people—including black women—could be heard.

### CINEMATIC CONVERGENCES: DE-SEXED, DE-RACED—MOMS, WHOOPI, AND AGENCY

Although Jackie Mabley made her big-screen debut in the small role of Marcella in the 1933 version of *The Emperor Jones*, starring Paul Robeson, her big-screen time was minimal. She made only six films in her career of almost six decades, three of which were race-film versions of skits in her vaudeville act, *Big Timers* (1945), *Killer Diller* (1948), and *Boarding House Blues* (1948), and all were made before the beginning of the civil rights movement. In these early films, as well as in the concert film of a 1969 black music festival held in New York's Yankee Stadium, *It's Your Thing* (1970), where Mabley delivered a particularly poignant version of the pop homage to slain American leaders, "Abraham, Martin, and John," Moms performed time-coded versions of her comic persona.

Only in her first and last films was Mabley actually asked to play a role: as Marcella (uncredited) in *The Emperor Jones* and as Grace, the title character in Stan Lathan's *Amazing Grace* (1974). The latter film is more memorable as a final

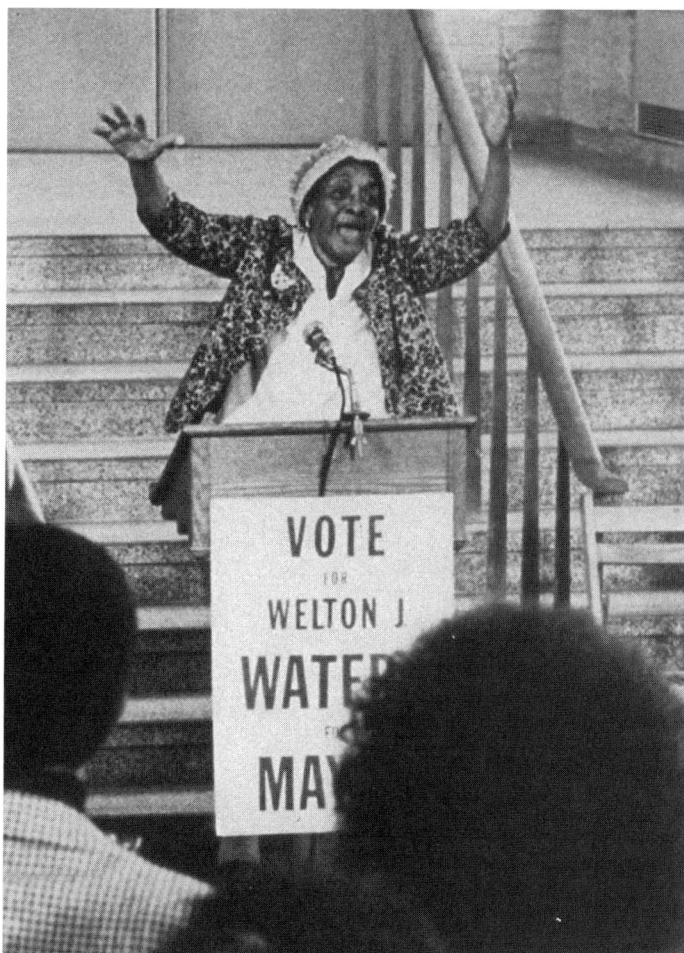

19. Moms Mabley's first starring role and her final performance as *Amazing Grace* (1974). Directed by Stan Lathan. Photo from Photofest. Reproduced with permission from United Artists.

showcase for the mugging and preaching aspects of Mabley's persona[27] and for
the appearance of black stars from the cinematic and vaudeville past like Slappy
White, Butterfly McQueen, and Stepin Fetchit than as an uneven social comedy about inner-city politics (with the system eventually "working" because
Mabley's Grace *reminds* the parties in question how the system should work).
Perhaps more significant is Mabley's positioning of both herself and the film
made during the blaxploitation age: "I'm not a Black moviemaker. I'm everybody's moviemaker all nations and all colors. I don't want to make any of my
brothers and sisters angry so I can't say what I want to say about a lot of
those Black films. But Moms don't make that kind of movie. Ours is a family
movie."[28]

By the time Mabley made it back to the big screen, both her comic sensibility and her notion of blackness seemed slightly out of step with the post–civil
rights era. Grace, unlike her previous constructions of the randy granny/
mammy, was full of hopefulness and certainty that the sociopolitical ills of the
black community could be solved by working within the existing institutional
structures—absent was any edge or cynicism embedded in either the film's narrative or in the nuances in Mabley's performance. Furthermore, the ethos of
color-blind family entertainment puts Moms squarely in the integrationist
camp—particularly given the contrasts she makes between her film and the
films associated with black power–informed agency (*Foxy Brown* or *Truck Turner*,
both 1974), as well as those that worked with a post–civil rights culturally
specific comedic framework, like *Uptown Saturday Night* (also 1974). While it is
not surprising that civil rights era sentiments informed the notion of black
activism and identity in terms of Mabley's comedic social discourse, the language of her differentiation between her film and the seventies black cinematic
fare, in this instance, seems oddly deferential. As though aware that this color-
blind assertion was somehow controversial at a decidedly not color-blind time
in the nation's history, Moms Mabley, comic diva, seemed reticent to speak her
mind.

In its previous stage and small-screen iterations, the Moms persona utilized
"mammy"-like dress and, to a lesser extent, behaviors (speech and gesture) to
present herself as one who could not be seen as a sexual object and, as such,
gave this familiar figure license to speak about sexual desire and acts because
there is no (perceived) possibility of her achieving sexual autonomy. Furthermore, Mabley, with her race simultaneously centered and elided because of the
randy granny/revisionist mammy construction, was able to speak to and of
aspects of the African American experience—without causing undue discomfort to mainstream audiences. On the cusp of the post-soul era, which begins
after both the civil rights and black power movements, the cultural, political, and
economic realities of life in the African American community problematize the
notion of overcoming someday when integrationist rhetoric did not assuage
fears and hostilities in Boston in 1976 anymore than it had initially in Little

Rock over two decades before.[29] Thus, one might assume that the notion of color-blind comedy coming from a desexualized black woman, one that seemed dated in the seventies, would have undoubtedly passed out of cinematic favor—one would be wrong.

Goldberg, in her dramatic roles, has played her share of revisionist mammies: the Jamaican housekeeper who heals the wounds left by the loss of her son by transforming the coming-of-age experience of her young white charge in *Clara's Heart* (1988); the stoic maid whose decision to respect the bus boycott transforms her white employer's understanding of the civil rights struggle in *The Long Walk Home* (1990); the musically adept babysitter who transforms the lives of her white family by fulfilling their professional and emotional needs in the first of Goldberg's interracial romances, *Corinna, Corinna* (1994); and even as a free-spirited lesbian singer who is transformed by her (unrequited) affection for her uptight white former real estate broker, for whom Goldberg's character becomes caretaker as she is dying from AIDS in *Boys on the Side*. In her comic roles, however, as previously mentioned, Goldberg's persona was often constricted in roles that were not intended for her and, as a result, the films featured a desexed and deraced Goldberg.

Even in her Academy Award winning supporting role as Oda Mae Brown in *Ghost* (1990), Goldberg, as the spiritualist conduit for the recently deceased

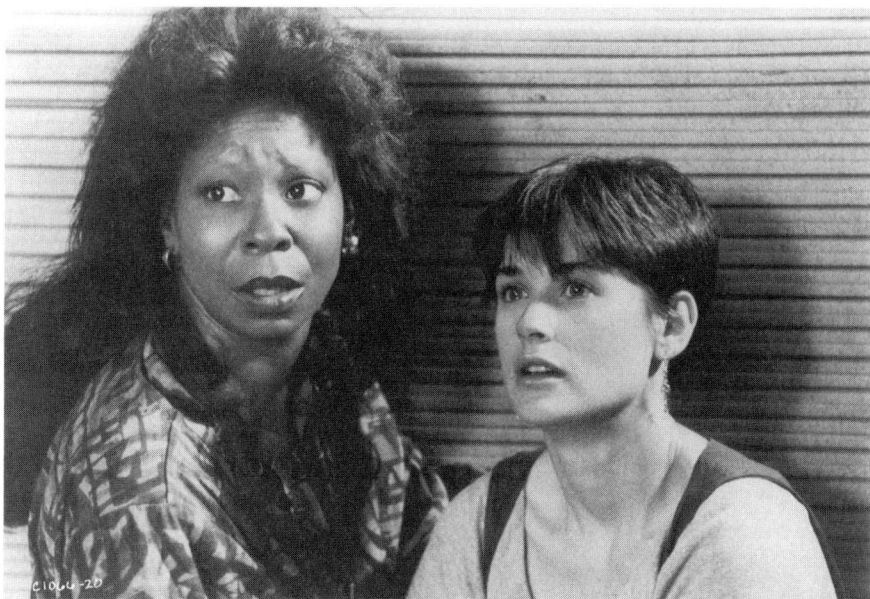

20. Whoopi Goldberg in her Oscar-winning role as Oda Mae Brown, the medium for yuppie love, with Demi Moore (as Molly Jensen) in *Ghost* (1990). Directed by Jerry Zucker. Photo from Photofest. Reproduced with permission from Paramount Pictures.

Sam and his grieving lover, Molly (played by Patrick Swayze and Demi Moore, respectively), besides providing comic relief in what would have otherwise been a supernatural weepie, gives her body in service to the tragic white couple. Interesting opportunities to play with both race and sexuality are squandered: play with this visual of Goldberg, in a big bad bouffant hairdo (rather than her usual dreadlocks), kissing Moore, in her eponymous pixie cut, could have been a means to question the nature of love (à la *Prelude to a Kiss*). Taking the easier, softer route, the hug and kisses shared between Molly and Sam via Oda Mae begin with Goldberg leaning in to Moore only to cut to Swayze touching Moore. Direct references to race were minimal and were not about being nuanced: Oda Mae, clad in one of many garish outfits (even by early-nineties' standards), bellows about "white men trying to kill me" as she beats a hasty retreat. Given the narrative's less-than-adventurous spirit, the lion's share of the film's comedy comes from Oda Mae's antics, which, although not the "Oh, Lawd" full-body tremors of Mantan Moreland, still hearken back to those all too familiar cinematic constructions of black folks and spooks. Donald Bogle describes the sequence in which Oda Mae, who has become a spiritual entrepreneur rather than a charlatan after her initial encounter with Sam, is occupied by an impatient spirit. Oda Mae, with great mugging effort, expels the spirit, and Bogle, while appreciative of the "funny," notes with some degree of resignation "the truth of the matter is that while we might have hoped that blacks terrified of ghosts would now be consigned to the era when Willie Best popped his eyes as Bob Hope's servant in *The Ghost Breakers* in 1940, Oda Mae Brown is yet another readily excitable creature, often lit up with comic fear. . . . Goldberg warmly modulates her reactions, giving them human dimensions. But an old set of stereotypical responses has simply been revamped for a new generation."[30]

The way in which Oda Mae's body is used in service to white happiness shows more than a passing similarity to the function of the mammy, as does the almost absurd desexualized physical appearance of the character, a fact that neither the warmth nor the humor of Goldberg's performance can negate. Goldberg's comic persona was repeatedly positioned within narratives that cut any possible sociopolitical edginess with integrationist sentiments in color-blind comedic morality plays. Nowhere was this more apparent than in the 1992 vehicle penned with Bette Midler in mind, *Sister Act*.

Like Moms' Grace, Goldberg's Deloris Van Cartier's construction was informed by a color-blind comic sensibility that seemed out of sync with both post–King beating America and Goldberg's own stand-up comic discourse. *Sister Act* is fundamentally a fish-out-of-water comedy in a nun's costume. First shown as the bespangled Diana Ross wannabe in a budget version of the Supremes, playing to a single unenthusiastic patron in a Reno casino, Goldberg is made to look intentionally absurd—and of questionable musical talent. The ill-fated romance between Deloris and Vince LaRocca, which ends when the former sees the latter directing a hit, is the plot device that hurls Goldberg's fish out of water; however, "it is worth noting race is a subject that *Sister Act* assumes is of no importance to the audience," and "nothing is ever made of the fact that white actor, Harvey Keitel, plays Goldberg's boyfriend."[31] The purposeful avoidance of any recognition of racial difference is undeniable: the only line that makes even passing reference to race is when Deloris questions the origins of her new name, Sister Mary Clarence, inquiring whether "Clarence" refers to Clarence Williams III, who played Linc, the black member of television's *Mod Squad*. At times, the color-blind ethos strains credulity—in the frantic casino chase climax of the film, no one thinks to cite the race of the only black nun in the convent as an identifying detail.

Given that the film was not written for Goldberg, when "race as subtext" appears in the narrative, it goes uninterrogated. For example, one can easily read the other inhabitants of the convent's immediate fascination with Sister Mary Clarence as a racialized moment—although their fetishizing of the activities of her fictional "progressive" order acts as the unwitting signifier for the "hipness" factor of black culture. When put in charge of the order's abysmal choir, Deloris/Sister Mary Clarence makes them into "chorus girls" with choreography and song styling influenced as much by gospel production numbers (their sanctified version of "Salve Regina") as those found on the Reno strip (their retooling of the Motown Classic into "My God")—although the influence of the former is never recognized. Furthermore, as critic Janet Maslin noted, race continues to inflect the audience's reading of the film: "[Deloris/Sister Mary Clarence is] scorned by Mother Superior (Maggie Smith), who disdains loud clothes and vulgar manners. Scenes that might have played as mere snobbery with Ms. Midler have the hint of racism, which might have been dispelled if the film had only addressed it head on."[32]

The elision of race is further codified with the progressive desexualizing of Deloris. A nun's habit serves even better than a frumpy housedress to establish the character as fundamentally asexual. Despite protestations to the contrary (throw-away lines like "and they don't even have sex"), the adjustment to convent life was not rooted in a sexual being's forced celibacy but rather in one who loves the night life being forced to be good and go to bed early. The transformation is complete once Deloris has the priorities of Sister Mary Clarence—willingly endangering herself (and, unintentionally, the rest of the convent) in order to perform the "big show" for the Pope, no less. While, Sister Mary Clarence initially exhibits flashes of chutzpah (moments of archetypal Whoopi), there are fewer such moments as the film progresses. Once rendered asexual and colorless, Goldberg's persona in Deloris/Mary Clarence is comfortably contained—and that made for good box office. Reaping $232 million worldwide, *Sister Act* is the highest grossing film in which Goldberg has starred and was, arguably, her last film to win popular, though not critical, acclaim. Ironically, the color-blind credo of *Sister Act*, released in May of 1992, was diametrically

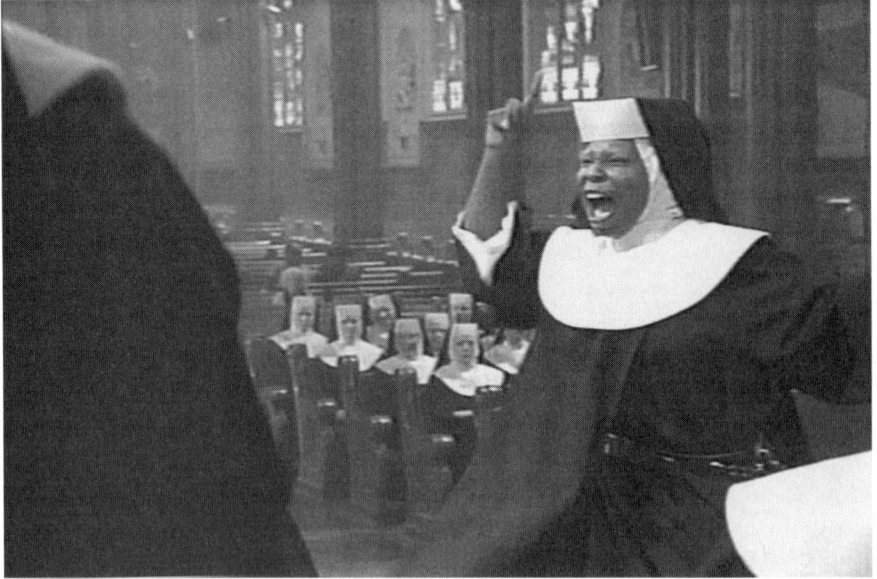

21. Whoopi gets the spirit and gives a little Motown-infused inspiration in *Sister Act* (1992). Directed by Emile Ardolino.

opposed to the comedic sociopolitical diatribe Goldberg had delivered onstage at Comic Relief earlier the same month. Although the times were decidedly not color-blind, the comic narratives that got big grosses, on some fundamental levels, needed to be for mainstream popularity and consumption. It must be noted that "for African American audiences, [Goldberg's] movies are also funny but possibly alienating. Goldberg herself endows her characters with an ethnic definition . . . through language, intonation, inflection and attitude. . . . But it becomes frustrating that such cultural distinctions are often used only as points of derision in these films."[33]

Bogle's frustration notwithstanding, given the success of this film (and Goldberg's willingness to conform her comic persona to mainstream cinematic imperatives), one would think that she would have no difficulty in continuing to be one of the few black female comic actors able to open a film. That has not always been the case—and the reasons why are by no means transparent. On one hand, the disparity between the comic film roles and her outspoken comedic sociopolitical discourse, although apparent, might not necessarily account for a decline in her cinematic popularity. On the other, her undeniable comic prowess and the purposeful construction of her comic personae may be, at times, in contentious conversation with the sociopolitical moment. Unlike Mabley, who read such moments warily and tread gingerly in positioning herself and her responses to those who positioned her, for Goldberg, as the lines between person and persona began to blur extratextually, her outspoken nature gave greater license (and fodder) for criticism and scrutiny.

### REMEMBRANCES OF DIVAS PAST, PART II: PEARL BAILEY

The kinship between the personae of Pearlie Mae and Whoopi may seem a bit more tenuous than ties between those of Goldberg and Mabley. While Pearl and Whoopi occupy opposite ends of the political and comedic spectrum, the comic personae of Goldberg are clearly inflected by her unabashed liberalism (which, only on occasion, actually informs her cinematic construction) just as Bailey's Pearlie Mae, while not directly addressing her unapologetic conservative political beliefs, invested heavily in the creation of idyllic constructions of Americanism, where the discussion of race was simply deemed unnecessary. Their personae were honed in their early stage performance—for Goldberg in small theaters before heading to Broadway and for Bailey in Chitlin' Circuit theaters and, quite early in her career, white, as well as black, nightclubs before becoming the unequivocal star of a Broadway show.

In their debuts on the great white way, as originators of roles—Whoopi in her retooled *Spook Show* debut and Pearl as the first Aunt Hagar in *St. Louis Blues*—each caused a sensation on Broadway. Whereas the former tapped into the wellspring of her multiple personae, the latter, despite high critical praise, only sampled a narrow swath of hers. Interestingly, each was involved in "non-traditional" casting coups when they took over roles in Broadway musicals from white actor predecessors. In each case the "fact" of race was downplayed. When Goldberg followed in Nathan Lane's role of Pseudolus in the revival of Stephen Sondheim's *A Funny Thing Happened on the Way to the Forum*, the casting controversy was as much about the fact that a woman was taking over the role as the fact that a black actor was playing the role of a "smart slave." Playing the role with equal parts broad vaudevillian style (utilized by both Lane and the original Pseudolus, Zero Mostel) and sly androgynous trickster, Goldberg fit with the bawdiness of the show's humorous tone. When Bailey followed Carol Channing in the role of Dolly in a black-cast version of Jerry Herman's *Hello Dolly*, a production that was seen as a risky venture in 1967, the character was remade into an ideal vehicle for the Pearlie Mae persona. The ad-lib prone Bailey enhanced the original with a swagger and sassiness that Channing's effusive Levi (and Streisand's Fanny Briced-Levi) lacked. Interestingly, Bailey bristled when the show was referred to as "all black," maintaining that she viewed it "as being all [read multi] colored."[34] However, although the Pearlie Mae persona made its way into her stage roles (although not, for the most part, into her screen roles), the nightclub was its perfect habitat.

The nightclub Bailey, captured best on her "For Adults Only" albums, used her act to establish her persona, which was described as "a girl who knew the

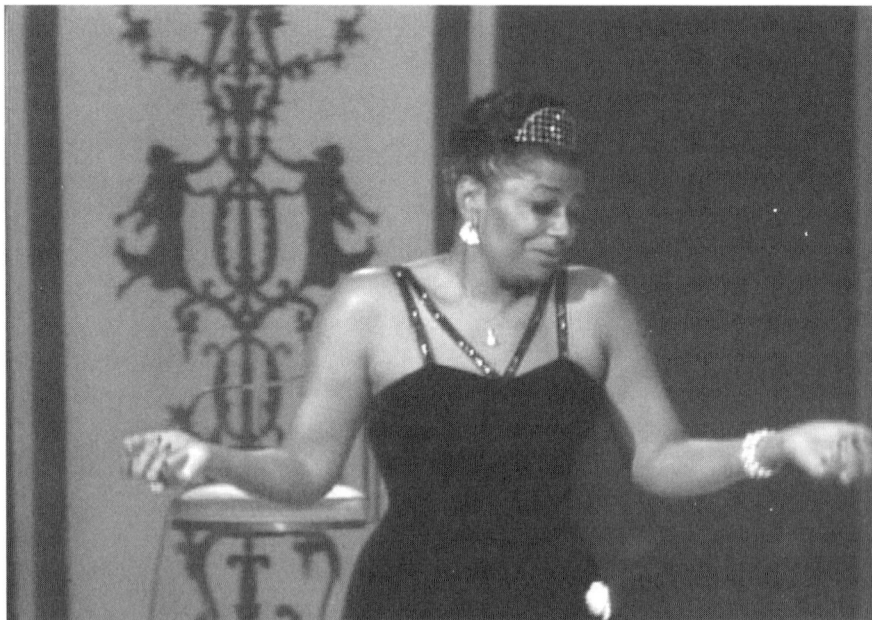

22. Pearl Bailey, sassy onstage and screen for decades. Photo from *Carol Channing and Pearl Bailey: On Broadway* (1969). Directed by Clark Jones.

facts of life but inevitably got her facts all mixed up."[35] This portrait of Pearlie Mae as a woman who been done wrong (and has done wrong, too) comes through, not only in the double entendre–filled songs but also in the asides and ad-libs that play with audience sensibilities. More naughty than genuinely blue, Bailey's act, when brought to the small screen, retained many of the mildly provocative elements that had won her mainstream popularity. By the late forties Bailey, already a nightclub veteran and having won raves for her supporting role in *St. Louis Woman*, was performing on television variety programs like *Cavalcade of Stars: Starring Jackie Gleason*. Described by Gleason as "the star that outshone the rest," when she came onstage, more than traces of divadom can be seen in Bailey's performance style. Her mannerisms were the same in 1949 as they would be in 1970 onstage in her own television variety show—she is sassy. Clad in a very feminine black strapless dress with jeweled bodice, tight waist, and full skirt, Bailey is definitely not desexualized nor is her song selection, "Good Enough for Me." Alternately singing and *talking* her way through the number, Bailey crosses musical theatrics with down-home earthiness:

> There are lots of girls who will stay out late.
> *Why do they do that? They think they are being very bright.*
> *But, not I. I say to myself Pearl be a lady. Be a lady.*
> *That's why I always come home every night except*
> *Saturday, Sunday, Monday, and sometimes it's slow getting in on Thursday.*

When I settle down and get married
I want all of my in-laws to be
*Simple country folk like the Vanderbilts, the Whitneys, the Morgans,*
*That's not a bad selection there.*
They're good enough for me
*You know the trouble with the world today is the women.*
*Women are selfish, they're greedy, so mercenary . . . I hear a man*
*They want mink coats. They want sable coats. Can you blame 'em? Do they*
*    get them? NO! they never get around to them. But I'm not like that.*
*    When a gentlemen gets me a gift I want him to get me something with*
*    sentimental value—something with a lot of heart to it that you can hold*
*    onto like a parking lot or something like that.*

Watching Bailey perform on her ABC variety show almost two decades later, the shtick is very much the same—although the content has been made even more family friendly. Her interactions with the audience, with asides and free-floating "darlings," create a sense of small-club intimacy in a large auditorium. Moreover, by her series premiere in 1970, both her clothing and her act had become more modest: with higher necklines replacing strapless fare, pants replacing full skirts, and Pearl's pearls of wisdom replacing rampant double entendre. One need only see the opening number of her series premiere to see the convergence of personae (Pearl as Dolly as Pearlie Mae), particularly when Bailey makes the kind of entrance one expects from a diva: with a chorus singing her praises. Reminiscent of Dolly's descent into that show's production number, "Hello Dolly," Bailey stands at the back of the house in gold lamé gown, diamond jewelry, and a chinchilla coat as an integrated group of chorus boys, dressed as ushers in red jackets with gold braid, sing, "Here comes joy, here comes love, here comes Pearlie Mae." An usher hands her roses as she saunters down the center aisle. Singing the chorus from another diva musical, "Applause," Bailey ad-libs freely between the lines of lyrics. Even a flubbed line becomes an opportunity for engaging the audience. Bailey throws an aside directly at one woman in the front row: "Can you ever believe this? . . . I just blew the first two words"; she sings, "Applause, Applause, Applause," adding, "Come on, honey, I'm live," before going on with the rest of the song. With "honeys" and "babys" sprinkled throughout, the song, this version belongs to Bailey as completely as the single roses she tosses out to the audience—and they appear enraptured by her presence. The presence is diva but a comforting kind of diva—making her audience at home in *her* theater. "Pearl never pushed her humor to the point where it might disturb an audience. [Whereas] Moms or Redd [Foxx] . . . seemed bent in driving up the wall with their incisive barbs, Bailey . . . was always a soothing figure."[36] Her guests were her musical contemporaries, past and present: Andy Williams, Bing Crosby, and Louis Armstrong. With the exception of a touching duet with Armstrong (clearly in his waning years), which was filled with reminiscences about "the old days" on the club circuit, Bailey's divadom was dimmed by deference to her "star" friends. Bailey literally gushed about the A-list talent she had proffered for her series premiere to such an extent that it almost seemed sycophantic. While this audience was clearly enthralled by the onstage Pearlie Mae, the viewing public did not appear to be; the show lasted only one season.

While one might argue that this was due to the waning popularity of the variety show, there were regressive aspects of the Pearlie Mae persona that some found troubling. Whereas her moments of self-aggrandizement were normal diva fare, her moment of deference, as well as her complaints about her aching feet as part of chronic lamentations about fatigue from performing, like her drawling version of "Tired," which she sang in her film debut, *Variety Girl* (1947), has more than just a trace of minstrelsy—acting as yet another spin on the revisionist mammy, in this case, one whose "people" are working her too hard. The coexistence of the diva and the mammy in the Pearlie Mae persona, in actuality, corresponds with the extratextual construction of Bailey in American popular consciousness: comforting to and comforted by the sociopolitical status quo, Bailey manages to occupy her own color-coded yet color-blind space in terms of her persona and social and industrial position, respectively. When one begins to examine how Bailey's espoused ideologies and her personal politics were received on the broader stage of popular opinion, one sees surprising correlations between the star's mediated construction and that of Goldberg, the comic diva on the other end of the political spectrum.

### EXTRATEXTUAL CONVERGENCES: PEARL, WHOOPI, PERSONAL POLITICS, AND (INTER)RACIALIZING WAYS

As with many performers, like Goldberg and Mabley, whose strong onstage personae define the popular conception of both the performer and her relationship to the era, the later iterations of Pearlie Mae, in the late sixties and early seventies, became a de facto poster girl for a conservative form of integration: like the version utilized on network television during the same time period, it meant there was only one persona of color. For those in the African American community who begrudged Bailey the "mammying" in her act, "her penchant for hamming it up with Republican presidents" was even more disturbing. As Dorothy Gilliam states in her review of one of Bailey's books, *Between You and Me: A Heartfelt Memoir of Learning, Loving, and Living*, "Sure, she's an ardent Republican, but many blacks wondered why she flaunted it with Nixon and Reagan—presidents many blacks and whites considered downright hostile to black advancement."[37] Not only was Bailey a welcomed visitor in the Nixon White House; she was also appointed special ambassador to the United Nations by Ford in 1975 and was awarded the Presidential Medal of Freedom by Reagan in 1988. Her friendships (particularly with First Lady Betty Ford, with whom she did a song and dance in Kraft's *All-Star Salute to Pearl Bailey*) established her affinity with Republican administrations in much the same way that Goldberg's presence on the campaign trail and in the 1992 Inaugural Celebration did with the Clinton White House. In both instances the comic divas maintained their allegiance to their presidents, regardless of the changes in the political climate—Bailey through Nixon's resignation and Goldberg through Clinton's impeachment.[38] While one can find other female comics—black and white—for whom the identity politics of their personae impact the way audiences do or do not embrace them—from Ellen Degeneres's coming out across media (on "The Puppy Episode" on her series, as well as in *Time* magazine) to the explicit discussions of sexual practice by Margaret Cho and Sommore in conversation with the sociocultural position of women of color in American popular culture. For Bailey and Goldberg, from opposite ends of the political spectrum, the rejection of the prevailing racial label and the commitment to interracial relationships, which was considered controversial back in each of their days, play different roles in how both comic divas were seen inside and outside of the black community.

Bailey's insistence that she had "never been hemmed in" by racial labels, and her refusal to use them, seemed comparable to the declarations of racial autonomy annunciated in later years by Republican stalwarts like Ward Connerly or Condoleezza Rice. Her "colorless" identity politics was rooted in a rehistoricized and very individual notion of race relations and an "up by your own bootstraps" American Dream ethos: "Growing up in the coalfields of Pennsylvania—You can't tell me that there was a problem with Blackness. . . . I don't wallow in the pity of what I am. . . . [Those who feel] 'I am mistreated because I am this color' then I feel sorry for them. . . . I am looking for this Blackness because I don't use the word, I don't think it's necessary. I think that's a fad to go along with 'I need my identity, baby.'"[39] Like many of the remarks made by Bailey on the CBS interview series *Signature* in 1982, the content of her commentary and its rejection of blackness as a designation is not as significant as her unapologetic and unwavering tone. Even during the early Reagan era the assertion of blackness had cultural and political resonance—particularly within the black community. Her "dismissal," not only of the word but of both the recuperation and agency embedded in the naming process as part of the "identity fad," denigrates myriad efforts within the black community to have some sense of history and cultural pride—something about which Bailey seemed fundamentally unconcerned. Associated with civil rights struggle and racial pride, *black* was the term that was used to signify both solidarity and empowerment in the days before *African American* became the (ostensibly) preferred expression. Thus, Bailey's rejection of the term seemed fairly consistent with her individualistic ideologies.

Interestingly, Bailey's vocal aversion to *black* is matched in intensity by Goldberg's aversion to *African American*. The chapter entitled "Race" in Goldberg's *Book* begins:

> Call me an asshole, call me a blowhard, but don't call me African American.
> Please. It divides us as a nation and as a people, and it kinda pisses me off.
> It diminishes everything I've accomplished and everything every other

black person has accomplished on American soil. . . . Every time you put
something in front of the word *American*, it strips it out of its meaning. The
Bill of Rights is my Bill of Rights, same as anyone else's. It's my flag. It's my
Constitution. It doesn't talk about *some* people. It talks about *all* people—
black, white, orange, brown. You. Me.[40]

Goldberg's association of hyphenated American terms with the denigration of
national identity presents an interesting thesis. Written in 1997, long before the
post-9/11 "patriotic" elisions of race, Goldberg's chapter presents a separation
of national and racial identity that speaks to the complex construction of clearly
delineated racial and national identities. While no more problematic than other
discourses around the ideological power of naming and the significance of the
recuperation of blackness, the expansiveness of her assertion (that the term
diminishes her accomplishment and every other black person's) adopts a tone
that is both unequivocal in its stance and condescending to those who view
things differently. Yet unlike Bailey's feeling sorry for those swept up in the
"identity fad" of blackness, Whoopi's rejection of "African American" also
encompasses a sense of both group identity and group oppression. One could
argue that the naming process is intensely personal, informed and inflected by
lived experience, as well as by multiple ideologies—clearly this is the case for
both Goldberg and Bailey. What is far more significant, for the purposes of this
study, is the way they defiantly frame and privilege their assertion of identity—
not in terms of highly personalized statements, which, given their personae, one
might expect, but rather as clearly annunciated ideological directives. One
should also note that Goldberg's annunciation of blackness and the fact that her
comedy addresses the continuance of racism also makes her discursive case on
a social and political level. Nonetheless, both Bailey and Goldberg were telling
it, not necessarily like it is, but as she feels it should be.

As celebrities involved in interracial relationships, one might expect that
both Goldberg and Bailey have received their share of criticism from black and
white communities and one would be correct. What is far more interesting is
the disjuncture between the level of ferociousness of the criticism and the time
period in which Bailey and Goldberg's life experiences actually occurred. It
seems that popular opinion, or at least the impressions given by the popular
press, reveals that during Bailey's day, which was not necessarily hospitable to
either interracial relationships or the celebrities who engaged in them, her marriage to drummer Louis Bellson did not carry with it industrial or sociopolitical ill will. Yet during the eighties and nineties, when interracial relationships
were on the significant upswing (as was the almost fetishistic entertainment
press coverage of celebrities), Goldberg's relationships with white actors Timothy Dalton, Frank Langella, and Ted Danson often fueled controversy and served
to delegitimize her position within the African American community.

Bailey and Big Band drumming virtuoso Bellson were wed in 1952, six
years before Mildred Jeter and Richard Loving, a black woman and a white

man, would marry in Washington, D.C.; seven years before the Lovings were convicted of violating antimiscegenation laws in the state of Virginia, where they had hoped to make their home; and eleven years before the Warren Court held that the Virginia statutes banning interracial marriage violated the equal protection and due process clauses of the Fourteenth Amendment. While Bailey's stardom, which was, for much of her career, established in nightclubs and theatrical venues (as well as in the recording industry), appeared to be unhindered by her status as part of a "mixed" couple, other black female contemporaries were not as fortunate. Lena Horne, singer, film star, and iconic black beauty, famous for her films like *Stormy Weather* and *Cabin in the Sky*, married musical arranger Lennie Hayton in 1947 but kept the marriage secret for three years for fear of the backlash from blacks and whites. One might hypothesize that it was the elegant Horne's status as one of the only black sex symbols of the pre–civil rights era, referred to as the café au lait Hedy Lamarr in her early years in nightclubs and in her numerous USO appearances during World War II, in contrast to Bailey's Pearlie Mae persona, constructed as a down-home girl, that offended both blacks and whites to the extent that the couple received hate mail and threats of violence.[41] If Bailey experienced this kind of animosity, she chose not to share it in public venues; rather, similar to her discussions of those who felt discriminated against based on race, she talked of the acceptance that she and her husband had received and positioned it as the norm, thus refuting notions of intolerance: "Lou and I got to sleep in Lincoln's bed—a mixed couple. Oh, dear."[42] Like much of Bailey's discourse on race, she framed her interracial marriage, and public reactions to it, as an issue only if someone, misguided by the "identity fad," wanted to make it an issue. While the extratextual construction of her life as part of an interracial couple may have challenged the race-relations status quo simply by its existence, *no* status quo was ever the target of her Pearlie Mae persona, which might explain why, in a decidedly less-tolerant time, she fared so much better (industrially and personally) than did Whoopi Goldberg.

Goldberg's interracial relationships have become comic fodder for black comedy, so much so that in Spike Lee's *Bamboozled* the character of Junebug (played by veteran comic Paul Mooney) jokes that the Hollywood blockbuster that he would make would be a sci-fi film called *The Last White Man on Earth* and that "Whoopi Goldberg and Diana Ross will be fighting over him." While jokes about the personal lives of celebrities have become progressively more common in American comedy, in Goldberg's case this extratextual reality is often mobilized to critique her onscreen choices and the reading of her comic personae. Nowhere is this more apparent than in the furor over the public aspects of her relationship with Ted Danson and their romantic comedy, *Made in America* (1993). As Jacqueline Genovese's article highlights, the fact that Goldberg was, at that point in 1993, "the highest paid woman in Hollywood . . . [was] not what's making headlines these days. Goldberg's rumored affair with her

*Made in America* co-star Ted Danson has forced its way from the tabloids to *McCall's* and *Parade* magazines."[43]

Although in numerous interviews Goldberg tried to turn the focus back to *Made in America*, her first romantic comedy, the subtext often dealt with her relationship with Danson as well: "You know, when I said [to studio executives in the past], 'Gee, I'd like to, you know, act with Dustin Hoffman,' they'd go, 'Well, you can only do a comedy. You can't do a love story because nobody's ready for an interracial love story.' . . . I think there's been enough interracial couples around. With a war in Bosnia, am I really going to worry about it?"[44] Like most of her comedies, *Made in America* was not written with Goldberg (or any black actor) in mind. At Goldberg's behest the revisions in the script attempted to embrace both her race and comic style, as well as the resurgence of Afrocentric sensibility emerging in the early nineties. As a result the interracial relationship is not constructed in the conventional impossible-love context (the *South Pacific* or *Patch of Blue* variety, for example), but it is not exactly endorsed either. *Made in America* follows Goldberg's Sarah Matthews—the owner of an Afrocentric bookstore called The African Queen and the widowed mother of Nia Long's Zora—from her discovery that the sperm donor for her conception of her now-eighteen-year-old daughter was not the ideal specimen of black manhood that she had requested but, rather, the local, very white, faux-cowboy car dealer Hal Jackson (Ted Danson). As is the case with most romantic comedies, creating verisimilitude is not necessarily a guiding factor in the story. The mixture of

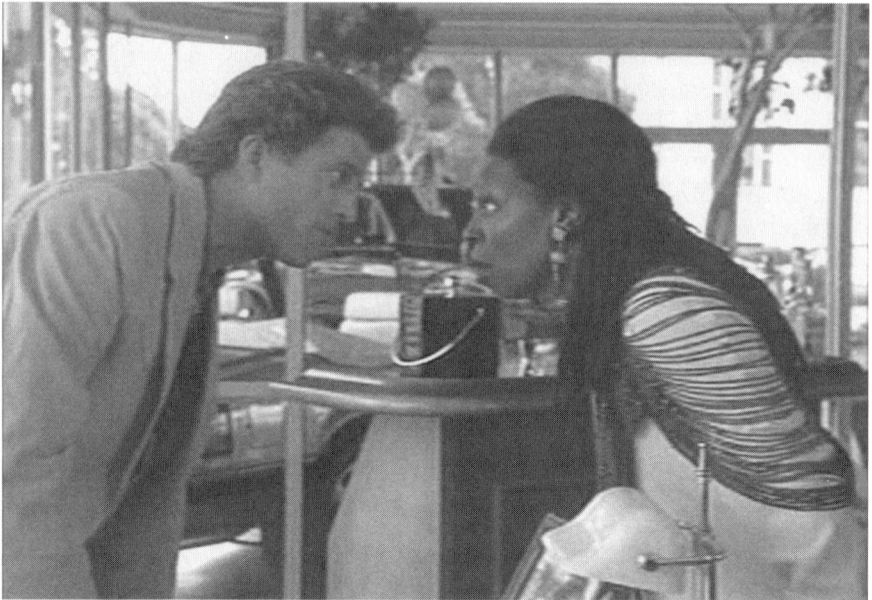

23. When Whoopi met Ted: *Made in America* (1993). Directed by Richard Benjamin.

budding romance between Hal and Sarah (from their initially hostile banter in his office about his role in Zora's life and the flirtatious discussion of "how good she smells" on a late-night walk after their first "date") to the broad physical comedy in the filming of Hal's television commercials (first by a desperate Zora and an angry bear, later by an angry Sarah and a desperate elephant) are not the stuff of which classic romantic comedy is made; then again, the same might be said of Matthew Broderick's and Annabella Sciorra's *The Night We Never Met* or Nancy Travis's and Mike Myer's *So I Married an Axe Murder,* two other romantic comedies from the class of 1993 that attempted to put an unusual spin on the boy-meets-girl generic paradigm. However, neither of those films was subjected to the critical vitriol heaped on the Danson-Goldberg vehicle—even before the stars' extratextual activities drew less than rave reviews.

*Made in America,* although by no means a perfect romantic comedy, garnered more attention—particularly after its release—because of the flood of press coverage given to the high profile of Goldberg and Danson as a couple. The extratextual construction of Goldberg and Danson offscreen and that of Sarah and Hal onscreen were in a fascinating dialogue with the times—the early nineties, when interracial marriage appeared to be on the rise—and a genre, romantic comedy, that continues to fundamentally ignore these couples. *Made in America* is an interracial romantic comedy but one that, as Donald Bogle notes, takes "precautions not to scare away any patrons with too explicit an interracial couple."[45] Nonetheless, the reviews of the film—in the black and white press— were decidedly mixed. *Boston Globe* critic Jay Carr lambastes the film for its "lack of self awareness," "off-putting manipulation," and for "Goldberg and Danson go[ing] at one another gratingly until it switches gears and turns goofily sentimental."[46] Janet Maslin's *New York Times* review saw the chemistry of the couple as the film's greatest asset, stressing the way in which the pairing of Danson and Goldberg yielded "a funny, disarming and believable screen romance, the first such movie role in Goldberg's career."[47] While what Maslin refers to as Goldberg's seeming "warmer and more comfortable" in the role of Sarah, the narrative seems to work against allowing the couple to slip into what I like to call the "sparkable period," when the romance of the romantic comedy becomes apparent—not only to the audience but to the characters as well. There seemed to be an ongoing deferment of this period, as Bogle notes: "The audience is led to believe that Goldberg has had Danson's child through artificial insemination, certainly not physical contact! Just when it appears that Goldberg and Danson will actually have a love scene, their romantic interlude turns into an unconsummated comic romp."[48]

Although the reviews in the mainstream press might have hinted at the extratextual realities of the coupling, the black press seemed to focus more on Goldberg, critiquing her choices not only in the film but in her personal life as well. Yuseef Salaam's review for the *New York Amsterdam News* is rooted less in the film's quality than in its ideological agenda: "Whoopi Goldberg's new

movie, 'Made in America' is a continuation of Hollywood's offer of racial assimilation to Black women. . . . The plot, like all of the white men–Black woman
romantic tales, has no Black men in Sarah's life. Her husband, a Black man, is
dead . . . [and] the remaining ones are clowns—a clowning eunuch [Will Smith
as Zora's best friend] and a silly homosexual [Jeffrey Josephy as James, Sarah's
flamboyantly gay employee at the bookstore]."[49] Like Salaam, who, despite his
disappointment with the film, praises Goldberg as a "beautiful woman . . . one
of the few Black women stars who has rejected fake hair weaves and wigs in
favor of her natural kinky hair and has refused to castrate her nose and lips (to
get white features)," Abiola Sinclair felt Goldberg's appearance was significant in
terms of her acceptance as a romantic lead for slightly different reasons: "[Gold-
berg] is Black enough [in terms of] Afrocentrism and commerce, mind you. It's
not that Whoopi Goldberg is Black but how Black! If she were a Denise
Nicholas or Mariah Carey, who is, as to be expected, marrying a wealthy white
man; if she had her hair straight, by nature or nurture, if she looked like Halle
Berry, the visual contrast would not have such an effect."[50]

Her allusion to the role played by color politics inside and outside of the
black community reveals a certain quandary for black women in the industry—
and in the black community. According to Sinclair's logic, one might assume
that it would be just as acceptable for Denise Nicholas, a light-skinned black
woman considered beautiful in Eurocentric terms, to act as the love interest of
Carroll O'Connor on the television series, In the Heat of the Night as it would
be on the big screen. I would contend that the answer is yes and no. While Halle
Barry has gone on to star in roles with varyingly problematic interracial relationships, like her Academy Award–winning role in Monster's Ball, the realm of
romantic comedy—the date movie and, arguably, the most easily digestible
genre for American audiences—remains the domain of same-race coupling. In
Goldberg's case the process of judging just "how black is she?" has double
meaning—as her extratextual existence bleeds into the reception of the filmic
text and its iterations of her personae. In 1993 Goldberg was in a no-win situation—seen as too black, in relationship to her constructions as a romantic lead,
and not black enough, because of her relationship with a white man, which was
considered more than tabloid worthy. The tenuousness of her position was only
exacerbated by the events at the Friar's Club Roast of Goldberg in October the
same year.[51]

Using material written mostly by Goldberg, Ted Danson, in blackface, gave
a profane, racial epithet ("Nigger" and "Whitey") filled tribute to Goldberg,
spending a great deal of the bit discussing "whoopie with Whoopi." Neither
Danson nor Goldberg anticipated the fervor of the outcry against their minstrel-
parodying antics. Those who were offended took the stunt as a personal affront,
and the tone of their criticism—as well as Goldberg's response—reflected this.
Talk-show host Montel Williams and Mayor David Dinkins were present at the
Friar's Club roast for Whoopi Goldberg and were among the first to speak out

against the "open insensitivity" of Danson's performance. Dinkins—New York's first black mayor, who only attended the roast to honor native daughter Goldberg—felt "embarrassed for Goldberg," calling the material "very vulgar" and stating that the jokes "went way, way over the line." The most vehement condemnation came, however, from the talk-show host, who stated, "I was confused as to whether or not I was at a Friars event or at a rally for the KKK and Aryan Nation."[52] Williams, who is married to a white woman, with whom he has a child, expressed the greatest offense at the jokes about "racially mixed kids" and stormed out of the building after the first seven minutes of Danson's tribute.[53] The black press also took Goldberg to task, not only for the incident but also for the aspects of her persona/person that had been previously considered "suspect," as exemplified in the *New Pittsburgh Courier:* "Goldberg, who is Black but has taken on a Jewish name and white boyfriends, apparently to bolster her career, finds nothing disturbing about racial jokes being made, the casual usage of the pejorative 'nigger' or a white man appearing blackface at a function in her honor. . . . Goldberg should not allow her seeming assimilation into white culture [to] give her amnesia as to how blackface, a longtime staple at minstrel shows, is a gross caricature of Negro people."[54]

The *New York Amsterdam News's* Abiola Sinclair was one of the few voices that put the incident in relationship to larger trends in comedy (particularly black comedy) in the early nineties: "As for these two comedians being stupid and tasteless, they are not alone in that description. Too many so-called comics are willing to resurrect the lowest in blue humor and negative imagery to embarrass the Black race."[55] Her reference to the emergence of the black comic content on *Def Comedy Jam* and the netlet black-block programming emerging on Fox (particularly with *Martin*), while not lessening the impact of Danson's performance and Goldberg's complicity does seem to recognize that there was a lot of "cooning" going on in comedy in the early nineties. Goldberg was unprepared for the reaction when she felt she had been "'roasted' with humor and a great deal of affection."[56] Not surprisingly, Goldberg's defense came in the form of offense. Citing the no-holds-barred history of the down-and-dirty Friar's Club Roasts, Goldberg questioned not the content of the comedy but the sensibilities of the audience: "If people on the dais and in the audience were not aware of what the day was supposed to consist of, they should have checked to see what the tenor of these roasts are, and then made a decision as to whether or not they wanted to participate."[57] While one might question the wisdom of the blackface stunt, Goldberg's reaction seems absolutely consistent with her sense of humor, of loyalty and of what free expression actually means to her. In this instance the impact of Goldberg's personal politics on the public perception of her celebrity, and, by extension, her film work, reveals how blurred the boundaries between the person and the personae had become for her.

While Goldberg's public personae—outspoken, unabashedly liberal, and resistant to being "niched"—often seemed to struggle with the roles that seemed only to utilize narrow swaths of "Whoopi" contained in fairly conventional narrative framework, it seems both telling and ironic that when a role appeared (Sarah Matthews in *Made in America*) that did afford a certain degree of convergence between the personal and personae, the reception of the text and of the extratextual controversies—the film itself and what one reporter referred to as "Whoopi and Ted's excellent adventure," respectively—were tied inextricably one to the other. Moreover, the event at the Friars Club and the subsequent outcry obscured the popular and critical opinion regarding Goldberg playing a role that challenged the ways that she had previously been constructed in film comedy: with all of its flaws, in Sarah Matthews, Goldberg had been presented with the *possibility* of playing a multifaceted character: a smart, funny, black woman, who was allowed some degree of sexual agency and personal autonomy. There was clearly liberatory potential in the Matthews character, for Goldberg and, arguably, for the comic representation of black women when viewed within the context of a genre in which black women were traditionally relegated to the periphery of the narrative as either the perpetual "Rhoda" (the less-feminized "friend" in the boy-meets-girl paradigm, to which Oda Mae is, at least spiritually, linked) or as the desexualized and distanced observer, who might offer comment but is essentially removed from the romance of the comedy (like Pearl Bailey's role as the musically inclined maid, Gussie, who wryly comments on the lives and loves of others in the Bob Hope vehicle *That Certain Feeling*).

Yet one wonders whether, even without the Friars Club debacle, Goldberg's reception as a character like Matthews would have been more than tepid at best. The extratextual construction of Bailey and its impact on her persona did not have a negative impact on her stage and screen presence, since, arguably, her iterations of Pearlie Mae, regardless of venue or medium, never posed a significant challenge to her audiences. Goldberg, on the other hand, seems simultaneously trapped and empowered by her personae, her personal politics, and the public perception of them both. Both Bailey and Goldberg, in true diva style, clearly annunciated their personal ideologies in relationship to their interracializing ways—and faced the implications of doing so. In the end Bailey's ways had minimal impact on either audience affinity with Pearlie Mae or her growing industrial cachet in the fifties and beyond, while for Goldberg they facilitated a color-coding of the popular conceptions of her personae more thoroughly than at any other point in her career during the burgeoning multicultural moment of the early nineties.

In *Black Looks*, published in 1992, the year of the LA uprising and the year before Goldberg's Friar's Club debacle (and the release of her first romantic comedy), bell hooks outlined directives for the radical empowerment of black women: "When black women relate to our bodies, our sexuality, in ways that place erotic recognition, desire, pleasure, and fulfillment at the center of our efforts to create radical black subjectivity, we can make new and different representations of ourselves as sexual subjects. To do so we must be willing to transgress traditional boundaries. We must no longer shy away from the critical project of openly interrogating and exploring representations of black female sexuality as they appear everywhere, especially in popular culture."[58]

I would argue that, at that same historical moment and the years that followed, Whoopi Goldberg has endeavored to present and represent a radical black subjectivity—with varying degrees of success. One might even argue that the most recent iterations of Goldberg's personae endeavor to simultaneously embrace and subvert the parameters of their politicized nature while recognizing change—in social and political mores and her lived experiences. Undoubtedly, the extratextual construction of Whoopi Goldberg's personae has resulted in a certain mitigation of their significance to the development of black comedy—particularly in relationship to women in black comedy. In the age of the narrowcast and the niche Goldberg's crossover capability continues to separate her from other black comic sisters. Nonetheless, as Adele Givens states, "Without Whoopi, there would be no 'Queens of Comedy.' . . . I'm just grateful that she was there before me, because without her there would be no me."[59] Moreover, there are other black female comics for whom crossover is both a goal and a possibility—one of whom, as will be discussed in more detail later in this chapter, is Wanda Sykes.

NEW MILLENNIAL DIVADOM

In the first decade of the new millennium Goldberg has garnered high praise and intense criticism—which actually describes the previous decade as well. In 2001 Goldberg joined the ranks of Richard Pryor, Carl Reiner, and Jonathan Winters when she was awarded the Kennedy Center's Mark Twain Prize for American Humor. The honor was bittersweet; it was presented a little over a month after the events of 9/11, and the native New Yorker expressed the national sentiment with great candor and sensitivity: "The events that hit our nation hit us all hard. . . . I didn't know where what I did fit into the fabric of the nation anymore. Tonight, all the people who came here to this show remind us that along with the tragedy, we must exist. We must be a part of life."[60]

In the years that followed 9/11 Goldberg's activism went into full throttle—nowhere more significantly than in Democratic Party politics. Goldberg found herself at the center of controversy and criticism after her now-infamous monologue at the Kerry/Edwards fund-raiser in New York in the summer of 2004. It is not surprising that Goldberg's statement at the campaign fund-raiser, which played with the double entendre and President Bush's name, in many ways, could be seen as vintage Whoopi—irreverent, funny, pointed, and, for some, of questionable taste. When she appeared on *Hardball with Chris Matthews* in January of 2005, Goldberg stressed that, because the text of her talk had not been made public, people were commenting on what "people would think I would say." Although on the program to promote a new project, when asked about her controversial use of double entendre, Goldberg recounted, "I said that I loved bush and that someone was giving bush a bad name.... I think it's time for bush to be in its rightful place, and I don't mean the White House"; when Matthews questioned Goldberg as to whether she thought the joke appropriate, she replied simply, "For a comedian, yes."[61]

As a result of the way her words were mobilized in the opposing party's camp, Goldberg, from which the Democratic campaign and party pundits distanced themselves, gained (temporary) quasi-pariah status in the party and lost her endorsement contract with the Florida-based Slim-Fast company. As had been true in the past, Goldberg remained steadfast in her claims that it was her right to freedom of expression, not the content of her comedy, that was at issue here. Slim-Fast's punitive measures did not chasten Goldberg's activism nor her tongue. By November of 2004 Goldberg was able to reflect not only on the actions of the company that had fired her but also on the party that had abandoned her. "Slim Fast knew who I was when they hired me and made its move without having the facts. Everyone else made the decision to back away—including Kerry and Edwards. It's indicative of what's wrong with our party."[62] It is striking that, once again, in the face of public controversy, Goldberg chose to take the offensive and make her position clear—no matter whom it might serve to anger or berate. Always outspoken, Goldberg has continued her divadom in the new millennium, although, one might argue that her choices of roles and venues mark both departure and return for Whoopi.

### CINEMATIC WHOOPI: PORTRAITS OF RESTRAINT

Goldberg's choices of roles in films like *Kingdom Come* (2001) and *Good Fences* (Showtime 2003) can be seen as significant departures in terms of character and in terms of the industrial construction of the films. As she stated in an interview with Kam Williams, "It may be true that there is some clout behind the name 'Whoopi Goldberg' that wasn't there before. But that doesn't mean that I can green-light a movie that I want to star in because my tastes are sort of out there."[63] Interestingly, one could make the argument that the black-cast dysfunctional-family comedy and the Showtime black melodramedy are the first in Goldberg's career that are actually niched—targeted for black audiences. Both Raynelle, the not-grieving widow and matriarch of the Slocumb clan, and Mabel Spader, a wife and mother of two, who slides uncomfortably into suburban assimilation, are almost the antithesis of the hyperverbal comedic roles often associated with Goldberg's big-screen personae. Deliberately seeking to play comic roles that differ from those in the past, with the subdued Raynelle in *Kingdom Come*, Goldberg challenges audiences—particularly black audiences' previous assumptions about the comic Whoopi: "They wanted more and said 'put some more "Whoopi" in it.' But if I had wanted more I would've taken another role—she's the mother."[64] As Stephen Holden notes, "Her devoutly religious widow, Raynelle, has harbored so much pent up anger at him that she calmly insists that the engraving on his headstone read 'mean and surly.' Ms. Goldberg, giving one of her more restrained performances, projects an appropriate mixture of long-suffering wisdom and curdled sanctimony with her Mona Lisa smile."[65]

The same can be said of Mabel Spader, the female protagonist of the Showtime film, who slides into isolation and alcoholism as she is taken from her comfortable working-class neighborhood to the tony suburb of Greenwich, Connecticut. Set in the late seventies, the film depicts Mabel as being pulled into the upper middle class by her black attorney husband, Tom (Danny Glover), who is determined "to end the colored man's losing streak" by any means necessary—initially by taking (and winning) a high-profile case in which the firm's rich white client has set two black vagrants on fire. The progressive disintegration of the family—daughter, Stormy, struggling to pass; son Tommy Two, struggling to (covertly) find some sense of blackness; and Tom, becoming more obsessed with power and status—and delineating himself from the "failure" of blackness—drives Mabel to the couch and the bottle (watching daytime television with scotch in hand). Again, the performance is restrained and contained; as Mabel loses her sense of self and her connection to a community of color, Goldberg plays the pathos with a light touch.

Interestingly, her female counterpart and antagonist is Ruth Crisp, played by Mo'Nique as a derivative of Nikki Parker, her television sitcom character, which in itself is a derivative of her stand-up persona. Crisp wins the lottery, moves in next door and brings half of the hood with her, which inspires fear and dread in Tom, seeing her as a threat to his "comfortable black" status and causes Mabel to initially ignore her to avoid racial "guilt by association." Mabel's budding friendship with Ruth, at the film's end, brings her back to (black) life and acts as a call for solidarity among black women. Goldberg's choices to play these repressed characters—in a supporting role in the broad comedy of *Kingdom Come* and in a costarring role in the melodramedy morality play *Good Fences*—speaks to her desire to redefine herself on film and, perhaps, with the very community that she is seen to represent in American popular cultural consciousness.

### Not Ready for (Network) Prime-Time Sisters: Whoopi and Wanda

On returning to television in her NBC sitcom, *Whoopi* (2003), Goldberg was adamant that the sitcom set in Manhattan actually be filmed in New York rather than Los Angeles, thus providing a literal and figurative return for the comic diva.[66] In some significant ways, however, Goldberg was not the only black comic diva making her way to prime time as part of television's class of 2003. While Goldberg's choice of recent film roles played against her personae, the character of Mavis Rae, the one-hit-wonder songstress turned hotelier, seemed to be the distillation of the most extreme aspects of Goldberg's comic persona: the hard-drinking, self-righteous, opinionated, outspoken, chain-smoking, intolerant of intolerance, unapologetically liberal (and anti-Bush) Mavis Rae is Whoopi to the tenth power. Not insignificantly, there was another hard-drinking, outspoken, opinionated black woman in the televisual class of 2003: Wanda Sykes in *Wanda at Large* on Fox. Although dissimilar in terms of premise—Mavis as the Manhattan hotelier and Wanda Hawkins as the Washington, D.C., stand-up comedienne turned political pundit—the convergences between the character constructions, the series' sociocultural milieu, and the ways in which the series are infused with the comics' personae are striking. Both series present milieus that act as a microcosm of their city setting. Whoopi's hotel is like a model UN, with Nasim (Omid Djalili), the Iranian handyman/bellman; Jadwiga (Gordana Rashovich), the Eastern European maid; Courtney Rae (Wren T. Brown), Mavis's Republican, unemployed former-Enron-executive brother; and Rita (Elizabeth Regen), his white girlfriend, who provides a caricature of what it looks like to "try to be black." In *Wanda* the milieu is black, white, and biracial: with Bradley Grimes (Phil Morris), Wanda's black conservative colleague, foil, and possible love interest; Keith (Dale Godboldo), her black dreadlocked cameraman/buddy; Jenny Hawkins (Tammy Lauren), Wanda's widowed white sister-in-law; Max (Mark McKinney), the high-strung station manager; and Barris and Holly Hawkins (Robert Bailey Jr. and Jurnee Smollett), Wanda's biracial niece and nephew.

Each series is purposefully bawdy—the sexual innuendo is a dialogue staple; each plays with notions of political correctness and defiance of imposed values systems; each provides a sister-friendly iteration of a black woman protagonist; each has been helmed by impressive creative teams. For *Wanda* the list of writers and creator/writers includes Sykes, along with another alum of *The Chris Rock Show*, Lance Crouther, Les Firestein, and Bruce Helford. For *Whoopi*, Goldberg enlisted heavyweight producers from some of the most successful sitcoms of the previous decade (*The Cosby Show, Roseanne, The Bernie Mac Show*), including Marcy Carsey, Caryn Mandabach, and Larry Wilmore. While one might think that these qualities would assure success, the final salient link between the shows is that neither survived past its first season.

Nonetheless, examination of the series reveals convergences between the narratives and the comic personae of their stars. Two particular episodes of the series illustrate the spiritual connections between *Whoopi* and *Wanda at Large*: each dealt with the personal politics of the central protagonist and her unwillingness to alter her beliefs or her actions in response to outside pressures. In "Vast Right Wing Conspiracy" Mavis's hotel becomes an unscheduled stop on the presidential motorcade and, through a series of miscommunications (Nasim tells Mavis that the Boss is in their W.C. and she assumes he means Bruce Springsteen), Mavis is labeled a Bush supporter and provides a photo op for the president. Like much of the series, the political content rests in the one-liners sprinkled liberally throughout the twenty-two-minute show. After realizing that it is Bush and not Springsteen, Mavis is horrified at having him in her hotel—and by her unknowing comments to the press:

MAVIS: Bush is in my can?!!! I can't believe he's doing to my bathroom what he's doing to the economy.

After being invited to a reception for the president, Mavis initially decides not to go, despite Courtney's pleading that this would mean that he gets to meet his hero. An argument ensues between the brother and sister about what the Republican Party has done for black folks:

COURTNEY: They freed the slaves.
MAVIS: You had to go back 140 years to find that.
COURTNEY: They have African Americans in the cabinet.
MAVIS: That's two hired, what about the other 37 million?

The rest of the episode offered more opportunities for Goldberg to be an equal-opportunity offender of conservatives. On being congratulated by an African American couple at the reception for "coming out," she responds, "Black republicans make about as much sense to me as Jews for Jesus." The black Republicans vocally object to Mavis being given "face time" with the president, and both she and a heartbroken Courtney are escorted from the hall. Despite Courtney's earnest admission of disappointment and anger with Mavis, she remains unrepentant, saying, "I had to speak my mind." The three-jokes-per-page structure of the series and the construction of Mavis as hyperliberal afforded Goldberg, albeit briefly, a weekly forum to "speak her mind" and to disseminate her brand of comedic social discourse. While the show played with moments of political incorrectness, particularly in the dynamic between Mavis and her "help," the show's tone, like Goldberg's personae, forwarded a liberal agenda addressing issues from racial profiling to the inadequacies of the current administration (with a side preoccupation with ridiculing the New York smoking ban).

In her stand-up act Wanda Sykes, who has graduated from headliner in the club circuit to headliner in theatrical venues, does not shy away from pointedly political and anti-Bush sentiments. In her Comedy Central special, *Tongue Untied*, Sykes addresses Bush's 70 percent approval rating in the early years of his first administration: "A majority of us were satisfied with the job the president was doing. Which makes sense to me because he pretty much did everything I expected him to do. The economy is in the toilet. We're at war and everything's on fire. He's met all my expectations." The Washington, D.C.–based local political pundit show in *Wanda at Large*, however, seems fairly apolitical. For the most part the critique is based in station politics, interpersonal conflicts, and Wanda's general intransigence. In "Clowns to the Left of Me" the episode veers into Sykes's stand-up act (and her politics) as she tangles with fanatical animal rights activist leader Charlotte Rankin (Jenny McCarthy). After settling their initial difficulties, Rankin feels she has bonded with Wanda: "I know you. . . . You're an African American woman, I'm a liberal. We're practically twins" and, in turn, asks Wanda to introduce her at a banquet in Rankin's honor and to "come and share

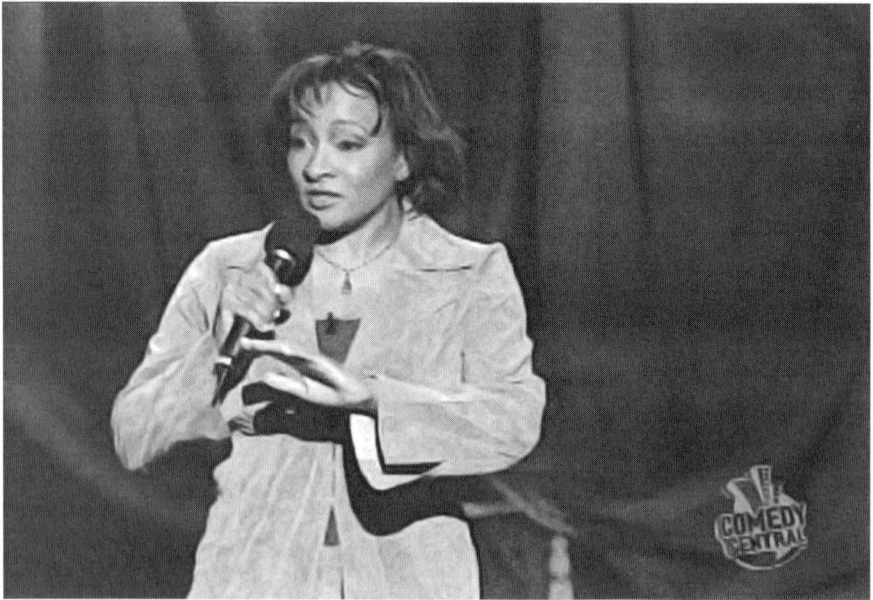

24. Wanda Sykes from *Tongue Untied* (2003). Directed by Paul Miller.

your struggles." The remainder of the episode is derived from an anecdote in her first half-hour Comedy Central special—with the exception of a brief passage in which Wanda and Jenny, her sister-in-law, are almost dying of ennui as the archetypal speaker drones on about how "she is woman." In the stand-up version of this story Sykes recounted doing a feminist event ("for free"), where she began by calling everyone "girls" and asking them to give "a big hand to the men who let them out of the house tonight" and ended with her having to be home in twenty minutes because her husband expected to "have his dick sucked after dinner." In the series version the blow job reference was replaced with an impromptu salute to someone who has done more to bring women into the public eye than just about anybody else: Hugh Hefner. Putting the cherry on the offensive sundae, Wanda introduces Rankin à la the WWE: "And now, the lightweight feminist of the World, Charlotte 'The Uterus' Rankin."[67] Under her breath onstage, Rankin forces a smile and calls her "just plain evil"—Wanda responds, "Now you know me."

One might argue that these series represent fairly traditional sitcom fare. It could also be said that, in sociopolitical terms, *Whoopi* and *Wanda at Large* provide comic fare that is pedantic and pedestrian, respectively. Despite these narrative flaws, however, both series, inculcated with the comic voices of their black female comic stars, are industrially significant—perhaps more so for Sykes than for Goldberg.

*Wanda at Large*, which was given a fatal Friday-night, 8 p.m. timeslot, was the first network sitcom venture for Sykes, whose humor may well be better suited for cable. Her guest appearances on HBO's *Curb Your Enthusiasm*, while sporadic, have received rave reviews and have positioned her within a highly successful piece of "quality television" programming. Larry David's wry, offbeat humor that informs *Curb Your Enthusiasm* allows guest star Sykes to play herself on the celebrity reality sitcom, which provides a hospitable environment for Wanda's comic exasperation at the neuroses of both Larry and her television best friend, David's onscreen wife, Cheryl (played by Cheryl Hines). The same is true of her feature segments on HBO's *Inside the NFL*, which may have acted as the inspiration for the offset, stunt-driven sequences of the Fox sitcom. Nevertheless, Sykes's presence on HBO and in her current Comedy Central quasi-reality series, *Wanda Does It*, which showcases its slightly egocentric star declaring her ability (and willingness) to do just about any job, reveals an important aspect of Sykes's comic personae—her crossover capability.

Whereas Goldberg, from the very beginning of her career, was engaged in crossover, Sykes's early association with *The Chris Rock Show* (as a writer on the Emmy Award–winning creative staff and as cast member) positioned her within a black comedy elite, thus providing her with a degree of cultural cachet and legitimacy with black audiences that (arguably) continues to elude Goldberg. Sykes's comic persona with its candid conversational and contentious sociocultural critique has the edginess of Goldberg's early work, but the ease of delivery is strangely reminiscent of Moms Mabley's when she took on the role of storyteller as truth-teller. Capturing the nuances and inflections of black vernacular speech, Sykes's voice, often brassy and a bit curt, speaks across cultural boundaries without seeming to make an effort to do so. Sykes emits a comfortable sexuality and self-assurance that shows no sign of either self-deprecation or self-denigration—neither too grateful to be in front of an audience or too haughty to play to the crowd. Like the comic with whom she is most closely associated, Chris Rock, and her comic diva predecessor, Goldberg, Sykes has crafted a distinct comic persona that, onstage, has the potential to reach and appeal to multiple audiences without contorting her voice or diluting the content of the comedy. However, as can be seen in the perusal of Goldberg's comic filmography, even the most distinctive persona can be the square peg shoved into the round hole of mainstream American comedy; Sykes's performances in supporting roles in mainstream comedies, *Monster-in-Law*, with Jennifer Lopez and Jane Fonda; and *In the Pink*, with Tim Allen, Cher, and Bette Midler, will provide a better indication of how she will survive the comedic middle passage. Nonetheless, one can safely assert that Sykes is a crossover comic diva-in-training.

## CONCLUSION: WHOOPI RETURNS

When one looks at the comic personae of Goldberg, now a veteran of crossover divadom, in the latter half of the millennium's first decade, it appears to be in both an introspective and retrospective period. It seems somehow appropriate to have endeavored to reassess and reread Goldberg's comic personae, her body of work, and its reflection and refraction of blackness and womanhood in the same year that Goldberg returns to the text that marked the moment of *Whoopi*. Goldberg's return to the Lyceum Theater in November of 2004 marked the twentieth anniversary of her landmark one-woman show. In *Whoopi Live* Goldberg revisited the characters that she had embodied in the retooled *Spook Show* in 1984. Along with the Surfer Girl, the Crippled Girl, the Little Girl with the Long Luxurious Blond Hair, Goldberg added Lurleen, "a menopausal Texas matron, who provides personal hygiene products and reflections on a suicide attempt."[68] The longest monologue of the new *Whoopi Live* belonged, as it did before, to Fontaine, Goldberg's male junkie alter ego. In this iteration of Fontaine the ex-junkie is a junkie again. Speaking through Fontaine, Goldberg immediately launches into an attack on the Bush administration, which acts as his justification for his relapse: "We had a president who lied about getting some and we impeached him. We got a president who lied about all kinds of shit. And people are dying. And we put him back. And I thought, 'I need more drugs.'" In his review Charles Isherwood noted that Fontaine's friendly discourse with the audience "evolves into a preachy lecture, and long before its conclusion, the pretense that we are being treated to the character's opinions rather than the performer's becomes transparent."[69] While admittedly saddened by the thought that the Fontaine/Goldberg persona that had previously acted as such an ideal vehicle for her comedic sociopolitical discourse was no longer effective, I was not surprised by Isherwood's conclusion. Given that the boundaries between Goldberg's personae and person have been in varying levels of collapse for over a decade, how could Fontaine/Goldberg escape unscathed? Whereas, in his earlier iterations, Fontaine had afforded Goldberg an anonymous voice through which to speak, unencumbered by gendered or personalized presuppositions about his/her political agenda, he now seemed to be entirely separate from her. Like the *New York Times* critic, most in the audience at the Lyceum, or who watch the special HBO presentation of the performance, will not be able to see Fontaine— rather, it will be Whoopi doing Fontaine. Although this may seem like a semantic difference, it underscores the quandary in which Goldberg has been placed; it seems that, in achieving the status of "Whoopi," a single name recognizable to supporters and detractors alike, the conflation of the personae and the person is complete. The actor who stated two decades earlier, "I can play anything," is now always playing herself playing a role.

What may seem like an existential dilemma is actually rooted in Goldberg's status as crossover comic diva in the industry and in her communities. When I began this study, I believed that by tracing the convergences and divergences between Goldberg's personae and those that came before (Mabley and Bailey) and those who came after (Sykes), I would be able to discern how and why Goldberg had achieved the status of crossover black comic diva while, at the same time, being socioculturally and industrially disempowered. The analytical path was far from linear, and the shifts in her personae were not simply causal.

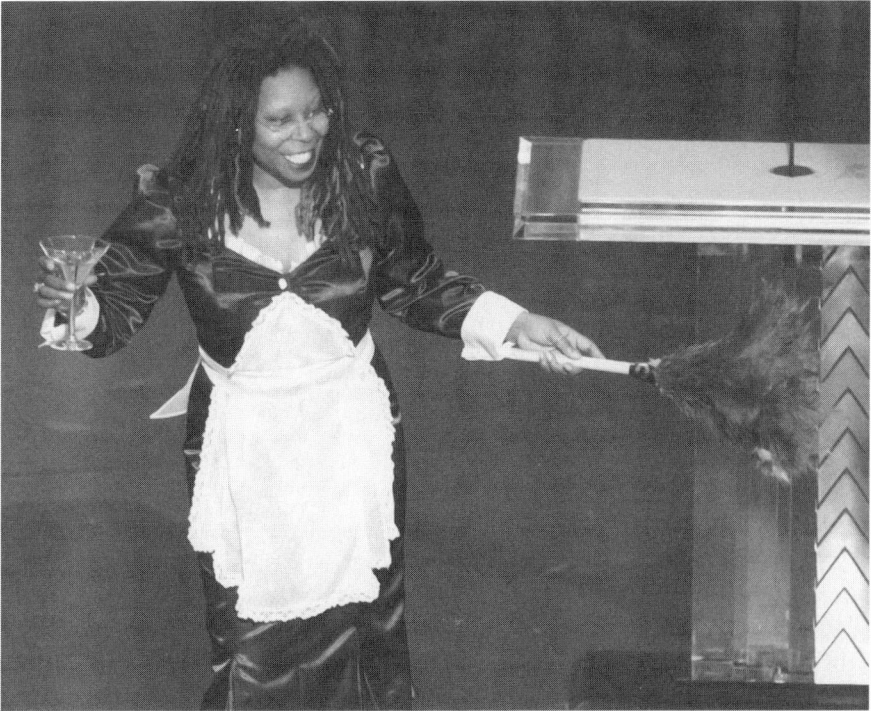

25. Whoopi Goldberg, hosting the Oscars, gives a shout-out to the "help" in her parody of *Gosford Park*. Seventy-fourth Annual Academy Awards (ABC), March 24, 2002. Photo from Photofest. Reproduced with permission from Academy of Motion Picture Arts and Sciences and ABC.

The individualistic, idiosyncratic, and overtly political nature of her comic personae, for which she was known (and, in some circles, revered), combined with the sociopolitical predispositions—about interracial relationships, political activism, purposeful androgyny, personalized gender and racial identities—frame aspects of the personal as culturally, politically, and racially suspect. In so doing, Goldberg is put into an even more problematic version of the representational bind faced by many black women in the entertainment industry. The view of her blackness, from inside and outside of the African American community, from inside and outside of the entertainment industry, colored the lens through which her personae and her work were viewed, judged, and classified—which is exactly what Goldberg had consistently fought to avoid. In the end Goldberg is a black comic crossover diva, but she also remains an anomaly—celebrated by both the mainstream entertainment industry and the black community yet fully embraced by neither.

# CHAPTER 5

# Dave Chappelle

## PROVOCATEUR IN THE PROMISED LAND

THE COMIC PERSONA OF Dave Chappelle is the logical end point for this ongoing study of African American comedy. In many ways Chappelle represents the intersections of multiple comic trajectories in black comedy. His act is often observational, like Cosby's, or perhaps more aptly, he's like Bob Newhart, if Newhart were black and had come of age in Washington, D.C., during the crack epidemic of the late eighties. Although Chappelle is a storyteller, who, with casual and almost lackadaisical candor, pulls you into his world and his logic, the content of his humor often has the sly righteousness and progressive radicalism of Gregory and the outlandish insider truism and gut-busting honesty of Pryor. Yet Chappelle's comic voice—and the dualities in his comic persona—reflects the dynamic, complex, and conflicted nature of sociopolitical discourse in the post–civil rights moment.

While this study has made the repeated distinction between person and persona, the dual nature of his upbringing—in a household that he has described as the "broke Huxtables,"[1] one that had pictures of Malcolm X on the mantel and Dick Gregory records on the stereo[2]—seems particularly instructive in terms of understanding how his emergent black comic persona plays into and, some would argue, determines "new" terms of crossover and, in turn, sets a new trajectory in black comedy. Chappelle is a late-phase post-soul baby, who grew up and learned to rock the mic in Washington, D.C., in the late eighties—after experiencing early adolescence in rural Ohio.

By the time Chappelle returned to Washington, D.C., after attending middle school in Yellow Springs, Ohio, the culture of Washington had changed significantly for its black residents: "crack had come out." In an interview with Terry Gross on *Fresh Air* in 2004, Chappelle recalled, "Selling drugs was like a legitimate job in the high school that I was going to. . . . It was that context [that] kind of isolated me—initially, and then when I started doing stand-up, it was like I thrived all over again."[3] Stand-up proved to be Chappelle's outlet— and a way out. Tricia Rose described hip hop as "a cultural form that attempts to negotiate the experiences of marginalization, brutally truncated opportunity and oppression with the cultural imperatives of African American and Caribbean history, identity and community."[4] Chappelle's emergent persona, inflected by his experiences at this pivotal moment of the post-soul era, reflects the inevitability of struggle expressed in Rose's words. Embedded within his comic discourse, there is a sense of wary hopefulness, self-determination, and self-aware black pride. However, there also seems to be a sense of fluidity in Chappelle's persona that embodies the movement in his life across communities and regions.

The dual nature of his black experience—identity formation in predominantly black and predominantly white spaces—also informs his comic persona. Chappelle enjoys a sort of dual credibility—his comic persona is inflected by both the Afrocentrism of the black hip-hop intelligentsia and the skater/slacker/stoner ethos of suburban life. This dual cred allows him to speak for and to Gen X and Gen Y subcultures in both the black and white communities. Chappelle is simultaneously a part of and at odds with integrationist mythologies, overtly political and involved in established notions of social action yet wary of the machinations of the political process. The comic is capable of incredibly incisive media and cultural critique, as well as humor that is at times more akin to *South Park* than to *Boondocks*.[5] He is also committed to a multiculturally specific worldview and a fully articulated black voice. Of course, this description could probably describe many of us at this post-soul moment. Seemingly today, when the fringe has been centered—hip-hop is mainstream American popular culture—Chappelle has become the poster boy of black comedy. However, it is vital to understand that Dave Chappelle, arguably the hottest comic on the planet in the new millennium, has been in the crossover game for a long time—whether by accident or by design.

Having begun doing stand-up as a teen in the late eighties on the comedy club circuit in Washington, D.C., which was "restrictive" in terms of the comic color palette (with no "blue" and one black as a de facto booking guideline), Chappelle learned to play within the limitations of the venue while not limiting his opportunity to connect with his audience on his terms. His big-screen debut in Mel Brooks's *Robin Hood: Men in Tights* (1993) set the trajectory for a film career split evenly between "black starring" comedies (*The Nutty Professor* (1996) with Eddie Murphy, *Blue Streak* (1999) with Martin Lawrence), mainstream films (*Con Air* [1997], *You Got Mail* [1998], and the indie cameo fest *200 Cigarettes* [1999]), and cult favorites with de facto crossover appeal (*Undercover Brother* [2003], with Eddie Griffin, and the quintessential Gen-X/Y stoner comedy *Half Baked* [1998]). As will be discussed later, Chappelle's choices in film roles map the development of a comic persona entrenched in both the black urban experience and the latent slackerdom of Gen-X and early Y. His broad—and overwhelmingly male—fan base cuts a wide swath through the lucrative eighteen-to-thirty-four demographic, which affords Chappelle a wide comedic playing field within which to hit *and* miss with his comedy.

It is impossible, however, to discern Chappelle's relationship to the day without connecting his comic discourse to the aesthetics and politics of hip-hop. Chappelle is like a comic MC. His comic oeuvre (film performances, stand-up sets, and television sketches), varied and conflicted, progressive and regressive, enlightening and embarrassing, parodies, samples, and remixes sub-genres and styles of comedy. By examining the construction of Chappelle's persona, his comic articulation of his African American experience, and its relationship to the popular notion of blackness at this historical moment, his relationship to the entertainment industry across media, and the tone, style, and content of his comedy, one can begin to understand how this provocateur in the promised land—the popular culture mainstream—marks a departure from and a return to the tenets of black comedic discourse in the post–civil rights era. It is always about keeping it *real*. The question is how is this *real* being read across the American racial and sociopolitical spectrum?

### As Hip-Hop as He Wanna Be

Just as scholars, critics, and folks on the street have all supplied myriad definitions of hip-hop, the comic persona of Dave Chappelle defies simple definition. Like hip-hop, it gives voice to this post-soul moment. Like hip-hop, it is wildly popular—across lines of class, culture, and, to a lesser extent, generation. Like hip-hop, it is always in danger of being misunderstood and misappropriated. One can see the ethos of Chappelle's comedy in both Ice T's assertion that hip-hop is "everybody's story . . . about capitalism and struggle . . . based on a certain culture. And if you don't like it you can kiss our mothafuckin' ass,"[6] as well as in Chappelle's self-espoused modus operandi of not holding back and "danc[ing] like there's nobody watching."[7] Chappelle's comic persona undeniably embraces the insolence and defiance embedded in much of hip-hop, but the style in which it is presented (particularly in his stand-up) is marked by an easygoing amiability. He slides social critique to his mixed audience in an easy, genial manner: it is just part of the story he's telling.

In Nelson George's seminal text, *Hip Hop America*, he compares the ways in which Public Enemy and De La Soul convey their political agendas not only in the lyrics but in the choices of their sound: "While P[ublic] E[nemy] looked for sounds that articulated anger and contempt, De La Soul sought bemused off-handed noises and deceptively childlike melodies."[8] In many ways Chappelle is to Rock as De La Soul was to Public Enemy: they are all talking about the African American condition, and they are all reaching beyond the boundaries of black popular culture for their samples (especially in terms of genre); they are all articulating their experiences of blackness in the post–civil rights era. Interestingly, as a result of doing it to a different "beat," as it were, they end up playing to and being embraced by different audiences.

Chappelle's affiliations with hip-hop go beyond the fact that his entrance music—on television and onstage—is an instrumental version of Dead Prez's

"Hip Hop." Rock had Grand Master Flash for his HBO series, Chappelle had Ahmir "?uestlove" Thompson of the Roots. The connection with "?uestlove" and the Roots goes beyond professional ties; Dave Chappelle is strongly affiliated with Okayplayer, a Philadelphia-based online community and collective of hip-hop artists cofounded by Thompson. In September of 2004, three months after signing on for an additional two seasons of *Chappelle's Show* with Comedy Central (in reality, its parent company Viacom) for an unheard of amount for basic cable—a reported $50 million—the comic hosted a "block party" in Brooklyn. Chappelle envisioned the filmed version of the concert as the *Wattstax* for the new millennium. The comic, who also produced the event, expanded on the role Pryor had played in *Wattstax*: providing the comic narration between acts. According to mtv.com "Chappelle dropped a poem ('Five thousand black people chillin' in the rain—nineteen white people peppered in'), challenged a Mohawked man to an MC battle, and sang two songs as R. Kelly, satirizing the infamous sex tape that show the R&B singer's ritualistic kinky side."[9] For this Brooklyn version of the 1972 Watts celebration of black pride (which had featured R&B, soul, and gospel greats of the era), the entertainment was provided by Okayplayers (Mos Def, Talib Kweli, Common, The Roots, Eryka Badu, and Jill Scott), Okayplayer cousin Kanye West, and one of the most militant of these conscious rappers, Dead Prez. Arguably, the highlight of the event was its finale: a reunion of one of the quintessential Afrocentric hip-hop acts of the nineties, The Fugees (Wyclef Jean, Pras, and Lauren Hill).[10]

Chappelle's block party, like his affinity for Okayplayers and his presence on the covers of hip-hop magazines *XXL* and *Blender*, is yet another way that the comic is becoming an advocate for the brand of hip-hop that might not make its way into MTV's *Total Request Live* (*TRL*). It should be noted that the love affair with hip-hop goes both ways. "I am music supervisor for the Dave Chappelle show simply because I am a fanatic for Dave Chappelle," stated ?uestlove Thompson, "He's a genius. He's a comic genius."[11] More than simply appreciating the significance of Chappelle's work, Roc-A-Fella mogul Dame Dash notes the contribution being made by the comic: "I think he's good for the community and culture. He's the truth. He knows how to be political in a funny way."[12] In addition, *Chappelle's Show* offers a space for diverse forms of hip-hop (beyond Usher, Outkast, Eminem, and Jay-Z) to be seen on prime-time television, which, in a televisual landscape without *In Living Color*, *Martin*, *The Chris Rock Show*, or *The Parkers*, is a significant contribution.

In his discussion of *In Living Color*, one of the first (and perhaps most critically significant) examples of netlet-niche programming in the nineties, Herman Gray teases out the series' "strategy of representation" and its heavy reliance on rap music and a hip-hop sensibility: "Rap and hip hop are used deliberately but quite strategically in the program to generate identifications across racial lines."[13] While one might make the same argument for *Chappelle's Show*, the connection is more endemic than strategic: the comic's persona is imbued with hip-hop sensibility—the aesthetic and the politics of musical genre are inextricably tied to his own. While *In Living Color* was informed by hip-hop, it must be noted that the series' cred is solidified because hip-hop is like a character on the show—often personified by the key figures who have become either recurring players on the series—or recurring gags.

The enjoyment of sketches featuring Mos Def or the Rza and the Gza of the Wu Tang Clan, and, indeed, the series as a whole, is not predicated on any particular knowledge of hip-hop culture. It is here that the negotiation between insider/outsider humor is complicated in some fascinating and, arguably, unique ways. In this comic text, as in Chappelle's stand-up, there exists another level of pleasure rooted as much—if not more—in cultural savvy than in solely racial affinity. This fosters a sort of de facto crossover, where the appeal of a distinct culture product (like Chappelle's comedic work or hip-hop, for that matter) crosses racial and cultural boundaries because of, among other things, shifts in taste culture or industrial reframing.

In referring to Chappelle's comedic discourse, I would argue that it was the shift in taste culture that led to industrial reframing. He was the right comic for the right moment and seems to purposefully interweave multiple threads of American popular culture—black and white. Speaking specifically to *Chappelle's Show*, which will be the subject of analysis later in this chapter, all sketches were penned by Chappelle and his longtime writing partner Neal Brennan, who is white. Thus, one must consider whether the comic strategy that informs the series and taps into various bases of knowledge and experience—mining all facets of popular culture—is purposefully multiple. In other words, one must ask how and why *Chappelle's Show*, like his comic persona, is uniquely suited for consumption by multiple audiences—all of whom have found a degree of affinity, at best, or uninterrogated attraction, at worst, with the content and/or style of his comic discourse.

Before undertaking a close analysis of his two premium cable specials, *Killin' Them Softly* (HBO 2000) and *For What It's Worth* (Showtime 2004) as a means of understanding his stand-up persona, which is fully articulated and yet still evolving in the new millennium, one must look at the comic's relationship with the entertainment industry and how that inflects and shapes the construction and execution of his comic modus operandi.

### BRIEF, STRANGE TRIP FROM BIG SCREEN TO SMALL

For most comics the path from local celebrity to national prominence goes through television. Whether in an appearance on *The Tonight Show with Johnny Carson* or on *Showtime at the Apollo*, television has allowed emergent comic personae to reach beyond the club circuit and into America's living rooms. The idyllic path for a comic goes something like this: the initial appearance leads to other guest spots, then a pilot, and then a series; the series leads to movies (and, sometimes, back into television). Although Chappelle's path to national prominence does converge with this idealized comic trajectory—having made stops at many of these same way stations on the stage-to-screen-to-screen trek—his journey has been both more circuitous and more direct.[14] When one industrially contextualizes the cross-media movement, Chappelle's popular culture and media status becomes even more intriguing.

Chappelle's trek from stage to screen was relatively direct: at nineteen (four years after he began doing stand-up ) he was tapped for the sidekick role in the least successful of Mel Brooks's film parodies, *Robin Hood: Men in Tights*. Although the role of Ahchoo, the Muslim second in command to Cary Elwes's Robin Hood, was neither the most progressive nor most challenging role that Chappelle has played (it mostly seemed to involve channeling Cleavon Little's "Black Bart" persona), it did establish him as a young black comic with *possible* crossover appeal. In fact, for the next decade Chappelle's film roles crossed back and forth between mainstream and black-oriented film. Although his turn as the wannabe bad guy in *Con Air* served as a generic departure, Chappelle's film oeuvre is, for the most part, filled with "buddy" roles—and not necessarily the "lead" buddy. Whether as the skittish former partner to Martin Lawrence in *Blue Streak* or the smart-aleck employee to Tom Hanks in *You've Got Mail*, Chappelle became known for making the comic best of small supporting roles. Interestingly, this ability to "work the material" can be seen as being (at least in spirit) similar to Pryor's engagement in mainstream comedy—particularly films like *Silver Streak*. Like Pryor, Chappelle's ability to give performances that (however unlikely the actual character constructions) appear to fit seamlessly with his comic persona: thus allowing him to utter lines that would normally elicit the rolling of eyes rather than laughter.

In *You've Got Mail*, as Chappelle and Hanks stroll through a construction site of the latter's new Borders-esque chain bookstore in Manhattan, Chappelle's observations—and deadpan delivery—resonate beyond the thirty-second sequence, which culminates with the comic's line, "This is the Upper West Side, man. We might as well tell we're opening a crack house." The "hipness" quotient in a Nora Ephron romantic comedy is relatively low—and Chappelle's presence, albeit brief, positions the film temporally—and culturally—not in a mythic, timeless (and homogeneous) Gotham all too common to the genre but rather in a city that could possibly be "in the world." While Chappelle's small and supporting roles in *Blue Streak* and *Showtime* were variations on the theme of "buddydom," they provide samples of different iterations of the comic persona that would later fill twenty-two minutes on Comedy Central. Even as the archetypal mean-spirited, abusive comic in *The Nutty Professor*, the heartless antagonist of Murphy's Professor Klump, Chappelle moves with self-celebratory ease through a rampage of insults with a kind of reckless abandon, making his performance memorable in a film that, on all other fronts, celebrates Murphy's comic versatility.

The salient feature in all of these performances is Chappelle's snarky, street-soft delivery. The quality often inflects roles that seem like stencils for "the black friend" in contemporary (mainstream) comedy,[15] transforming them into overdetermined and self-conscious parodies of those character types. This self-reflexivity in Chappelle's versions is played with a wink to the audience (sometimes literally) in his two most prominent big-screen roles, which also happen to be films that gained de facto crossover success, *Half Baked* and *Undercover Brother*. In the starring role of Thurgood Jenkins and the supporting role of Conspiracy Brother, the "buddy" persona qualities are combined with the innate insolence and sly subversiveness that, as we will see in the next segment of this analysis, inform Chappelle's stand-up comic persona. Neither film will be remembered as revolutionary comic cinema. *Half Baked* is a reenvisioning of the Cheech and Chong stoner films of the seventies, replacing the two Latino leads and low-rider iconography with a multicultural ensemble and a cross between Dead Head and hip-hop culture; and *Undercover Brother* is a blaxploitation parody starring Eddie Griffin as the eponymous brother.

A product of Clinton America in the post–civil rights era, *Half Baked*'s Thurgood, the good-natured stoner/custodial engineer (who clearly did inhale), acts as the poster boy for Gen-X slackerdom in an urban space that is mythically benign: the "real world" threats—even to the friend in prison—are offset by a sort of stoned idealism in a chemically altered fairy tale. Within a film that provides taxonomies of "weed" users (played by popular culture hipsters like Jon Stewart as the "Enhancement" Smoker, Janeane Garofalo as the "I'm Only Creative When I Smoke" Smoker, and Snoop Dogg as the "Scavenger" Smoker) and his literal partners in crime, Brian (Jim Breuer), the Anglo deadhead; and Scarface (Guillermo Diaz), the Cuban wannabe gangsta, Thurgood is the everyslacker, *who happens to be black*. In the film's cultural milieu lines of race and ethnicity are constructed as less significant than those of smoker and nonsmoker. By articulating that "in our world" these are the rules that apply, *Half Baked* others the mainstream, "straight" world.

Less libertarian than libertine, the politics of the film reframe notions of difference along its implied insider-outsider paradigm, thus "naturalizing" racial and ethnic difference in this Gen-X dominated world. This is not to say that *Half Baked* is bereft of broader social critique—it just appears in flashes, embedded in the "weed" humor shtick. In the film, penned by Chappelle and Brennan, Thurgood's throwaway jokes reveal how racially and sociohistorically aware a slacker can be—in a fairly sardonic and self deprecating way. For example, when "Scientist" (the name given by Thurgood to the researcher in his facility in response to being called simply "Janitor") tips the latter in high-intensity "weed," Chappelle's character volunteers to be a guinea pig for the medical marijuana study, adding, "My grandfather was a Tuskegee Airman, you know." This seeming non sequitur, which actually invokes the unethical Tuskegee Research project rather than the barrier-breaking freedom flyers, is delivered with a certain degree of insolence for authority, in general, and white authority, in particular, and purposefully provides an off-kilter condensation of African American history.[16]

Thurgood, the literal voice of the film, is posited as an insider in multiple subcultural contexts (African American, stoner, slacker), whose actions, including this moment of historical misinformation, are emblematic of a consciously nontraditional ideological agenda. Selling drugs to liberate (bail out) their compadre, Kenny (Harland Williams), the only member of the quartet who actually serves an active purpose in society (an effusively positive kindergarten teacher), is hardly a "Just Say 'No'" message; rather, it is countercultural. I would argue that Chappelle's character actively defies a singular positioning; after all, a sympathetic drug dealer is fairly hard to pull off—and Thurgood pulls it off. As figures in a lackadaisical rebellion, Thurgood and his buddies exist outside of mainstream culture—happily fringed. This construct, the subcultural insider who revels in his outsider status, inflects Chappelle's comic persona—regardless of the comedic and discursive intensity of the role.

As Conspiracy Brother in *Undercover Brother* Chappelle is provided with a character that is as self-indulgently subversive as he is paranoid—militantly unhappy in his fringed status. Again, Chappelle approaches the role with a sort of unbridled fervor, playing the paranoid Brother as a cross between a Black Panther wannabe and a refugee from a late-night AM radio conspiracy talk show. While purporting to question the actions of the Colin Powell–esque general, who has suddenly transformed into the archetypal Uncle Tom (including abandoning political life in order to open a fried chicken franchise), Conspiracy Brother's rant turns into an indictment of the ruling (Republican) party:

CONSPIRACY BROTHER: Name one thing that the Republican Party has ever done for the black man.
SMART BROTHER: The Emancipation Proclamation
CONSPIRACY BROTHER: Okay . . . Name two.

Again the play with the notion and knowledge of history emerges as a key element in the construction of Chappelle's character, whose knowing and unknowing actions undermine and underscore the claims by the black nationalist–informed character. Within the protectorate of the "Brotherhood," the fictional institution entrusted with protecting black folks from "The Man," Conspiracy Brother is seen as an extremist—and his hypotheses are suspect.

While further examination of *Undercover Brother* could tease out some fairly schizophrenic notions of black empowerment elaborated on in the film parody, let it suffice to say that the humorous ferocity of Conspiracy Brother's tirades about the white poaching of black culture, conspiracy theories (that prove in some cases to be correct in their cinematic world), and unabashed (albeit stereotypical) celebrations of black pride provide character traits, sociohistorical contexts, and comedic devices that would serve Chappelle well in his future Comedy Central series. Obviously, any comic, much less one who began working as early in life as Chappelle, would continue to evolve over the course of fifteen years in the business; what is so interesting about the development of

Chappelle's comic persona is the ways in which his screen comic persona is condensed and refined to serve his televisual comic persona. Of course, at the beginning of the postnetwork era that was not the case.

For many comics the situation comedy acts as segue from stand-up to big screen—which was more than slightly problematic for the black comic. One alternative outlet for the black comic was provided by the surge of social sitcoms (including the ghetto sitcoms of the seventies starring established black comics like Redd Foxx on *Sanford and Son* and new talent like Jimmie Walker on *Good Times*), which initially showcased comedic social discourse before degenerating into a resurgence of televisual minstrelsy and typical examples of the workplace comedies of the mid-seventies. However, the virtual prohibition on *more than one black* per any given mainstream sitcom made the conventional route to the big screen more circuitous for the African American comic.[17] Another established route, through *Saturday Night Live*, which over its twenty-eight years has launched the careers of John Belushi, Bill Murray, and Mike Myers, to name a few, and is widely considered the comic's access road to the entertainment's A-list, did not serve the same function for its African American "Not-Ready-for-Prime-Time Players": only Eddie Murphy and, to a lesser degree, Chris Rock have successfully made that cross-media passage *as a result* of their *SNL* tenure. With the dawning of the postnetwork era the increased opportunities for the second wave of post–civil rights era comics came from changes in television industry that were more industrially than aesthetically driven. Again, this was not *exactly* the path that Chappelle took.

As a result, the flow of talent into cable comedy programs, netlet, and network programming in the early nineties was unprecedented—that's the good news *and* the bad news. The increased interest in comedy performance and the subsequent programming needs of burgeoning cable outlets coincided with Chappelle's early days on the comedy circuit in the late eighties and early nineties. *Russell Simmons' Def Comedy Jam* on HBO and BET's *Comic View* were at the forefront of the stand-up boom and gave much-needed national exposure to the hordes of young black comics inspired by the work (and the high-profile successes) of Murphy, Arsenio Hall, Robert Townsend, and Keenen Ivory Wayans, Hollywood's new "Black Pack." Chappelle was a beneficiary of this surge, appearing on *Def Comedy Jam* multiple times in the mid-nineties. As Chappelle noted in a 2001 interview about the realities of black comedy in the early nineties, "Before Def Jam, Black comics were not getting a lot of exposure, granted it did portray a narrow audience of comedy, but it got so popular the demand became bigger than the supply of talent."[18]

At this juncture one needs to view Chappelle's persona in relationship to those of his *Def Comedy Jam* peers.[19] While Chappelle's comedy is clearly informed by a "post-soul aesthetic," so, too, was *Russell Simmons' Def Comedy Jam*. The series, the brainchild of hip-hop impresario Simmons, gave a venue for stand-up comedy that spoke to an emergent black cultural moment when hip-hop moved from the fringes of American popular consciousness slowly but surely toward the center. What emerged from this black comic space was a Def Jam persona, the embodiment of the comedic conventions that moved from the main stages of black comedy clubs to the niched market of a mainstream venue, HBO. Like the great nephews of Redd Foxx and Rudy Ray Moore (aka "Dolemite"),[20] the godchildren of Richard Pryor, and the kid brothers of Eddie Murphy, the Def Jam comics spoke, in purposefully outrageous tones, with acts designed to challenge the limitations of what could be said on televisual main stages. The Def Jam persona, driven as much by a "oh, no he didn't" sense of outlandish content as a comic self-determination, seemed intent on "flipping the script" on the racial politics of comedic discourse. In this brave new comic world the politics of racial differentiation were key in not simply bringing the periphery to the center but shifting the center—making the margin the main-stream. Thus, the litany of "white people be like" jokes acted not simply as a reversal but rather as a mechanism for asserting that "this is our world"—at least in certain venues and certain media outlets. The performers of *Def Comedy Jam*, from Martin Lawrence, Chris Tucker, and Eddie Griffin to future "Kings" and "Queens" of comedy (Cedric the Entertainer, Bernie Mac, Steve Harvey, D. L. Hughley and Adele Givens, Miss Laura Hayes, and Sommore, respectively) embodied bawdy (and often physical) humor that reaches back beyond the Chitlin' Circuit into the conventions of minstrelsy—tropes that have historically inflected *mainstream* comic representations of blackness.

Both Chappelle, who appeared in the waning years of the *Def Comedy Jam* era, and Rock, who acted as guest (and guest host) during the series' early years, share with their Def Jam brethren the black-centered comic sensibility (and a boundary stretching sense of decorum). However, neither their stand-up nor their film and television roles carries with them the same stylistic (and, some-times, regionalized) cultural specificity or the sexual bawdiness (often tinged with misogyny) tied to multiple iterations of the Def Jam persona. For both Rock and Chappelle the sociopolitical and sociocultural base of their humor overshadows the blueness of their comedy. In other words, the "oh, no he didn't" component of the humor is rooted in their sociopolitical critique.

Nevertheless, the flood of black comics into the aforementioned cable ven-ues (and the stand-up programs on Comedy Central after 1991), as well as their slow trickle onto network and netlet television on series like *Hanging with Mr. Cooper*, with D. C. Curry (ABC, 1992–97), and *Martin* (Fox, 1992–97) con-tributed to a (slightly) increased black presence on television—but only in comedy of course. However, it was the netlet's "black block" programming strategies, first utilized by Fox and later adopted by both the WB and UPN, that reset the trajectory for numerous black comics. The 1998 WB Thursday-night block (*The Wayans Bros.*, *The Jamie Foxx Show*, *The Steve Harvey Show*, and *For Your Love*) and the 2003 UPN lineup (*The Parkers*, with Mo'Nique; *One on One*, with Flex Alexander;[21] *Girlfriends*, and *Half and Half*) mirrored the counterprogramming strategies used in the early nineties by the fledgling Fox netlet—exemplified by its Thursday-night alternative to *Must See TV* with *Martin*, *Living Single*, and *New York Undercover*. Initially, Fox had allowed series to defy conventional generic boundaries in comedy—as seen in the dysfunctional domcom *Married with Children*, the landmark animated series *The Simpsons*, and the colorized sketch comedy series that revitalized the variety genre, *In Living Color*. However, by the fall of 1998, all of those series (with the exception of the flagship show, *The Simpsons*), as well as black block comedies *Martin* and *Living Single*, were lost in the passage from netlet to network, from "urban" audience base to "broader" demographic. As Keenen Ivory Wayans noted, "Fox changed the course of Black television unintentionally. They didn't go out to make Black shows, they went out to make alternative programming."[22]

Even as one traces the movements of other comics across media, the sitcom remains the primary televisual vehicle within which the African American comedian can gain national attention. Throughout the nineties, black-oriented situation comedies like *Martin*, *The Hughleys*, *The Steve Harvey Show*, *The Jamie Foxx Show*, and *The Parkers* exemplified how the stand-up persona was filtered through the weekly series into mostly *black-oriented* American film comedy over the decade (*Big Momma's House*, *The Brothers*, *Booty Call*, *Barbershop*, and *Soul Plane*). The fact that the dual construction and dissemination of Chappelle's stand-up persona differed from his fellows also speaks to the multiple reading and multiple constituencies that existed—and exist—for his comedy.

For Chappelle it was film, not television, that afforded him the opportunity to develop his comic persona. Although as early as 1996, when black block counterprogramming strategies had taken hold on the netlets (and some enthusiasm still existed for singular black comics on network television), Chappelle had signed a series of deals with Disney (Touchstone Television) to develop sitcoms for network consumption, none of his offerings proved palatable either to the comic or to the networks. Chappelle developed eleven pilots during the decade of the nineties—only one made it to the airwaves. That singular "success," *Buddies*, was an interracial buddy comedy that had a thirteen-episode run on ABC. The show treated the professional partnership and buddydom of the two leads, Chappelle as Dave Carlisle and Christopher Garlin as John Butler, as a monumental feat—a victory of the civil rights era. *Buddies*, which presented a "we are the worldist" narrative, complete with parental characters who depicted the black and white regressive social forces (bigoted "white trash" mom played by Judith Ivey and rigid "black pride" dad played by Richard Roundtree), was a spin-off of *Home Improvement*, a sitcom hardly known for its progressive racial or gender politics. "It was a bad show," said Chappelle on a *60 Minutes* interview. While there are numerous examples of this not preventing a show from running a full season (after all, how long did *Suddenly Susan* run?), the problem with this series (and the other eleven pilot attempts) was an inability to find an appropriate vehicle within the genre to allow Chappelle's burgeoning comic to be showcased. The fact that Touchstone continued to make pilots starring Chappelle attests to the company's belief that he was marketable (on network as well as netlet television). However, Chappelle's inability to find a "niche" in the age of "niche-marketing" signaled that his comic persona was not ready for sitcom prime time.

By the late nineties the changing network/netlet climate made it even more difficult to find an appropriate vehicle for Chappelle's comic persona. By 1998 Fox had virtually gained network status and was, for the most part, out of the black-block business. The WB and UPN were still looking toward black comedy programming to open up the "urban" (read nonwhite) audience. Both broadcasting entities catered to black viewers—seeking to fill a niche not adequately served by the major networks—at least in terms of the sitcom. A. J. Jacobs's prediction in his 1996 *Entertainment Weekly* article that "the bigger UPN and the WB get, the whiter they become" (15–16) has certainly proven true for Fox: nearly three-quarters of the network's programming has no black series regulars.[23] The programming tides are shifting at the WB and UPN: the WB's teen wave appears to have peaked, and it has lost one of its only critically praised programs (*Buffy*) to UPN, where *WWF Smackdown* has become its cash cow.[24] While one may wonder about the fate of the black sitcom once all the netlets "come of age," the question of whether or not Chappelle could find a place within the sitcom schema would soon be answered.

Chappelle, with Peter Tolan, who had also worked on *The Larry Sanders Show* and Denis Leary's short-lived and critically acclaimed series, *The Job*, developed a series for Fox television based on *his* life as an up-and-coming comic in New York City. With six episodes ordered and the show slated as a midseason replacement in 1998, negotiations between Chappelle and the network fell apart when Fox executives, seeing the Touchstone-produced sitcom as "too black," suggested that the lead female character be changed from black to white, in order to "broaden" audience appeal. Chappelle and Tolan walked away, and the former spent the better part of the next year (and multiple appearances on *Late Night with Conan O'Brien*) venting about Fox's network practices: "This network built itself on Black viewers . . . [This network view of 'universalizing' appeal] tells every Black artist no matter what you do, you need whites to succeed."[25] The Fox debacle, like Margaret Cho's experience with the network dictating what her Asian American experience should look like,[26] soured Chappelle on both the genre and the networks. In many ways, given the restrictiveness of the genre and the openness and fluidity of Chappelle's comic persona, the lack of "fit" between the two is not surprising. As Chappelle himself noted, "I tried sitcoms before, and it's something about the way I'm funny that is not for that venue. People [would] never know the extent of how funny I was. I'd be Urkel. I'd be rich, but I'd be Urkel."[27]

Ironically, the same year that Chappelle walked away from the Fox deal because of its desire to "universalize," his autobiographical sitcom, *Half Baked*, which provided a multicultural stoner world, was released and received limited but definitely de facto crossover success. While clearly the issue of artistic freedom was at stake, Fox's prescriptive required Chappelle to falsify the cultural milieu he was trying to present. Unwilling to play the "tokenism" game with Fox (and making the details of his dispute with the new number-four network public), Chappelle spent the next half decade honing his comedy on the road and in a wide variety of film comedies, waiting for the aesthetic and industrial opportunity in which his kind of comedy could flourish. Chappelle and Brennan had a vision for a series but no clear venue: "The idea was that I wanted to do a variety show that was very personal, almost as if you know . . . you could bring somebody's joke-book to life."[28] The generic switch—from sitcom to sketch comedy—was pivotal in terms of allowing Chappelle to pull together the myriad aspects of his comic experience into a televisual text. With the choice of genre in place, a venue was needed—enter Comedy Central. As an article in *Entertainment Weekly* proclaimed, "In a universe that measures audiences in hundreds of thousands rather than the network tens of millions, [Comedy Central] has . . . provid[ed] the most nurturing environment for comedy's most daring minds."[29] Chappelle's brand of comedy seemed an ideal match for the eighteen-to-thirty-four male demographic that had been established during *South Park*'s tenure at the network. The meteoric rise of *Chappelle's Show* was tied to a changing of industrial needs, as well as changing tastes and expectations for comedy in the postnetwork era; the key element in series—the blend of the sophisticated, the sophomoric, and the subversive is Dave Chappelle's comic persona. By *Half Baked*'s release in 1998, Chappelle's stand-up persona and his "buddy" persona were in the melding process; by *Undercover Brother*'s release in 2002, the process was (seemingly) complete.

Chappelle's comic persona can be compared to the best reduction sauce: yielded by slowly "boiling down" the cinematic iterations of his comic character traits—the likable, quick-witted observationalist (the "buddy"); the lackadaisically subversive outsider (the slacker/stoner/X-er); and the radical, institutional/tradition-wary cultural critic (the "brother")—the comic concoction is a result of a process inflected as much by the times and by the elements themselves. The cinematic iteration of Chappelle brought him into the comedy mainstream, while the Comedy Central series, which will be discussed in great detail later in this chapter, made him (albeit temporarily) the basic cable's $50-million man. However, to understand the significance of this comic's work, ideologically, culturally, and aesthetically—and the de facto crossover appeal that makes this particular cultural production as problematic as it is promising, it is necessary to understand where it all began: it had been established long before *Robin Hood: Men in Tights* or *Chappelle's Show*, when he was onstage rocking the mike.

### A Nice Guy Can Say Just About Anything

You can tell a lot about a comic by the way he or she comes onto the stage in a theater show. In *Bring the Pain* Chris Rock, dressed in black, walks on like an M.C. getting ready to battle. Eddie Murphy, clad in an elaborate black and purple leather ensemble, begins *Raw* posed in silhouette like a rock star. Decked out in red-suited regalia, Richard Pryor strolls onstage in *Live in the Sunset Strip* like the coolest cat in the neighborhood—and you're lucky that you get to see him. Chappelle's entrance, for his first hour-long HBO special, *Killin' Them Softly* (2000), is markedly different—more like the guy who's going to see the show than the guy who's doing the show. The chorus to DMX's "Party Up in Here" thumps through the hall as Chappelle saunters onto the stage at the Lincoln Theater in Washington, D.C., in a t-shirt and jeans. The chorus booms: "Y'all gon' make me lose my mind / up in HERE, up in here . . ." Chappelle enters like the guy on the block who everybody likes, coming into a party that's in full swing. This air of casualness immediately fosters an intimacy with the audience—and the crowd responds to his innate likability. Chappelle is keenly aware of the advantages he receives as a result of his demeanor: "I get away with a lot of stuff because it's not mean spirited. People can tell the difference."[30]

In the sixty-minute set that follows, a plethora of penis and weed jokes, commentaries on race and police, and a seemingly apolitical take on the political landscape, all freely peppered with obscenities and the *N* word, does not alter that initial impression: he remains likable. Unlike Rock, who hits the stage with warp drive critique of many of the same subjects, Chappelle, utilizing amped-up versions of the naturalistic sound effects or broad gestures that anyone might use in everyday exchanges, is the funny guy on the corner, telling you "some shit" about life. Although there are jokes in Chappelle's act that speak to serious issues like police brutality and overt racism, as well as other social and political maladies plaguing the urban black community, he does so in a way that is not directly accusatory. His idiosyncratic and meandering storytelling style has an undercurrent of wry incredulousness. In numerous interviews, Chappelle maintains that he "likes telling stories" and that whatever social commentary there is in his comedy is not deliberate—and that times we live in quite simply offer "fertile ground" for comedy.[31] Thus, Chappelle does not come off as the archetype of "the angry young black man"—although, given the content of his later comedic discourse, there is some anger there . . . underneath.

In *Killin' Them Softly* Chappelle's opening series of jokes positions him *with* his audience—as if he is sharing something that he knows they already know—by commenting on the "new" D.C.: "D.C. has changed—it's different now. [Pause] There's a lot of white people walking around. . . . I left D.C. in the eighties when crack was going on. White people were looking at D.C. from Virginia—with binoculars. [In white voice] It looks dangerous. Not yet." The prospect of a black comic using "white voice," a process that, for Chappelle, involves "taking all the rhythm out of my voice and speaking as monotone as possible," isn't in itself unique: doing the "white guy" has become a common tool in the "white people be like" subgenre of black comedy. However, despite the broadness of some of his humor, Chappelle's politics of differentiation in discussions of racial inequality always, at least seemingly, displaces blame. The white Virginians waiting for the D.C. to not be "too dangerous" are not vilified even as he makes a statement about how crack ensured D.C.'s de facto segregation.

Not so surprisingly, Chappelle's politics of differentiation are part of a "friendly" setup—quite literally—in his stories about his white buddy, Chip. As the white slacker/stoner everydude, Chip is constructed as Dave's counterpart, who exists without the burden of race. As Dave describes an evening with Chip when both are high and under the influence in New York City, he is simply incredulous at Chip's ease with the cop he asks for direction—after admitting to being "a little high" as well as the cop's somewhat genial reply. The initial punch line to the bit—that this story may not be "amazing to you but, ask any of these black fellas, that shit is incredible" provides anecdotal commentary on the differences in black and white relations to the police. Of course, the final payoff to the story acts as mitigating factor, using the obligatory "weed" joke to take the edge off, as it were: "a black man would never do that, it would be a waste of weed."

This discursive two-step or comedic misdirection play is often a part of Chappelle's humor and that of many comics (black and white) on the circuit today. However, when Chappelle does it, the function it serves seems to be managing the audience's comfort level: push them, pull back, challenge them, and assuage their misgivings. Rather than go straight to the social commentary, like Rock's full-throttle ideological assault or even Bernie Mac's simple statement of "truisms," the few declarative statements about social issues are simultaneously matter of fact and a little bit detached. What else would you expect from a Gen-X black comic? "Black people are very afraid of the police. That's a big part of our culture. It doesn't matter how rich you are, how old you are. We're afraid of 'em. [Pause] And we have every right to be." The strong declarative statement that deals somewhat indirectly with notions of racial profiling—the dangers of driving or even walking when black regardless of (or perhaps because of) celebrity guides the audience into the realm of cultural critique. To further personalize this process, Chappelle approaches a white female audience member about *her* experience of being pulled over by the cops: "They ask for your license and registration? [Pause] I'm just guessing. That's not what they say to us." The pointedness of his "commonsense" assertion of the differences between a black man's experience of the police is immediately undercut by a somewhat sophomoric insertion into the bit regarding *his* exchanges with police: "O.K. nigger, spread your cheeks and lift your sack." While the crassness of the anatomical I.D. required of him also speaks to notions of harassment (a cavity search for a speeding ticket), it also plays into the kind of gross-out humor that often elicits laughter and a "that's wrong" (as in "that's outlandish") response rather than actually considering the wrongness of racial inequality underscoring the joke. These mitigating factors make it easier for his multicultural audiences to laugh at one part of the joke and leave the critique to the side.

As Chappelle regales the audiences with further travels with Chip, he continues to utilize comedic misdirection to discuss how law enforcement functions for blacks and whites. Chip's ability to explain away erratic drunk driving (Dave was in the car but he was smoking weed) by saying simply, "I'm sorry, Officer. I didn't know I couldn't do that," has Dave, who backs away from the mike, in the throes of the kind of incredulous laughing that one might have when telling a story at the club. His shift to the "real" is both striking and effective: feigning ignorance is no defense for a black man: "[Black guy couldn't do that.] They know we *know* the law. Every black dude in this room is a qualified paralegal."

Again this story says something "real." For a black man, who grew up in D.C., this very definitely expresses a very real condition. Fifty percent of black male residents of D.C. have been incarcerated and, despite the cleanup that the city has experienced since the days of Mayor Barry, the prospects for young black men are limited, to say the least. The implication is that interfacing with law enforcement is not a choice for black men—it is an inevitability. Furthermore, the notion that this threat to black males is nothing new is historicized by the second payoff to the bit. Chappelle voices an old black man, wise to the realities of black males and the justice system, who acts as both conscience and legal counsel: "Nigger, don't do that—that's 5 to 10." Chappelle adds wryly, "We know the law and the penalties."

The thing that takes some of the sting out of Chappelle's social critique is that there is never any *direct* blame—at least not for the people in the audience. While Rock may talk about the problems with white people and then say, "But you folk paid to see me, you're O.K.,"[32] thus making the exchange more about business than pleasure, Chappelle always gives the audience a different kind of out: he implies that he *knows* white people (for example, the story of his friend, Chip, among other anecdotes) and that makes it O.K.[33] Far from functioning as a reversal of the old "some of my best friends are black" integrationist adage, Chappelle's observations reflect his worldview that portends not to being color blind but rather color *conscientious*—aware of the state of race relations but not necessarily determined by them. In the discussion of police brutality he points to the fact that what was common knowledge in the black community— multiple incidents of police brutality—was looked at warily by the white community: "Not that you didn't believe us, you were just a little [pause] skeptical . . . Then *Newsweek* printed it, you knew it was true. [Slipping into white voice] 'Honey, they seem to be killing negroes like hotcakes.'"

In post–Rodney King, post–Amadou Diallo America, the existence of racialized police brutality—since the tape that was seen around the world and the shooting that had Amnesty International calling for a review of the

NYPD—and the dangers of driving or just walking while black have become visible issues in mainstream media outlets (like *Newsweek*), not just in the black press, on Pacifica Radio, or National Public Radio.[34] Chappelle purports that there is a singular response to all police "indiscretions." After describing an incident of unwarranted violence, he mimics the older officer explaining the process to his partner, "No paper work, just sprinkle a little crack on him and let's get out of here." This is actually fairly biting; however, by leaving the indictment of the system out of the joke, he just asserts that it is not what it should be.[35]

In *Killin' Them Softly* Chappelle directly addresses overt racism in some clever but fairly nonconfrontational ways. He recounts his dinner in Mississippi, when chicken was ordered for him because, as he says in southern white voice, "Black people and chickens are quite fond of each other." Chappelle's response to this not-so-subtle moment of racism is to be "*upset*, not mad" for unexpected reasons: "All these years, I thought I like chicken because it's delicious. Turns out I'm genetically predisposed to liking chicken. I got no say." While the joke could have simply been read as another reminder of racism "down South," Chappelle complicates it by adding an anecdote that after this incident he felt embarrassment over people seeing him eat chicken in public. Chappelle, speaking as a white passerby, who is definitely *not* southern, points in the direction of the imaginary Chappelle eating chicken, and says, "Look at him. He loves it. Just like it said in the encyclopedia." This subtle commentary on the fact that racism stereotypes don't reside solely "down South" may be the closest that Chappelle comes to blaming anyone in this 2000 version of his stand-up routine.

That is not to say that some of Chappelle's comedy doesn't meander toward the more direct Def Jam model—particularly when the politics of differentiation is used to show "what white people be like." Chappelle engages in gentle ribbing about white protectiveness of their political views, recounting that, in one particular conversation with a white friend (not Chip), the choice of candidate was not seen as polite conversation, but his sexual practices were fair game: (in white voice) "I'm trying to tell you about fucking my wife and you keep asking me all these personal questions." Chappelle follows up with assertions of black behavior in regard to their political affinities: "[Black people] will talk about beating up politicians. If I see George Bush, I'll kick his muthafucking ass for cutting my Medicaid."[36] Another example is playing with the "unhipness" of mainstream white folks like his lawyer, whose response to his madeup slang used as a good-bye ("Zip it up, Zip it out") is "Uh . . . O.K. . . . Zippity doo dah, bye-bye." The clever *Song of South* allusion aside, the joke is basically a throwaway.

Chappelle's best social critique seems almost incidental. In his hijacking routine he plays on dialects and expectations—constructing a Chinese terrorist who inexplicably has a Middle Eastern accent and the unlikelihood of seeing a black hostage reading the terrorist's statement on the news ("They is treating us good. We is just chillin' and shit . . ."). The focus of the bit is on a media-rooted misconception. On scanning the plane for black folks, he catches the eye of the only other black passenger on the international flight, "a fella from Nigeria," who was looking directly at him—the two exchange thumbs-ups. Chappelle explains that this exchange is woefully misread by white passengers: (slipping into white voice) "Oh my God, I think those black guys are going to save us." Chappelle's incredulous shake of the head to the audience conveys that the reality of the situation was quite different: the "thumbs-up" signified the recognition of the fact that *they* (the black passengers) were going to be okay because as he states simply, "Black people are bad bargaining chips." The joke series plays out in some interesting ways. After juxtaposing the white passengers' anticipation of a rescue moment similar to that pulled off by Wesley Snipes in *Passenger 57* (when the black body is utilized to ensure white safety) and the status (read value) of blacks to America, in broad institutional terms, Chappelle asserts that "[for once] racism [is] working in black people's favor."[37] In this instance he puts forth a complex comic sequence that can be read as rather sophisticated racial commentary.

Even Chappelle's description of his "accidental" trip to the ghetto, which is simultaneously absurd and startling, plays with this kind of commentary. It begins with his discovery of the location of his chauffeur's impromptu stop when he notices a distinct change in the urban landscape ("gun store, gun store, liquor store") and ends with his admonishment of a "hardcore" baby (yes, infant) for standing on the corner at 3 a.m., selling weed, to which the baby dealer replies, "Fuck you, I got kids to feed, nigger." The "accidental" journey doesn't directly critique the sociopolitical circumstances that make this particular urban landscape a comment on the lack of *other* businesses in the ghetto or tease out the reasons that *really* young kids are in the drug game. One might, however, read the baby's reply to Chappelle's admonishment—*from his seat in the limo*—as a commentary on comfortably liberal antidrug rhetoric. Chappelle would probably say that he just thought it was funny.

Chappelle, for the most part, avoids direct political commentary. In *Killin' Them Softly*, which was taped after the contested 2000 presidential election, Chappelle begins his discussion of politicians with a caveat: "When I go to vote, which I don't . . ." One might hypothesize that the source of his espoused apathy about the political process could have been rooted in either the disenfranchisement of blacks who did vote in Florida or in the belief that, in 2000, the two-party system had not generated distinct choices for the voter. Whatever the case may be, a definitive statement, one way or the other, cannot be easily discerned. Chappelle later states that he doesn't know anything about their policies, but he would choose politicians on "character." This might allude to the focus of the 2000 presidential campaign on the moral timbre of the candidates, as much as their espoused policies, but it is hardly incisive critique. Notably, Gore goes unmentioned as Chappelle states that he would vote for Clinton *again* and produces sympathetic references to the Clinton White House that rationalize away the core of the scandal and the impeachment by saying that "busy men fuck those close to them."[38] His characterization of Bush—as the crazy uncle who, "when shit goes down, says 'let's go kick their asses'"—seems to be painted with broad, indifferent strokes. The harshest criticism offered is encased in an absurdist vignette when Chappelle strongly asserts, "All I know about George Bush Jr. is that he sniffed cocaine—that might be fine for a mayor [referring to Marion Barry] but not in the White House." With Chappelle voicing a cokehead president in need of a fix, who sounds more like the stereotypical junkie from a seventies drug film than a head of state, the scenario he paints is of the president exhibiting cokehead behaviors while engaging in foreign policy (he offers a blow job in exchange for a signature on a treaty). This elicits hoots from the crowd—and from Chappelle too, who backs away from the mike laughing uproariously. Despite the fact that the joke "kills"—and foreshadows the kind of absurdist moments so commonly seen on *Chappelle's Show*—it doesn't resonate, in sociopolitical terms, beyond the laughter.

That is not to say that Chappelle's comic choices are not at times curiously inconsistent. Chappelle's sexual politics, like those of many contemporary comics, black and white, can be both regressive and sophomoric. Interestingly, the gender humor feels almost like material from an entirely different set—an add-on, if you will. The meandering storytelling becomes joke-telling. When he chastises the women in the audience for not feeling sympathy for Monica Lewinsky ("no one wants to be the most famous cocksucker in the world"), he says, "That's just jealousy," implying that Lewinsky's position was enviable. Furthermore, from his assertion that every woman in the audience had "at least one dick they regret," to his statement that "if pussy was a stock, it would have plummeted [because] you give it away too easy" appears oddly old-fashioned and judgmental, qualities that are virtually absent in every other area of his stand-up. Any possibility of a libratory space in his gender humor is lost entirely when he theorizes that had it been an older woman, rather than Lewinsky, who had been involved with Clinton, she would have used her "services" to secure policy and "sucked us into utopia"—in other words, when lacking in "virtue," whoring for the greater good is admirable.

As Chappelle further rebukes women for their complaints about men—"Yes. Chivalry is dead and women killed it"—it seems worse than reductive; it seems unoriginal. Women, in general, don't occupy a significant space in Chappelle's comedy except as occasional foils and punch lines. Interestingly, with all the talk of sex and penises sprinkled throughout the sixty-minute set, Chappelle articulated a different kind of male world—less boys club and more "lost boys," in a slacker Neverland where, despite their occasional usefulness, women (and their "issues") had no real place. While I would necessarily categorize it as sexism by omission—and there is certainly material out there that is far more misogynistic—in this comic world that seems extremely tolerant and "laid back" on every other front, the gender material seems, as previously stated, curious.

*Killin' Them Softly* is an appropriate title for this, Chappelle's first major stand-up special. Dave Chappelle's stand-up, for all of its outlandish moments, was fairly subtle—at least in terms of its social commentary. Sliding in and out of "white voice"—and between twin poles just south of gross-out humor and just north of scathing social critique, Chappelle's first stand-up special did "kill," to use the comic's terminology, but it did so with the soft touch that allowed for multiple audiences from multiple experiences to actively engage in his comic worldview. Interestingly, both of Chappelle's stand-up specials appear to have derived their names from popular songs from over thirty years ago—one, a play on African American popular songstress Roberta Flack's aching ballad of displaced identification (which was, in a stylistically contemporized version, recorded by Lauren Hill and The Fugees), "Killing Me Softly" (1973), and the other from sixties "stars-of-the-future"-studded white rock band Buffalo Springfield, "For What It's Worth" (1967).

In ways, the two songs can be seen as emblematic of two very different eras: the former a song-about-a-song that resonates too deeply with an audience member (and results in a recognition about various aspects of her life) comes from the early seventies—when the promises of the civil rights era were being replaced by inflation, de facto resegregation (failures of busing), and a sense that a golden moment had been lost; the latter a quintessential (and woefully over-used) anthem of emerging political awareness, also about recognition, and the acknowledgment that the times they *needed* to be changing both politically and socially—and that individual action was required. While the connection between these songs and the actual stand-up routines may seem tenuous, the variations on theme of recognition supply the essential differences between the 2000 and 2004 versions of Chappelle's stand-up comic persona. Industrial shifts aside, Chappelle's tone in the 2000 stand-up is informed by a certain casualness that might even be seen as indifferent; cynical but not quite sarcastic, the anec-dotal strategies of the set make it possible for the audience to take—or leave—that embedded social critique. It might resonate for some, but for others it's just about the funny.

By the summer of 2004 Chappelle's cachet, both in pop cultural and indus-trial concerns, had increased significantly. As previously mentioned, Comedy Central's $50-million man (or his comedic shtick) was everywhere—in person on late-night television, from *The Tonight Show with Jay Leno* to *The Daily Show with Jon Stewart*, and by proxy in the multitudes of "Whuuuuuts" and "I'm Rick James, bitches" that could be heard around the water cooler, in the club, and in the frat house. The only question that remained was how popular his Showtime (not HBO) stand-up special would be. However, the articulation of the comic's persona in *For What It's Worth* revealed that, since the emergence of *Chappelle's Show*, the soft-street sensibility associated with both his big-screen personae and his earlier stand-up had gotten harder.

Like Chris Rock's breakthrough comedy special *Bring the Pain*, *For What It's Worth* supplies a de facto lesson in comedy history before the comic comes to the stage. In voiceover Chappelle explains the choice of The Filmore in San Francisco, which he calls, "the most historic venue you've got as far as comedians are concerned." As Chappelle asserts, "All the best came through the bay," photos of Lenny Bruce, Richard Pryor, Robin Williams, George Carlin, and Paul Mooney are shown in quick succession as the jazz-infused theme from Minnesota acts as the soundtrack.[39] His final statement declares, "You don't have to be the biggest star—as long as you come with it and people [are] coming out." Of course, Chappelle is the biggest comic star at this post–civil rights moment; the semi-self-effacing comic persona of *Killin' Them Softly* (and the aforementioned opening passage) is replaced by the 2004 iteration.

From the opening bit, *For What It's Worth* demands the attention of the audience. More declarative, strongly worded, and extremely direct, the implied "You'd better *recognize*" seems a departure for Chappelle—as much a sign of the times as a sign of his changing industrial and cultural cachet. The young comic, who had sauntered in special number one, comes onstage with a decided sense of sly bravura: he stealthily creeps onstage, he stops and smiles slyly, with hands raised—clasped like a champion after a fight—he walks downstage and struts around the perimeter of the stage . . . giving high fives to the folks in the front row as he says, "Let me hear it." Chappelle is not just going to the party this time—he's well aware of the fact that he is the party. He exclaims, "I did it big this year. From cable, Nigger! Goddam ," signaling that he understands his unlikely position of power. Clad in goldenrod Zaire t-shirt (depicting Ali's punch that took Foreman out in the "Rumble in the Jungle"), jeans, and a hipster suit jacket, Chappelle seems uncharacteristically pumped up for the set in San Francisco. The difference in his demeanor in *For What It's Worth* signals that the tone of this set is going to be different—less everydude on the corner and more "the greatest," Muhammed Ali.

Arguably his first bits hardly seem revolutionary—including San Francisco being the "gayest place on earth" and borderline heterosexist jokes about Castro as "America's anus." However, as he chronicles his trek to the misnamed *Tender-loin* district ("there was nothing tender about the motherfucker, it was rough"), Chappelle eases into critique of the Bay Area: "I'd never seen crack smoked so casually." Chappelle's commentary is still encased in casual storytelling, but it is decidedly less meandering.

While one might argue the bit signifies that even in the often idyllically constructed San Francisco, the problems of the urban landscape—like crack and the social maladies associated with it—are still present, even if they might appear more genteel, the casual crack comment lays the groundwork for his usual comic misdirection that plays out over the course of the next few jokes. Chappelle espouses admiration for "San Fran" as a bastion of tolerance, but the comic's platitudes for the hometown crowd are short-lived. The self-congratulatory cheers are replaced with nervous (and, perhaps, even embarrassed) laughter as his take on the comparative politics of the region becomes clearer: ". . . I realized how you did it—put all the niggers on the other side of that bridge—it's not so happy on that side . . . [when you leave] people are like [in the surfer version of white voice] 'Bye. Bye. Thank you for coming to San Francisco' . . . soon as you get to the other side, 'Welcome to Oakland, bitch.'" With the click, click to signify the locking of the car doors, one cannot be certain whether Chappelle is speaking of his own impulses on exiting Bay Bridge or those of his audience—although his look at the audience seems to say, "You know that's what you do." While not directly confrontational, it is not comfortably ambiguous either.

Chappelle seems less concerned with the audience's comfort. Four days before the premiere of the Showtime special, he remarked on the differences between his experiences of stand-up before and after his newfound stardom: "When you're starting off in stand-up, it's like you're pit fighting—you've always got to win the crowd. And now that I'm the 'funniest man in America,' people will laugh at anything I say [titters from the crowd] even when I try to open up and say something sensitive. [The crowd laughs again.]"[40] Instead of playing *to* his audience in *For What It's Worth*, on some level Chappelle seems to be playing *with* them. More than a mere semantic distinction, the comic's friendly relation is progressively complicated by overtly cajoling, encouraging, and in some instances demanding that the audience own up to its own complicity in the sociopolitical absurdities of post–civil rights era American consciousness.

With the comedic raison d'être of challenging any uninterrogated assumptions, Chappelle's musings were replaced by pronouncements in a harder-edged mode of address. Although his use of "white voice" is not new in the post–Def Jam era of comedic differentiation, the ways in which he mobilizes his multiple forms of whiteness in his characterizations in *For What It's Worth* and, most definitely, in *Chappelle's Show* call into question how those of us in the audience constitute racial identity. The process of making meaning from these comedic texts is further complicated by the fact that these performances of whiteness are often juxtaposed with performances of varying types of blackness, thus urging one to look at and beyond stereotypical constructions to ask what it means to perform race.

One could never characterize Chappelle's humor as conciliatory, but this material verges on the confrontational. From his de facto anthropological study on food and culture to the "liberation" of Iraq and antiwar activities, Chappelle's stories take circuitous yet purposeful paths that veer from being nonsensical to crass to commonsensical to pointed and even radical. His food and culture material exemplifies this kind of comic movement between nonsensical and commonsensical. By asserting that cultural stereotypes based on blacks and Latinos are rooted in the fact that whites guard their dietary preferences, he seems to be channeling Conspiracy Brother, "I study white people—you don't know that? I'm writing a paper on you . . . not even for school, nigger, just to do it." Confronting stereotypical assumptions, he capitalizes on class- and race-coded dietary assumptions. Chappelle states that he learned of "juice," the coveted elixir consumed by white folks, during his study as he compares it to "drink," the sugary, colored, and vaguely fruit-flavored substance with no nutritional value consumed by black folks. Chappelle even ends the routine by invoking the Sunny Delight commercial in which a small multicultural cadre of boys comes to rummage through the fridge, with all others opting for Sunny D and the black kid seemingly eyeing "the purple stuff." Thus, the "drink" becomes a signifier for a literal notion of "taste" culture and dietary choices that are informed as much (if not more) by fiscal realities than culinary preferences.

This is an example of archetypal Chappelle storytelling. *After Chappelle's Show* his mode of address to the audience is very direct, complete with "mock" confrontation, and the implication that "I am surveying your culture" forces the recognition of whiteness and the disparities in relationship to their cultural counterparts, in this case, black people. Some might argue that the politics of juice might seem a bit benign, but I think there is more than a tangential "ketchup" connection in this story, if only on a subtextual level.[41]

At times the same sort of comic storytelling trajectory takes an even more direct and unexpected path, as in Chappelle's discussion of the "liberation of Iraq" and the elimination of what he called the "subtle psychological nuance of oppression" that took place when Saddam Hussein's image was erased from Iraqi currency in what appeared to be a rare "sincere" moment for the comic. However, almost immediately after, Chappelle, no longer choked up about this act of goodwill, queries the lack of the same actions domestically: "But, if you could do that for Iraq, what about our money? Our money looks like baseball cards with slave-owners on 'em." His subsequent disparagement of George Washington (and a bit of historical miseducation) calls into question myriad icons of American culture, which, historically speaking, have different meanings for African Americans—particularly when the father of our country actually could have been the owner of our forefathers.

Perhaps what makes the embedded moments of the strong social commentary even more effective is that they are intermingled with the comedic version of comfort food for the Chappelle fan base—namely "weed humor." As with much of Chappelle's humor, the route to the comedic payoff, even in "weed humor" takes time and is of course not solely weed humor. In his bit about Native Americans that begins in Wal-Mart in New Mexico and ends with buying weed with which to smoke the peace pipe and getting more than half-baked with Navajo tribesmen because "we have to celebrate, 'Nigger, I thought you were dead,'" Chappelle models how cultural insensitivity is not solely the province of white America: his remarks about Native American culture are products of an elementary school social studies class, "You're hunter-gathers." When he asserts that he has stopped smoking weed with black people, his race-based choices about whom he will get high with is based on the fact that black people talk about their hard times while white folks only talk about their other "high" times. However, implicit in this assertion, albeit tangentially, is a commentary on the need for this form of escapism for some segments of the African American community. Clearly not a "Just Say No" moment, Chappelle's story considers, for a split second, why young black males are not saying "No."

The spine for many of Chappelle's stories in *For What It's Worth* is the cult of personality, the interrogation of which serves multiple ideological functions. In his account of his family's ill-fated trip to Disney World his fellow travelers in the Magic Kingdom were unable to distinguish between Chappelle the celebrity and Chappelle the family man: "And . . . fucking everybody, [sliding into a surfer infused version of white voice—the 'dude' is implied] 'Hey! Hey! Rick James, bitch! Rick James, bitch!' [sliding back into his own voice, tinged with touches of annoyance and resignation] 'Hey, man. [Do you] mind not calling me a bitch in front of my kids?' Even Mickey Mouse did it."

His description of his subsequent burst of anger, which culminates in an uppercut that knocks Mickey's head off, is undoubtedly Chappelle's way of commenting on the problems with rabid (and often inebriated) fans, who chant the "Rick James" catchphrase ad nauseam. The hypothesis that Chappelle did to Mickey what he would have liked to do to some overly enthusiastic fans does not seem outside the realm of possibility. This story also serves to reposition Chappelle as the everyguy who happens to be a celebrity, thus reestablishing his "likability" in the face of challenging material.

In service of debunking the cult of celebrity, Chappelle actually works to convince the audience of his incredulousness at the attention paid to and the price in scrutiny paid by celebrities. Interestingly, in this material he employs a somewhat self-denigrating strategy, as in his references to his aborted impulses for antiwar activism: "If they'd do that to three white women [The Dixie Chicks]—they would tear my black ass up." Later he admits that he is not above reproach in terms of cashing in on his own celebrity; having been spokesman for both Coke and Pepsi, he declares "All I know is Pepsi paid me most recently so—tastes better." By admitting his fallibility, Chappelle maneuvers the audience into reacting to his candor rather than the admission of taking the easier softer path on both political and commercial fronts.

Noting that things do not bode well for the black celebrity at this historical moment, the comic points to a number of African American stars in very public legal struggles in post–O. J. America[42]—from Los Angeles Laker star Kobe Bryant (whose performance intensity, according to Chappelle, reads as though the judge had told him to "play for [his] freedom" in the NBA finals) to Michael Jackson's recurrent dipping into some racially coded conspiracy theory, Chappelle notes the strange coincidence between disruptions in the political status quo and recurring allegations against Michael Jackson. His equivocal sympathy for Jackson also serves as a cautionary tale about celebrity: "One day people love you more than they've loved anything in the world and the next day, you're in front of a courthouse dancing on top of a car."

By beginning this series of stories with, "I don't know why people listen to me," and thus appearing to speak with what seems like "utter candor," Chappelle disarms his audience by adding a quasi-confessional element to the set. Additionally, by using his own experiences in juxtaposition to other high-profile celebrities, Chappelle teases out the absurdities of worshipping celebrities while also using it as a set piece from which to discuss other issues as well. For example, Bill Cosby's statements about many of the problems facing the "lower-class" segment of the African American community caused a significant furor in the spring and summer of 2004. Chappelle's matter-of-fact defense of the comic icon's *right* to speak was resonant, as was his rationale for the "hard" nature of Cosby's critique: "Bill Cosby has some real shit to say and the whole world freaked out. . . . Just because he's been selling pudding pops for the last twenty years, people forget that he's a nigger from Philly and the projects and he might say some real shit from time to time." The Cosby controversy resonated across multiple registers of the African American community from symposiums on university campuses to the airwaves (*MacNeil-Lehrer News Hour, The Tavis Smiley Show*). One might be surprised by Chappelle's rather outspoken defense of Cosby; after all, Chappelle is aligned with the hip-hop culture, whose progress, at least indirectly, Cosby bemoans. Nonetheless, Chappelle's choice to defend Cosby's freedom of speech as an individual rather than as the voice of the community also inserts a reminder of the elder comic's experiential ties to the urban black community.

While one must note that Chappelle doesn't actively defend the *content* of Cosby's remarks, by referencing it as "some *real* shit," some modicum of agreement might be inferred. The bit is completely consistent with the ethos of Chappelle's comedic social discourse, in which multiple (and sometimes conflicting) ideologies and cultural experiences are articulated—as is the pointed comic misdirection that follows. In what seems to be even further implicit agreement, Chappelle describes the advice he had given to students at his old high school in Washington, D.C., about ceasing to place blame on whites for all black social ills: "and you've got to learn [pause] to rap, or play basketball or something, Nigger. . . . You are trapped. Either do that or sell crack. . . . That's the only way I've seen it work. Get to work entertaining these white people. [Chappelle ends the bit by doing a little dance.]"

The pleasure of this misdirection is twofold: the unanticipated shift from what appears to be positivist rhetoric of self-determination to a blatant assertion of the untenable position for black kids in the ghetto is a tried-and-true Chappelle comic device, and the content of the statement speaks to the fact that the civil rights era rhetoric (as annunciated by Cosby), on some level, does not and cannot necessarily apply in the lived experiences of black urban youth today. Imbued with a certain degree of fatalism, Chappelle's comment speaks to the notion that the same old problems facing black American youth (poverty, unemployment, substandard education) have been complicated by the current sociopolitical climate. Even so, the comment does not reject the possibility that there might be another way, but neither does it give any indication of what that way might be. The little dance also places a curious punctuation mark on the sequence—it signifies mock complicity and thus positions the comic, whose work is filled with libratory impulses, as one who is also cognizant of and trapped by certain realities of being black in contemporary America.

The utilization of comic misdirection within the context of casual story-telling to make an incisive sociopolitical point is the most useful weapon in Chappelle's discursive arsenal. If one believes that his most telling commentaries come at the moments when the incisive masquerades as the outrageous and relatively benign, Chappelle's routine that begins with the discussion of R. Kelly's alleged penchant for water sports, and the legal troubles that followed, is the Trojan Horse of *For What It's Worth*.[43] After briefly engaging in a discussion of Kelly's actions, which were caught on tape, Chappelle makes a startling pronouncement: the issue that people should be discussing is not whether or not Kelly actually "peed" on the girl. "The real issue is how old is fifteen—that America really needs to decide once and for all."

In one of the longest stories in the sixty-minute stand-up, Chappelle challenges the audience's reactions with multiple instances of comic misdirection, which at each juncture forces more social (and personal) introspection. Chappelle winds through a discussion of his experiences of being fifteen—when he had already begun doing stand-up, smoking a little weed, and watching his friends deal crack—and suggests that "getting pissed on" would not have been what posed the greatest threat to him. By inserting his own experience as a black teenager in urban America, Chappelle foreshadows issues of differentiation that will come into play later in the story. He calls into question why fifteen is seen as such a universally accepted age of innocence in his discussion of the public's concern over the kidnapping of Elizabeth Smart, who was held for six months eight miles away from her home. Contrasting the prolonged media frenzy over Smart's kidnapping with the virtual silence over the kidnapping of a little black girl, Chappelle recounts, "During this half a year that [Elizabeth Smart] was missing, there is this seven-year-old black girl who gets kidnapped in Philadelphia. Nobody knows her name [Erica Pratt] . . . talked about it on the news two or three times, she shoulda been the top story because she chewed through the ropes and had both of them motherfuckers in jail in forty-five minutes. [Moderate applause from the audience.] I'm not making this up."

In moving from Kelly (and the African American fifteen-year-old) to Smart to Pratt, Chappelle shifts the conversation from sexual fetish to media and societal culpability over whose innocence, safety, and story is valued. However, the critique is not complete. Responding to the audible cooling of the audience, Chappelle addresses the discrepancies between the views of a child of fifteen by telling the story of another fifteen-year-old black male in Florida, Lionel Tate, who accidentally killed his neighbor doing the wrestling moves that he'd seen on television. "Now was he a kid? No. They gave him life—they always try our fifteen-year-olds as adults [silence from the audience]. . . . If you think it's okay to give him life in jail, then it should be legal to pee on 'em, that's all I'm saying."

The discursive movement that uses the banal to somewhat titillating Kelly sex scandal as its beginning and end exemplifies Chappelle's process of stretching his comedic boundaries. At multiple points during this sequence he pushes the audience toward discomfort—and interrogation—thus risking both a degree of his "likability" and the friendly relations he enjoys with his multicultural audience. Far from opaque, these clear statements about inequity give a glimpse of the implicit pedagogy that I would argue informs the politics of differentiation in Chappelle's comic persona. By forcing audiences to interrogate the interconnectedness of a multiplicity of factors from daily life, from media, from our own long-held societal assumptions—about race, class, and ethnicity—Chappelle provokes the audience and puts our own notions of community, identity, and, of course, race, on the discursive table.

The tools employed by Chappelle to communicate his comedic social discourse—mobilizing anecdotal observations, literal shifts in voice and perspective, mining popular culture and media, comic misdirection—have been utilized by myriad comics from Pryor to Rock, and their comedic social discourse is shaped by the times and the medium in aesthetic ideological and industrial terms. Often one mediated persona seems in conflict—how else can you explain Pryor's appearances in *The Toy* and *Live in the Sunset Strip* in the same year. While Rock's rant-filled shtick informed his HBO series, none of his film roles have been able to capture the incisive and insightful nature of his stand-up—despite the fact that he had writing credits on both *Down to Earth* and *Head of State*. As we've seen throughout this study, something often gets lost in the translation of the stand-up comic's persona. Sometimes it is obvious—the network requirement to clean up language (prime-time Whoopi is not exactly HBO Whoopi) or the shift from one genre to another (Murphy in *Beverly Hills Cop* vs. Murphy in *Dr. Doolittle*, *Mulan*, *Shrek*). Sometimes it is more subtle—the tweaking of Wanda Sykes's persona from *Wanda at Large* to *Curb Your Enthusiasm* (all the personality, less critical bite). For Chappelle, his comic persona has been refined in this cross-medium trek—and not in the traditional sense. A condensation of his former selves, Chappelle's comic persona in *For What It's Worth*, less laid-back and more cynical than it was in *Killin' Them Softly*, exists to revel in spinning yarns full of social truths that audiences may not want to hear. This was a task with which, at least seemingly, Chappelle had become progressively more comfortable. After all, he had been doing it weekly on Comedy Central since 2003.

### Dancing Like Nobody's Watching:  *Chappelle's Show*, De Facto Crossover,  and the Postnetwork Era

In the winter of 2005 the last session of my television history course was dedicated to *Chappelle's Show*. I had chosen this particular text not because of the low-level spectatorial frenzy surrounding the series—and it was difficult to move around campus without hearing someone quote the series, and not even because of the complex intertextuality of many of the sketches. The lecture—and my motivation—could be summarized in one sentence: I know what I'm laughing at, but I don't know what you're laughing at. The sketch screened in class was an indirect parody of Antoine Fuqua's *Training Day*, with Chappelle in the position of Ethan Hawke, and Wayne Brady, former talk-show host, daytime Emmy winner, and one of the Anglo-friendliest black men on the planet, in Denzel Washington's Oscar-winning role. In what was a fairly diverse class by University of Michigan standards, one quarter of the students were people of color, a majority of whom had seen *Chappelle's Show* and many of whom had seen this particular sketch when it had premiered a few weeks earlier. While I was prepared for differing reading positions, I had not quite anticipated how what was read and what was not read would inform the discussion that followed. As I listened to their responses, which displayed varying levels of sociopolitical and pop cultural acuity, an ongoing internal monologue provided a sort of interrogatory Greek chorus regarding the comedic discourse that was *not* being addressed:

> If you didn't know it was a parody of *Training Day*, how were you reading the conflation of Brady and Denzel Washington, the most popular black actor on the planet?

> If you didn't see it as a parody, why was a pimped out Wayne Brady so funny? Why did the line, "Is Wayne Brady going to have to choke a bitch" get the biggest laugh?

> What about Chappelle in the Ethan Hawke role—trading one Gen-X slacker archetype for another one . . . of color?

> Do you get the need for black actor solidarity comments between Chappelle and Brady—when, in the arena of film comedy, historically, there could be only one?

When peeling back the layers of this sketch, one discerns a multifaceted critique on the place of black actors in Hollywood that encompasses everything from the intersections between cinematic tropes of black male sexuality and criminality to the query so eloquently stated by Jadakiss in his hip-hop hit

"Why did Denzel have to be crooked, when he took it." Then again, some saw a funny sketch with quintessential nice guy Wayne Brady playing against type—really against type. All of this in a five-minute sketch. I knew that there was something going on here—aesthetically, sociohistorically, and ideologically—and it needed to be unpacked.

*Chappelle's Show* was, arguably, one of the funniest and most incendiary series on American television in the early 2000s. The series' contentiousness, as well as its conflicting ideological and comedic impulses, position *Chappelle's Show* as the product of *our* sociohistorical moment, in the first decade of the new millennium, when duality seems the norm. Since 2003, the lines between taste cultures seem to blur easily, with the former fringe—hip-hop culture—soundly ensconced at the center. When the montage for the Boston Red Sox ALCS victory flashes on the screen and plays to the soundtrack of Public Enemy's "Welcome to the Terrordome" (the "Refuse to Lose" passage) or Outkast's "Hey, Ya" is used as theme music at the Emmys, the Grammys, and the Oscars, few stop to acknowledge that somewhere along the line a taste culture shift has taken place. But these are also the times when the illusion of national insulation has been burst by the events of 9/11. We live amid multiple wars—culture wars that divide Americans along red and blue boundaries, interpretations of constitutional and human rights and a vision for the future that seems diametrically opposed to our fellow citizens along color-coded lines. In these times a War on Terror has done for many of us what Vietnam did for our parents—turn anger into activism and/or the sense of national unity into national disarray. The devastation wrought by Hurricane Katrina on America's Gulf Coast forced the media, the nation, and an administration to confront issues of race and poverty. And although this may seem a difficult point from which to launch into an analysis of African American comedic social discourse in general, and sketch comedy in particular, I would argue that in profoundly ambivalent times, the forms taken by our humor—and the discourse embedded therein—provides telling measurements of the American psyche. For African Americans, laughing mad has always been a strategic approach to dealing with adversity, oppression, and ambivalence.

Since its midseason premiere in 2003, *Chappelle's Show*, which the comic describes as "hip-hop Masterpiece Theater," engaged issues of race, class, ethnicity, and popular culture with irreverence, candor, and a decidedly black sensibility rarely seen in prime-time television comedy. As *Chappelle's Show* cocreator, Neal Brennan stated simply: "We're trying to push the genre and make stuff that [is] more interesting and personal. . . . We went to a place, Comedy Central, that sort of needs us and gave us a lot of freedom. . . . We didn't get much money but that was the trade-off—you get control."[44] The duo that brought us *Half Baked* rejuvenated sketch comedy that they describe as "cultural rather than political"[45] and infused it with a hip-hop sensibility and the espoused creative ethos of "dancing like nobody's watching." However, given that the show averages a viewership of 3.1 million per episode *on basic cable*, people are turning to it in droves.[46] While the situation comedy is always about containment—within the twenty-two-minute format, within cultural norms, within certainties of narrative closure—sketch comedy is always about transgression, and in this particular postnetwork era, "edgy" is considered good for business—as long as it's not too "edgy."

By directly engaging performances of blackness and whiteness, *Chappelle's Show* rides the razor's edge of that category, which many, much to Chappelle's chagrin, find surprising, given the fact that the series, cocreator, Neal Brennan, is white. Chappelle expresses a certain degree of exasperation about the fact that "people think in terms of race. Because the show is so racially charged, they're amazed that a white person and black person can be cohorts."[47] In actuality, with an interracial writing team at the helm, specifically engaging in issues of race, Chappelle and Brennan model comedic social discourse where the unspoken is spoken—and the absurdities and hypocrisies that often inform "polite" conversations about race relations are laid bare. On one hand, one might argue that Brennan's and Chappelle's steadfast adherence to the notion that theirs is a "personalized" form of comedy, thus taking the ideological edge off of the racially charged nature of the humor, affords *Chappelle's Show* a greater degree of discursive freedom. On the other hand, the ideologically idiosyncratic ethos might also facilitate the view that the series neither endeavors to nor aspires to engage in more complex sociocultural critique.

By tracing the comic lineage of *Chappelle's Show* from Richard Pryor's abortive foray into prime time in the late seventies through *In Living Color's* emergence at the birth of the netlet era in the early nineties (which coincides with hip-hop "blowing up" and into mainstream popular culture), one can begin to discern how and why *Chappelle's Show* marks a point of rupture *and* a point of convergence for myriad often conflicting articulations of blackness in the post-soul era. One must also consider how the series' de facto crossover appeal problematizes its unique status as industrial and cultural phenomenon. The notion of blackness engaged in this study is an open fluid construct, neither fixed nor finite: in fact, *both* racialized tropes and nuanced fragments of multiple black identities are encompassed herein as articulated in media and in everyday life. The intertextual pleasures of the texts (especially those rooted in popular cultural referencing), at three very different points in the history of American television have provided viewers with a degree of cultural cachet as a reward for being "down"—meaning hip to the sociocultural positioning of black language, style, music, and humor embedded in the texts.

As with any form of cultural acuity, there are multiple levels of "downness." Insider/outsider, black/white, civil rights era/post-soul sensibilities—from these differing reading positions, segments of the audience discern cultural traces and treatises produced in these comedies, which, in turn, inform the notions of blackness in contemporary American society. *The Richard Pryor Show,*

*In Living Color*, and *Chappelle's Show* tell stories of blackness for mass consumption; however, in the process of mass consuming these movable cultural feasts, the spectatorial palates are not always sensitive enough to discern all the ideological ingredients. But, arguably, such is the nature of the subgenre of sketch comedy, where catchphrases are often appropriated while context is lost.

Sketch comedy is only vibrant when allowed to be transgressive, when it is permitted to prod, poke, and puncture the audience's comfort zone and otherwise tweak the social and political status quo. However, the libratory potential of the subgenre of sketch comedy in general and these African American comedy texts specifically, must be seen within the context and constraints of American television. While *The Richard Pryor Show*, *In Living Color*, and *Chappelle's Show* all exhibit—and realize—this transgressive potential, their pushing of aesthetic and generic boundaries takes place within, not outside of, the industrial constraints of American commercial television. Pryor's attempt at network prime time, Wayans's Fox series, and Chappelle's Comedy Central show, when understood in industrial, historical, and sociocultural terms, each embody conditional success and mitigated failure.

In September of 1977, *The Richard Pryor Show*, hailed by television critic Tom Shales as "the most perilously inventive comedy hour to hit prime time in years," began its regrettably short run.[48] As Paul Mooney aptly stated, "[*The Richard Pryor Show*] was way before *In Living Color*. I have nothing against *In Living Color*, I wrote for it. . . . [It] is a spin-off from *The Richard Pryor Show*. We were the first ones to land on the moon called color and provocative. We were the first ones to land there."[49] Mooney's assertion posits Pryor's show at the beginning of an African American comic lineage in relationship to *In Living Color* and, by extension, to the new-millennium series; given that Mooney's influence on each of the three texts is considerable—as head writer, staff writer, and comedic inspiration/recurring player, respectively—his positioning of *The Richard Pryor Show* as the black sketch comedy alpha to *Chappelle's Show*'s omega has considerable authority. Nonetheless, any examination of Pryor's show (and the comedy special that spawned it), alongside *In Living Color* and *Chappelle's Show*, while logical, is complicated by the fact of Pryor's significantly smaller televisual oeuvre than those of his comedic progeny, as well as by the markedly different sociohistorical and industrial context at the inceptions of each. After all, both *In Living Color* and *Chappelle's Show* were seen as good matches with media outlets that, for similar reasons, were in need of challenging material to fit into predetermined niches.

Given that these particular series must inherently be viewed as examples of cultural production, in the process of positioning each of these televisual texts historically one must also situate them within the context of black popular culture of their respective days. Because of the shifting industrial status of the players in each of these texts and the ability of the sketch/variety format to engage in deliberate practices of cultural production, one can discern how the different choices made, in terms of depicting their constructions of the African American experience in their particular televisual milieu, correspond to and conflict with both the aesthetic and cultural politics of their shows and their times. The theme music of each sketch comedy series offers views of *one* of the ideological directives embedded in the shows: The O'Jays' "For the Love of Money" for *The Richard Pryor Show*, Heavy D and The Boyz's "That's the Way You're Living When You're Living in Living Color" for *In Living Color*, and Dead Prez's "Hip-Hop" for *Chappelle's Show*.

While only the chorus of The Ojays' tune is used during Pryor's series ("Money, money, money, money. Money!"), the song was already associated with Pryor's televisual presence. On *The Richard Pryor Special?* as the theme song, Pryor's send-up of television evangelism featured the comic as the Rev. James L. Williams, a money-grubbing preacher/sex symbol with a chorus of "angels" and a personal style that was more Sly and The Family Stone than Reverend Ike. Arguably, in a larger cultural context the song's "bling" cautionary tale—and the fact that the Ojays' tune is a vestige of the Wattstax era (1973) rather than the disco-inflected music of the late seventies—speaks to the profoundly ambivalent black cultural moment in which *The Richard Pryor Show* premiered.

For both *In Living Color* and *Chappelle's Show* the theme songs resonated with differing segments of hip-hop culture. *In Living Color*'s "old-school" theme by Heavy D provided a utopian view of the emergent hip-hop culture as the cure for national ills in its unabashed celebration of a multicultural moment. While the song failed to fully capture the darkly sly sensibility possessed by the Wayans' first television outing, it acted as a virtual counterpoint to the rhymes of "gangsta" rappers—which did not predict a time when "prejudice was obsolete" and "safe to walk down the street." Nevertheless, In *Living Color*'s role as Hip Hop 101 for mainstream audiences cannot be ignored. As Kristal Brent Zook notes, "[*In Living Color*], which has had guest appearances of rappers Monie Love, Queen Latifah and, and Flavor Flav, is grounded in a definitive hip-hop aesthetic manifested in the dress styles, graphic art, music and language."[50] The role of hip-hop culture, however, while more than cosmetic, is less than ingrained in the series' narratives. The engagement of hip-hop culture, like the view of the multicultural moment, is presented simply and directly and fundamentally without any self-conscious critique.

Like "For the Love of Money," Dead Prez's "Bigger Than Hip-Hop" presents a cautionary directive. *Chappelle's Show* utilizes an instrumental version of a song that, like the series itself, simultaneously invokes and critiques hip-hop culture. While Heavy D's theme, pop-esque and positivist, celebrates the second golden age moment, Dead Prez's rant against how hip-hop's cultural capital is being spent, by whom, and on what is unlikely to be heard on *TRL*:

You would rather have a Lexus or justice?
A dream or some substance?
A Beamer? A necklace? Or freedom?

Still a nigga like me don't playa-hate, I just stay awake
This real hip-hop; and it don't stop 'til we get the po-po off the
     block.
They call it . . . hip-hop, Hip-hop. Hip-hop.

In some ways, comparing the tone of *Chappelle's Show* to that of *In Living Color* is roughly analogous to the comparison between the "fat lover" Heavy D and the "revolutionary but gangsta" Dead Prez. Just as the two series intersect with two different subcultures of hip-hop, so, too, do the series mobilize codes that speak to the *culturally* savvy. In his discussion of *In Living Color*, one of the first (and perhaps most critically significant) examples of netlet niche programming in the nineties, Herman Gray teases out the series' "strategy of representation" and its heavy reliance of rap music and hip-hop sensibility: "Rap and hip-hop are used deliberately but quite strategically in the program to generate identifications across racial lines."[51] While one might make the same argument for *Chappelle's Show*, I believe that the connection is more endemic than strategic: the comic's persona is imbued with a hip-hop sensibility—the aesthetic and the politics of musical genre are inextricably tied to his own. While *In Living Color* was informed by hip-hop, the series' cred is solidified because hip-hop is like a character on the show—often personified by the key figures who became either recurring players on the series or recurring gags: during the first two seasons the Rza and the Gza of the Wu Tang Clan, Dame Dash, Snoop Dogg, Method Man, Mos Def, and, first as the subject of and later as player in parody, Lil' Jon. The mogul of "Dirty South" hip-hop originated the callbacks, which are an integral part of the "crunk" sound; however, after Chappelle's parody of Lil' Jon, the imitations of those callbacks—"Whuuuuut? Whuuuuut? Whuuuuut? Oh-kaaaay!"—could be heard everywhere—from hip-hop radio stations to the front porch of the Beta house. These hip-hop stars were integrated as players in Chappelle's comic troupe, which supplied an additional level of pleasure for those who knew who was playing along here.

     One of the first examples of this comes from early in the first season of *Chappelle's Show*, when what appears to be a commercial for a Wall Street investment firm veers into comic left field: as the voiceover states, "Cash rules everything around us. Cream. Get the money—dollar, dollar bill, y'all," Smith Barney becomes Wu-Tang Financial. The pleasures of this skit are multiple. On one hand, the presence of two black men, the Rza and the Gza, looking more "corner" than corner office, speaking to white upper-middle-class suburbanites and giving them "hard" advice on investment strategies, is unquestionably fodder for humor. When the Gza says, "You need to diversify your bonds, nigger. . . . This isn't *Trading Places*, nigger, this is real fuckin' life," audience expectations are clearly being toyed with, thereby playing with and against stereotypes. Those who know hip-hop, however, also know that the Rza and the Gza are brilliant: innovative producers and savvy businessmen, as well as part of a legendary rap group; for these viewers Wu Tang Financial, however unlikely, is not outside the realm of possibility.

The enjoyment of this sketch, and, indeed, the series as a whole, is not predicated on any particular knowledge of hip-hop culture. It is here that the negotiation between insider/outsider humor is complicated in some fascinating and arguably unique ways. In this comic text, as in Chappelle's stand-up, there exists another level of pleasure rooted as much—if not more—in cultural savvy rather than solely racial affinity. This fosters a sort of de facto crossover, where the appeal of a distinct culture product (like Chappelle's comedic work or hip-hop, for that matter) crosses racial and cultural boundaries due to, among other things, shifts in taste culture or industrial reframing.

In all three of the series the engagement of stereotypes acts as the spine for sketch material; and, to borrow Chappelle's metaphor for series' sketch comedy style, in series that are like the bits in "a comic's joke book," some of them work, and some of them don't. There is a certain analytical quandary that one encounters in the process of examining sketch comedy—its inherent inconsistency—not only in terms of quality but also in terms of its ideological and aesthetic imperatives. The selection of any number of sketches could be used to make differing assertions about the ways in which the series' content speaks to the articulation of blackness at its given historical moments. Thus, in the spirit of full disclosure, when turning to the televisual texts themselves, I have selected what I believe to be the most *provocative* examples of each series pushing its own self-imposed (and industrially-imposed) boundaries in relationship to stereotypes (of class, as well as race), "insider" humor, and the performance of blackness *and* whiteness. In so doing, I hope to reveal a cacophony of sometimes dissonant articulations of African American comedic discourse that resonate across the span of the post-soul era.

In her analysis of *In Living Color* Norma Miriam Schulman reminds us that "appropriating a language of stereotypes in order to undermine the dominant order is an age old device employed by persecuted groups to subvert the status quo."[52] On each of the series the mobilization of stereotypes contains the potential to confront *and* conform to popularly, if silently, held racial stereotypes. The "Reparations" sketch, from the first season of *Chappelle's Show*, presents a litany of stereotypical constructions of blackness, mostly annunciated by the "white" media. Correspondents from Action News present stories of what happens when black people "get paid." On some level the pleasures of this particular text are based in (minimally) dual recognition—the laughter impulse rooted in the "that's just wrong" response to constructions of African American taste culture and another more self-reflexive commentary that speaks to playing with "their" (read outsider) understanding of our (read insider) cultural foibles. The line is hundreds of people long at the check-cashing liquor store because, as the perky blonde correspondent chirps, "There are no banks in the ghetto because banks hate black people," is the first of many reparations-induced news stories explained by a white-faced Chappelle (as anchorman Chuck Taylor), who "makes sense" of the phenomenon for the virtual and literal audience. The finance reporter's announcement of eight thousand new record labels being formed in the last hour, the market implications of Cadillac Escalades and gold going through the roof while stock in watermelon stayed "surprisingly low," and the newly merged world's largest company, FuBu/KFC, leave few stereotypes unstated. The litany of racialized tropes includes the transformation of Al Roker-esque weatherman Big Al, from one who jovially performs amenability to his "true" self, a "straight-up gangsta."

Perhaps the most interesting character is the individual who is said to usurp Bill Gates as the world's richest man, "a Harlem native known simply as 'Tron.'" In matching gray PNB Nation oversized basketball jersey and shorts, Chappelle plays Tron as a stylish street hustler with gold ropes hanging on his arms. Tron explains to the white female reporter that his new status was acquired by virtue of "a hot hand at a dice game, baby girl." After facetiously stating that he is going to put money back into the community (and then "Psych!"), Tron intones a simple financial plan: "I'm gonna spends all the money before you white people changes your minds." Tron also taunts Taylor—"I got your girl, Chuck"—just prior to asking the white female correspondent to give "a lap dance for the world's richest man." When, later in the season, Tron reappears in *Mad Real*

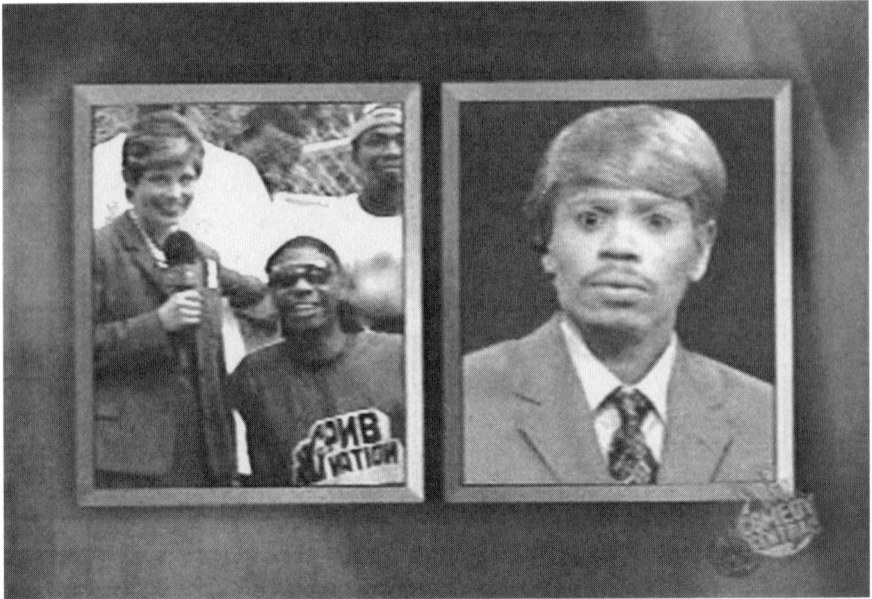

26. Getting paid: Chappelle as America's richest man and the anchor who disdained him on *Chappelle's Show* (2003). Directed by Rusty Cundieff, Andre Allen, Scott Vincent, Bill Berner, Bobcat Goldthwait, and Peter Lauer.

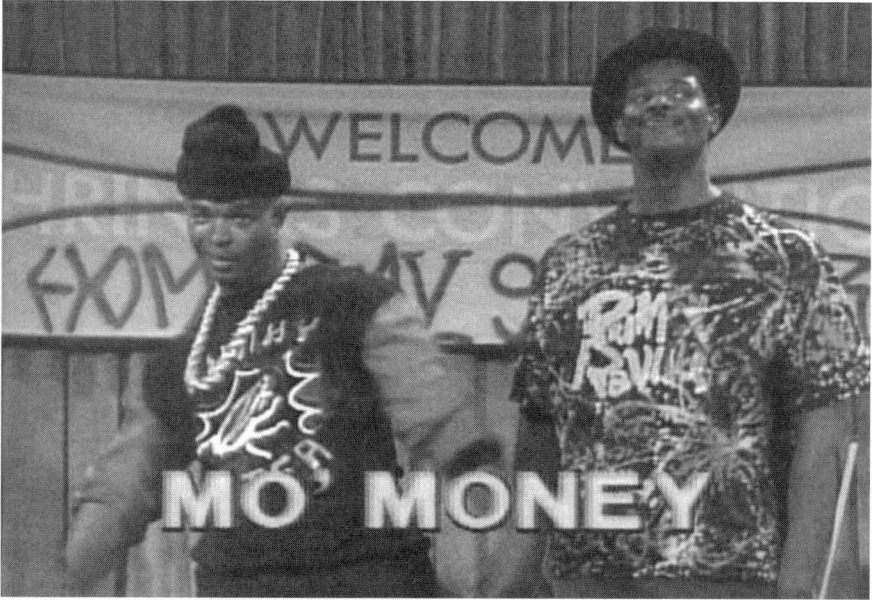

27. The other Wayans brothers, Keenen Ivory (right) and Damon, as "homeboys." *In Living Color* (1990). Directed by Terri McCoy, Paul Miller, and Keenen Ivory Wayans.

*World*, a racial reversal of the MTV reality series, he again acts the antagonist to whiteness—this time to the lone white "innocent," Chad, who is placed in the house with a cornucopia of characters who occupy "ghetto" constructions of urban blacks by constantly partying, never working, and, "without provocation," hating the white man. In this sketch Tron acts as a facilitator for the token's downfall when he beds Chad's not-so-virginal girlfriend (on film)—as does Charlie Murphy as Tyree, the prison-hardened thug who, over a "look," "shanks" the white guy's father—and makes the final house meeting pronouncement that Chad has to go (because, as one of the black female housemates says, they "don't feel safe" with him).[53]

In "Homeboy" sketches on *In Living Color*, popular mediated spaces are also utilized as a means of putting black urban stereotypes on parade. First introduced as proprietors of the Homeboy Shopping Network, a parody of the Home Shopping Network, Whiz (Damon Wayans) and The Iceman (Keenen Ivory Wayans) are like Tron, visually coded as hip-hopified hustlers. Given Whiz's Flavor Flav–inspired timepiece hanging around his neck and The Iceman's multiple Africa medallions, the Homeboy's images are conflated with notions of Afrocentrism rooted more in style than in ideology. Their mobile place of business operates first out of the back of a moving van full of clearly stolen goods ("televisions that are exactly like those in finer hotels" and "[gold] chains that have been broken in transit") and later out of the parking lot at

Dodger Stadium during a game (the seventh-inning stretch marks the used-car sale coming to a rapid end). The Homeboys use the language of HSN to move their "hot" properties: "Act now and get this complimentary gift," which might happen to be the Gideon Bible stolen from the same room as the aforementioned television.

While these sketches primarily engage the "black-male-as-criminal" trope, the segment for the Homeboy seminar provides a litany of Reagan/Bush era stereotypes of blackness. The seminar, which promotes their book, *How to Get Mo' Money without using Yo' Money*, offers a concrete plan for getting cash from an entity "who got more money than they know what to do with—the Gub-ment." Beginning with the kind of "intriguing fact" that often opens infomercial-like seminars: The Iceman states, "Did you know that food stamps cannot be used to buy alcoholic beverages?" to which Whiz responds, "How can I make this knowledge work for me?" Pointer in hand, they instruct the audience through a cartoon chart of a proposed food stamp scam that involves finding "an unscrupulous individual" (drawn as an older black wino) to whom you sell a six pack of beer (which cost $3.99 "or depending upon the security system") for $40-$50 worth of food stamps (which he doesn't need—"he's eating fine . . . he might even be in your family"), which the viewer can, in turn, sell for $25 to "a little fat lady named LaQuita with like 15 kids" (drawn as the archetypal "welfare mom," complete with curlers in her hair, cigarette in her hand, and kids on her hip). "What does that equal—mo' money, mo' money, mo' money."

As with both the "Reparations" and "Mad Real World" sketches, the over-the-top distribution of stereotypes in the short narrative of the "Homeboys" bits—and the condensation of the racist characteristics attributed to the central (and peripheral) players in these narratives—would seem to signal the inherent "unreality" of the scenario being depicted. However, after screening these sketches yet again, I am struck by the fact that the stereotypical tropes are simply not unfamiliar and not, therefore, startling to the viewer in and of themselves but rather by their placement alongside a series of similar constructs. It makes me wonder—and worry—about the perceptions being formed regarding the object of the laughter from different demographic spaces in the diverse body of the series' audiences.

No doubt you can see insider humor playing with outsider expectations throughout these sketches. Sometimes it comes like a wink to the audience—like the truck full of Kools driven by Donnell Rawlings, who models the black people's "love of the menthols" and supplies one of *Chappelle's Show's* all too familiar phrases, "I'm rich, bi-atch." At other times humor is written into the very texture of the sketch. The ways in which insider strategies are utilized on Pryor's and Chappelle's series provides counterpoints not only in terms of tone but also of the times. Although by virtue of its brief network run, a four-episode sample, one can sense the direction of comedic social discourse in Pryor's series and the potential for engaging the often problematic process of presenting insider humor to an audience of insiders and outsiders. Both series present constructions of a black president—one with Pryor as a fictional "40th President" and the other a "through-the-looking-glass" construction of the current administration with Chappelle as "Black Bush." One of the central differences between the two portrayals is the function played by "markers" of blackness, the most easily discernible of which is language. Pryor is playing presidential (read formal and proper) and slides into blackness, encouraged by black presence at a briefing, while Chappelle, as a "thugged-out" Bush whose posse supports his "keeping it real," gives the "straight-up" motivations for his actions.

The critique in the sketches engages both the performance of blackness and how the perception of these performances, more often not, comes through the lens of the media—the televised news briefing for Pryor's chief executive and the television news documentary for Chappelle's Black Bush. In "The 40th President," while Pryor dabbles in some degree of contemporary political commentary (addressing the SALT talks and the neutron bomb, which he states is "not in the cellular realm of reality" and, therefore, can be seen as a "neo-Pacifist weapon"), race is the centerpiece of the sketch. Questions from black reporters put Pryor's Prez at ease, and he begins to answer questions as "a brother": in response to an inquiry about his new FBI director (from a very young Marsha Warfield as a reporter from Jet), he responds, "I figure Huey Newton is best qualified—he knows the ins and outs of the FBI, if anybody knows the ins and outs of the FBI." The significance of the reference was quite possibly lost on a mainstream audience, who knew Newton only from either the anti-Panther rhetoric in mainstream media or the revolutionary prowess that had inspired the "Free Huey" campaign in the late sixties. In fact, the cofounder of the Black Panthers had, that same year, returned from a three-year exile in Cuba to face (and to be acquitted of) murder charges in an America that he believed had changed enough for him to get a fair trial. Those who knew got the double edge of the joke.

This was also the case with the black revolutionary-costumed, "Brother Bell" (Tim Reid) from *Ebony*, who begins his exchange with "Yo, blood," by which Pryor's president is taken aback. The recovery is quick, with Pryor responding "Alaikum Salaam" to the reporter's "As-Salaam-Alaikum." The Nation of Islam greeting and black nationalist coding from a reporter at *Ebony* might be read as a surprising moment of verisimilitude for white audiences, for black audiences (and others in the know), a politically *radical* correspondent for the magazine that, in some circles, has been criticized for being "more interested in showcasing the symbolism in black America" than "the critical substance in black America," seems unlikely, at best.[54] This contradiction is further underscored by Brother Bell's question: "Brother, about blacks in the labor force . . . What are you going to do about having more black brothers as quarterbacks and coaches?" While a legitimate question, it is decidedly less political than one

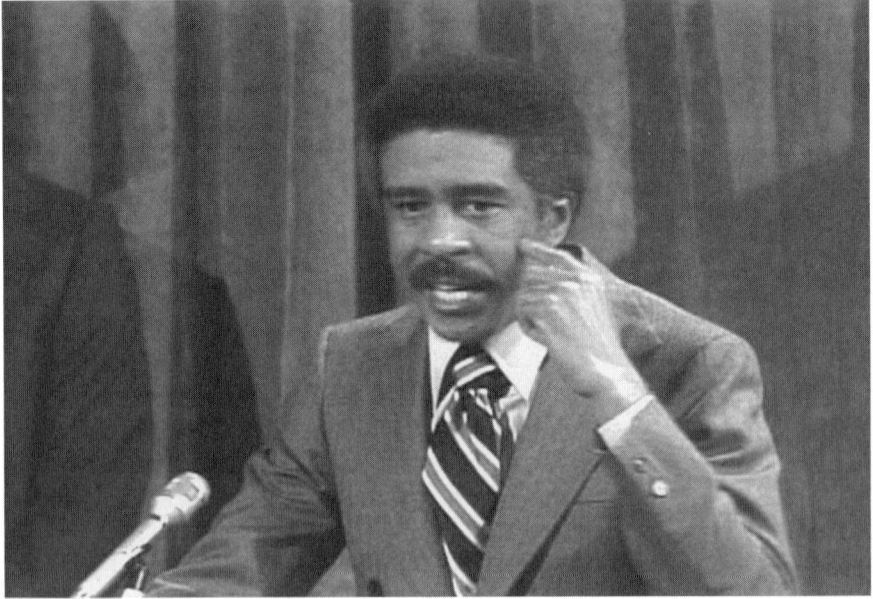

28. Pryor's fortieth president's jaws are tight. *The Richard Pryor Show* (1977). Directed by John Moffitt.

would expect from the way the character is presented—unless, of course, you actually read *Ebony*. In Pryor's series this subtle critique allows for the fact that some audiences will engage (read laugh at) the "affect" of blackness rather than its substance.

*Subtle* would not be a word used to describe the critique of "Black Bush." Chappelle introduces the sketch by immediately placing it in a "them vs. us" context regarding both perception and policy. "If our president were black, we would not be at war right now—not because a black person wouldn't have done something like that, because America wouldn't let a black person do something like that without asking them a million questions." Thus, the premise of the sketch becomes facetiously educational: making it clear to nonwhites why they wouldn't trust the government either if it was being run by "Black Bush." The broadness of the sketch (including Mos Def as a gangsta George Tenet, who assures the press that his napkin full of actual "yellow cake" proved that Saddam Hussein did, indeed, have WMDs) did not undermine the fact that Bush's actions (if not his rhetoric) had more than a touch of "street" sensibility. In a segment of the faux documentary entitled *Path to War*, Black Bush, momentarily, performs "presidentially" by discussing the times as being "ripe for regime change." This performance quickly fades as Black Bush gets "honest," with Donnell Rawlings (in another prime example of a supporting character citing/questioning cultur- ally coded expression) providing callback confirmations.

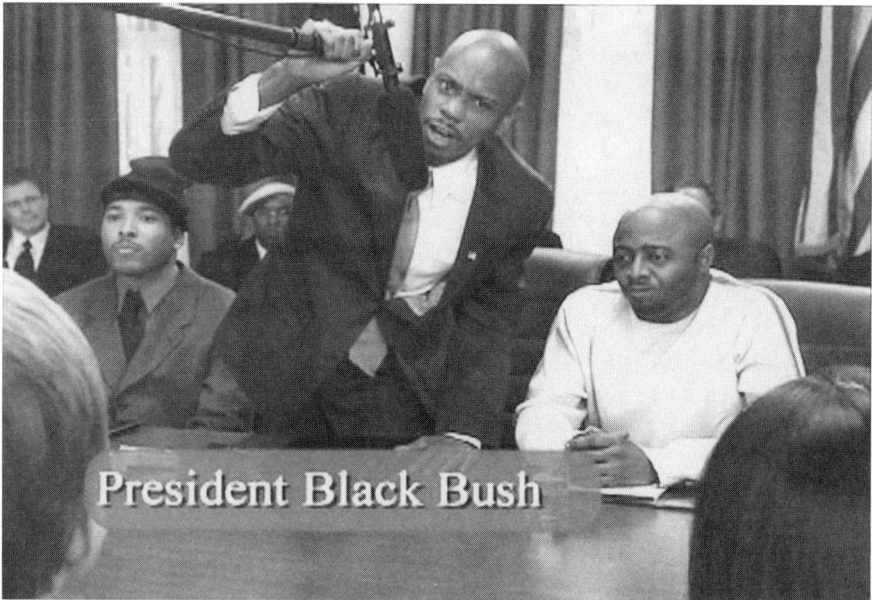

29. Keeping it real: Dave Chappelle (center), as straight-up President Black Bush (2003). Directed by Rusty Cundieff, Andre Allen, Scott Vincent, and Neal Brennan.

BLACK BUSH: But, if I can be real.
RAWLINGS: Be real, son.
BLACK BUSH: Can I be real?
RAWLINGS: Be "real" real, son.
BLACK BUSH: He tried to kill my father, man. I can't play that shit.
RAWLINGS: Say Word. He tried to kill your father.

Jumping up from his seat, Black Bush grabs the boom mike like an angry M.C. and says (in melodramatic outrage) directly to the camera, "The nigger tried to kill my father." To which Rawlings as his "backup" replies, "Word to everything we love. We're coming to see y'alls."

The image of Black Bush, in all its "thugly" nuance, and his Pentagon posse getting ready to roll, replicates any number of moments in black gangsta-inflected films—from *Menace II Society* to *Baby Boy*—particularly if one substitutes "boy" for "father." The pleasure added here for insiders is rooted in their knowledge of other black cultural productions—like Black Bush naming Afrika Bambaataa and his Universal Zulu Nation as part of the coalition of the willing. The central premise, however, that if one examines the actions of the administration, the emotional illogic of the foreign policy seems more about turf, pride, and "cream" than exporting freedom can be understood without one's being able to decipher the hip-hop currency in the text. In these sketches the conflation of race and culture provides at least two viewing positions from which to understand the comedy—but that does not prevent the viewer or this scholar from discerning the direction of the comedic discourse. That is not always the case.

Race is clearly not the only construct coming into play in these series. The intersections between race and class inform the positing of the street hustlers in the urban postindustrial American milieu: arguably, while the spectator may infer that these narratives position Tron, the Iceman, and Whiz as African American males utilizing the employment opportunities presented to them, in the end they are, nonetheless, the target of the laughter. Perhaps simply a sign of the times—an era where the notion of enlightened self-interest seems to have become progressively outdated, the sketches featuring *In Living Color*'s homeless guy, Anton, and *Chappelle's Show*'s crackhead, Tyrone, for all their media savvy and self-referential prowess are fundamentally media spoofs, with their respective fringed behaviors acting as the virtual comic rim-shot. In the parody of the PBS upscale fix-it series, Anton hosts "This Old Box," citing the home improvement possibilities for his place of residence. The sketch dabbles in presenting the realities of living conditions for folks on the street, but ultimately, Anton's pride in his ingenuity—the jerry rigging of electricity, heating, and plumbing, which constructs him more as a homeless version of MacGyver than Bob Villa—is the punch line.

While there is a touch of the Little Tramp in *In Living Color*'s portrayal of Anton, Tyrone lacks any redeeming qualities: driven entirely by his addiction— he is willing to do anything and to give detailed accounts of those actions. The archetypal crackhead, whose exploits have found their way into numerous stand-up sets (Chappelle and Chris Rock's included) and American popular memory (whether through "crack whores" and "crack babies" common in the rhetoric of the Reagan-and-Bush-the-elder era on the dangers of urban America or in devastatingly accurate cinematic constructions like Samuel L. Jackson's Gator in *Jungle Fever*), Tyrone's appearances seem to exist outside of a socio-historical sense of the crack epidemic's impact on urban America. The sketches are disturbingly funny: whether as the pro-crack "antidrug" lecturer for an elementary school class or the contestant for whom the most outlandish (and disgusting) tasks on *Fear Factor* seem like a Sunday brunch. Chappelle plays Tyrone, white-lipped and scratching, with jerky movements (and sometimes, old-school dance moves), as the character intones his status, happily outside of the mainstream, in an accent that is difficult to pinpoint in terms of region. When the host prepares the crackhead for each progressively horrifying task, Tyrone replied confidently with some variation of "Didn't tell you, Joe Rogan, I smoke rock."

The outlandishness of both Tyrone and Anton seems a stark contrast to the two-part sketch that introduced Pryor's underclass characters. In the instances when the black underclass is directly engaged, the result is often transgressive without necessarily mustering an ideological punch. Yet one must also consider whether the kind of bittersweet construction of comedic discourse dealing with class disparity, homelessness, and the sociopolitical roots of underclassness illustrated in Pryor's "Junkie and Wino" sketch could play in the contemporary comedy climate. The same might be said for a seriocomic two-act sketch from *The Richard Pryor Special?*, which chronicled a night in the life of Willie the wino, Pryor's construction of the barfly cultural critic, who made a striking and poignant debut on his special—and to whom he never had gotten the opportunity to return on his own show. First shown in his bar cultural milieu, Willie is depicted in relationship to a disaffected segment of society, which he proceeds to critique even as he positions himself as a part of it (before the bartender gives him his nightly escort to the door). While the barfly milieu seemed somehow outside of time—by virtue of the "integrated" crowd (there were two non-blacks, one patron and the bartender) and the not-surprising constructions that his fellow patron/alcoholics were out of step with society (regardless of the era)—the home space is historically situated across the civil rights and post–civil rights era. In the second part of the sketch we meet Willie's wife (played by Maya Angelou), who Willie says "is gonna kill me then she's gonna talk me back to life and then kill me again." In the soliloquy from Willie's long-suffering wife, Angelou gives Willie something that neither Tyrone nor Anton possesses, socio-cultural context.

Separated by a decade from each other (and at least two from Pryor), the most concrete examples of *In Living Color*'s and *Chappelle's Show*'s engagement of this segment of the black underclass reveal a comic strategy that is decidedly more explicit, undoubtedly darker and markedly less human. In the end, as Gray asserts, the construction of Anton—and I would argue Tyrone as well—leaves the black underclass "exposed . . . as television objects of middle-class amusement and fascination . . . amusing social incompetents with whom few can or should identify and for whom most have little if any feelings."[55] I believe this also raises questions about how comedic social discourse actually can and cannot function in contemporary society. The prescriptive implications of the Pryor sketch, although not overt, speak to the idea that understanding Willie's back-story—and, thus, educating the audience—can have a broader impact on popular consciousness toward the similarly downtrodden. There is no such educational directive in the sketches featuring Anton and Tyrone, no prescriptive about how to understand their plight—in fact those who come to either the aid or the defense are often cast as liberal suckers.[56]

While the word that best describes the tone of the humor is *unflinching*, when one returns to the repeated assertions about the "personal" nature of comedy on *Chappelle's Show*, there is some flinching going on. While *Chappelle's Show* clearly taps into both hip-hop flavored black thought *and* a generational ethos, the comic refuses to address why and whether it might be seen as "representative" of the ideologically informed within the subcultures he engages.

Whether this refusal might ultimately be used as a way of undermining the ide-ological work being done in the comedic televisual text, *Chappelle's Show* (and the popular cultural buzz it has generated) has slapped race back onto the dis-cursive table of sketch comedy with the kind of resounding and unanticipated thud not heard since Richard Pryor and Chevy Chase played "word associa-tion" on *SNL*. In this historic sketch, written by Paul Mooney for Pryor, *Nigger*, the key word in the sketch, which has been used "like aural wallpaper," to bor-row Elvis Mitchell's phrase on *Chappelle's Show* and in the stand-up work of Pryor and Chappelle, acts as the nexus for the problems and the potential for articulating the black experience in comic social discourse. It also underscores the fact that the use of and the response to the *N* word is always a commentary on both blackness and whiteness in post–civil rights America. As Chappelle maintained in a *60 Minutes* interview, "If you could sum up the story of Amer-ica in a word, ["nigger"] might be the word. It has connotations in it that soci-ety has never dealt with."[57]

Both *The Richard Pryor Show* and *In Living Color* reflect on whiteness in differing ways—but both do so indirectly, and their use or probation of the *N* word is also deliberate. One might argue that the never-produced Pryor sketch parodying the pathos on parade game show, *Queen for a Day*, by substi-tuting race for royalty—and having minorities play for all the subsequent priv-ileges that being "Whitey" affords—speaks directly to notions of white privilege without actually revealing how whiteness is constructed. The pathos on parade here are myriad tropes of downtrodden-ness associated with poor, disempow-ered, and otherwise disadvantaged people of color—as contestants vie for prizes including "a year's supply of believable excuses for utility bill collectors, a case of ripple . . . and a Beverly Hills mother of three to clean your house and do your windows." The privilege is the subject of the comedic discourse—the whiteness is not. Furthermore, the use of the *N* word is reserved for sporadic referencing—like a "nigger I knew in Detroit." Given the network climate in the days long before *Def Comedy Jam* and the struggles with the censors that Pryor and his writers faced, the politics of *nigger* were clearly a battle they were not willing—or able—to fight.

The *N* word was prohibited on *In Living Color*—as were discussions of AIDS, white supremacy, and crack—opting for a positivist if irreverent view of the moment of "multiculturalism" in the early nineties. The choice of method in engaging socioculturally packed issues was often contingent and ambivalent—in other words, they were testing uncharted netlet waters. In the "Toms" sketches on *In Living Color*, the performance of whiteness—and not the embedded privi-lege—is the topic. The "Toms" (Damon and Keenen Wayans) are played as the fully assimilated Negro version of the Smothers Brothers (sans any sense of politi-cal or racial awareness) hosting their own talk show. In response to being called "brother" by their African American guest, Tom (Damon) incredulously remarks on the other "brother's" confusion: "*We're* brothers [signaling to the other 'Tom']."

You're just an angry black guy." In this throwback construction of "good Negroes," the Toms perform "whiteness"—down to the processed hair, V-neck sweaters, and a song style and speech that fetishize the "whitest of white" cultural practices as the norms to which they aspire. The "Toms," by name and deed, present an overdetermined construction of black folk trying to be white, and when presented as the antithesis of the "stay black" sentiment of that day are not challenged to move beyond these essentialized notions of performing whiteness—as living racialized punch lines for "white people be like" jokes. In these sketches either privilege or performance of whiteness is the subject of the comedic critique, and this narrowing of the discursive focus limits viewing the oppressive structures of whiteness as ingrained, unspoken, and uninterrogated. In other words, in these comedic discourses, whiteness gets off easy, and audiences get to stay fairly comfortable. This is not *completely* the case on *Chappelle's Show*.

In *Chappelle's Show*, the strategic use of the N word, with its multiple contemporary and historical meanings, plays a prominent role. In *Am I Black Enough for You? Popular Culture from the 'Hood and Beyond*, Todd Boyd contends that "what is truly compelling about this word [*nigger*] and its resulting image is that many in contemporary society, in opposition to a large percentage of African Americans, have chosen to adopt a nuanced form of the word as a vital part of their own cultural identity. The modern-day 'nigga' . . . equally defies aspects of mainstream white culture, as well as the at times restrictive dimensions of status quo black culture."[58] In some ways I believe Boyd's assertion describes Chappelle's use of the word, but in other ways I believe something less successfully subversive is going on. On one hand, when asked about audience discomfort with his frequent use of *nigger*, Chappelle shrugs and replies, "To each his own . . . [*nigger*] used to be a word of oppression. But when I say it, it feels more like an act of freedom . . . for me to say that unapologetically on television," thus articulating the libratory component of using the N word.[59] On the other hand, the comic maintains that his frequent use of the N word has no greater significance than "that's just the way" and that "there are people who speak that way as one of the subcultures in America."[60] And while Chappelle admits that he would be furious if a white comic invoked the N word in his act, the subcultures for whom usage is acceptable seem vaguely defined as those "who know in what context to say it. They know who and when and why and where they're saying it."[61] Regardless, his use of the word *nigger* is tied to some form of rebellion—if only against those convinced of the negative power of the word, regardless of who uses it: "I'm not concerned when black intellectuals say the 'N' word is awful. If people stop saying the 'N' word is everything going to be equal? Is a rainbow going to come out of the sky, and all of a sudden things are going to be better for black people?"[62] By looking at two sketches from the first and second seasons of *Chappelle's Show*, we can begin to see how the show's articulation of blackness—in its myriad often conflicted mediated forms—forces the audience to recognize whiteness as a cultural construct as well.

In January of 2003 the sketch on Clayton Bigsby, the black white supremacist, appeared on the premiere episode of *Chappelle's Show*, which, according to Brennan, the network initially fought. "[Comedy Central didn't think it was exemplary of what the show is and that was the most vicious fight we ever had with them because we were like, 'This is exactly what the show is.'"[63] The *Frontline* parody was inspired by Chappelle's grandfather's story—in reverse. Chappelle describes his grandfather as "a proper dude" and fair skinned—"he could've been white, he was born in a white hospital in Washington, D.C., in 1911 so one of his parents had to have been white."[64] Like Bigsby, his grandfather was blind from birth; unlike Bigsby (who is played by Chappelle), he was cognizant of his race, even as he was put in the position to "pass" to avoid trouble during school. Following the assassination of Martin Luther King Jr., his grandfather, riding the bus in his D.C. neighborhood, became aware of a "ruckus" caused by a white person being on the bus—"Grandpa thought the white person was foolish until he realized that he was the white fellow in question"—his grandfather emerged from the situation safely when "he got real on 'em" and showed that he was a "soul brother."[65] This story became the source material for what is arguably the series' most provocative sketch—and it was on the show's premiere episode.

The first fifteen minutes of the show had been irreverently amusing, including a commercial parody of the annoying "club dancing" girl in the Mitsubishi television spots, faked archival footage of a Nat King Cole's Christmas special (which quotes both hip-hop language and the malt liquor pouring segment of Dr. Dre's "It's a G Thing" video), and an absurdist skit on having a "home stenographer." However, there had been nothing earth shattering about the series' premiere thus far. Chappelle's introduction to the sketch definitely led one to believe that something outrageous was to come: "I still haven't been cancelled yet, but I'm working on it. And I think this next piece might be the one to do it. This is probably the wildest thing I [have] ever done in my career. I showed it to a black friend of mine and he looked at me like I had set black people back with a comedy sketch. [Shrug.] Sorry. Just roll it.[66]

The filmed sketch, which appears identical to a segment in the PBS documentary series in terms of tone as well as visual conventions (identified "talking heads," voiceovers, slow-motion passages, setting the subjects in their respective environments), begins with a warning (white letters on a black screen) read in voiceover by longtime television character actor Bill Bogert, as journalist Kent Wallace:

WARNING

For viewers sensitive to issues of race, be advised that the following piece contains gratuitous use of the "N" word. And by the "N" word, I mean Nigger. There I said it.

The warning, which engages white liberal discomfort with the word ("there I said it"), is the first indication of the contentious nature of the sketch. The camera freezes on a long shot and pulls into a close-up of Chappelle as Bigsby, clad in large dark glasses, camouflage hat, overalls, and red-and-black flannel, rocking on the porch of his rustic homestead (loving, also blind, white wife at this side), as Wallace's voiceover, dripping with incredulousness, questions, "How could this happen? A black white supremacist." After supplying *Frontline* with an extensive list of the people he hates ("Niggers" leading the list), Bigsby ventures off of his lands (and out of the bubble wherein his "whiteness" is secure). When we learn that Bigsby and all of his classmates at the Wexler School for the Blind were told that Clayton was white, the performance of "whiteness" is called into question by the headmistress's reply to Wallace's inquiry ("and he never questioned it?"): "Why would he?" she stated, simply.

Furthermore, while Bigsby's construction and his tirades clearly illustrate the absurdities of white supremacist discourse, what I find more challenging is the way the sketch plays with the intersection between the word *nigger* and the performance of "whiteness." The image of Bigsby (Chappelle) slapping one of the locals on the back and joining in on the verbal hate-fest, which is in actuality being directed at the black white supremacist himself, is as startling as it is subversive. The locals stand in stunned silence as Bigsby continues to hurl epithets, ending with a fist clenched call for "white power." The white recognition of performing whiteness is further complicated when Bigsby encounters a car full of young white suburban males, constructed as co-opters of blackness (dressed in hip-hop regalia and blasting rap), who take the call of "Boogedy, Boogedy, Nigger" from the BWS as a sign that they are, indeed, "down." At his book signing, attended by Klan members, skinheads, and rednecks in full dress, Bigsby wears KKK robes, in order to, his bodyguard, Jasper, reminds him, keep his identity secret from those "unsympathetic to the movement" (and, thus, to keep him "useful"). After a vitriolic tirade against everyone from any marginalized group to the liberal media, Bigsby acquiesces to the crowd's calls to "Let us see your face, brother" and dehoods—literally blowing his followers minds.[67] While one might argue that these constructions are merely jokes—some broad, some subtle—playing with long-held stereotypes, I think something far more complex is going on.

In this sketch the question becomes, "Who *is* the Other, anyway?" The reception of this particular performance of whiteness, although absurd, represents a certain type of "authentic" voice, that of the unbridled, white supremacist—who happens to be black. Before dismissing this notion, as an intellectual stretch, consider how as Bigsby, Chappelle forces the viewer to see how "whiteness" is quite literally performed—not simply by his southern inflected "white voice" but also by depicting these forms of whiteness as "learned" constructs—whether by Bigsby, his supporters, or even the young suburban boys. Whiteness

is not invisible here; thus, the Clayton Bigsby sketch can be seen as comic discourse that pushes the viewer to acknowledge that "everyone in this social order
has been constructed in our political imagination as 'a racialized subject'" and
"to make visible what is invisible when viewed as the normative state of existence: the white point in space from which we tend to identify difference."[68]
Rather than refracting meaning from the "white point in space," the focus on
difference is on the white space—Clayton Bigsby may be black, but it is performing whiteness that is being interrogated.

Over the course of the nine-minute sketch, the word *nigger* and other racial
epithets against African Americans (including "coon," "jungle-bunny," and
"nigras") are uttered twenty times—which must be some sort of record for
broadcast television. The usage of the *N* word in the context of this sketch, for
the most part, simultaneously confronts and conforms to the historical construction of the term, which Todd Boyd asserts "connotes a racial hierarchy that
has been in America since its inception. . . . 'Nigger' remains a lingering example
of the culture defined by slavery and the world that grew up in its aftermath."[69]
(For the sketch's suburban boys, *nigger* was conflated with *nigga*—a distinction
to which I will return.) The use of the *N* word in this particular sketch—by
forcing an interrogation of whiteness and the sociohistorical baggage in accor-
dance with white supremacist ideologies—is positioned within a context of
libratory comedic discourse.

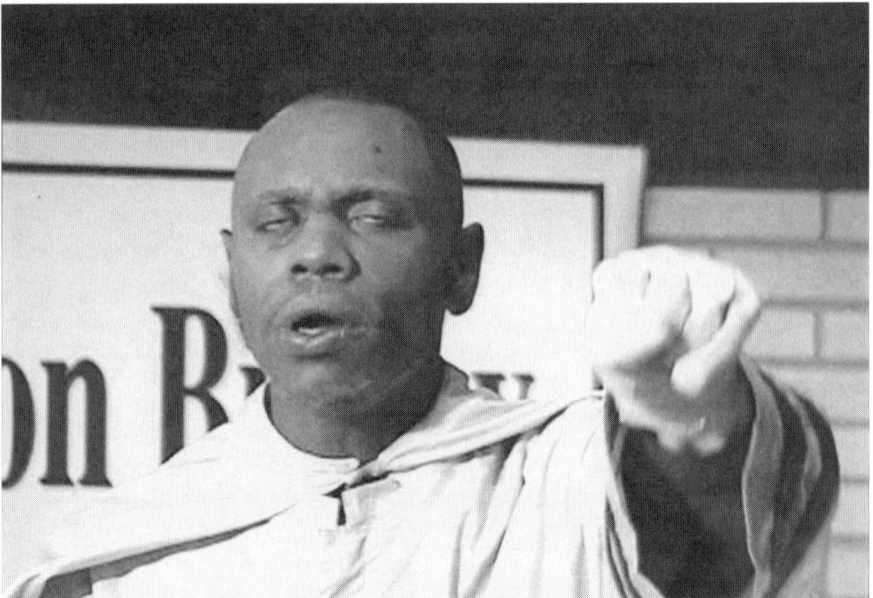

30. Clayton Bigsby, the black white supremacist, makes his debut on the series premiere
of *Chappelle's Show* (2003). Directed by Rusty Cundieff, Andre Allen, Scott Vincent, Bill
Berner, Bobcat Goldthwait, and Peter Lauer.

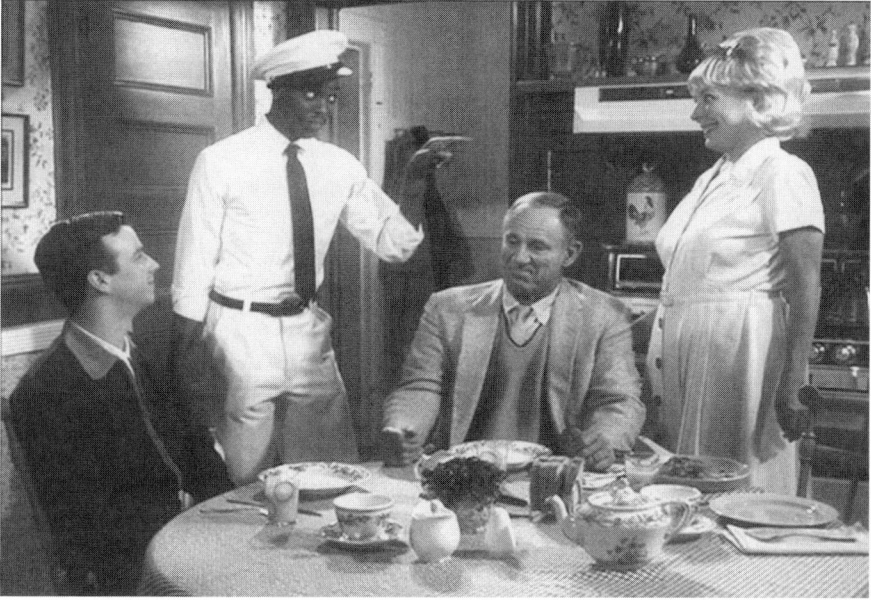

31. Not your typical fifties domcom: "The Niggar Family." *Left to right*: Tim (Johnny Pruitt), Clifton the Milkman (Chappelle), Frank (Dan Ziskie), and Emily (Margo Skinner) on *Chappelle's Show* (2003). Directed by Rusty Cundieff, Andre Allen, Scott Vincent, and Neal Brennan.

The same could be said for the much-discussed sketch from season 2 of *Chappelle's Show* about the family with an unusual last name.[70] Shot in the grainy black and white of a fifties' domestic comedy, a perfect suburban home, reminiscent of *The Donna Reed Show*, comes into view as do cutesy script letters, that spell out the name that is being sung to a tune that could have been on the Hit Parade in 1955: "N-I-G-G-A-R, it's the Niggar family." The introduction of the wholesome Niggar family, Fred, Tim, and Emily, who look like extras from *Father Knows Best*, continues as they wave from their front stoop and then as the parents run behind a teenaged Tim on his two-wheeler as the verse sounds, "Teaching Tim how to ride a bike, these are the Niggars that we like." Described as "deeply cutting and even subversive" by Bob Simon on *60 Minutes*, the sketch again uses the N word as a means to list every possible stereotype about "niggers" in this off-kilter context. While everyone, except the Niggars, seems to be aware of the other context of their last name, it sits in the center of the sketch like the elephant in the living room—spoken but unacknowledged. Whether in reference to their newborn niece's "Niggar lips" or the "Niggar boy" being "such a talented athlete and so well spoken," racial stereotypes are sprinkled on top of the narrative like jimmies on a sundae.

The most interesting interactions in the sketch are between the Niggars and their "colored" milkman, Clifton (who is introduced in just that way). Chappelle

plays Clifton as though he was channeling Eddie "Rochester" Anderson, with
the mixture of subservience and insolence in his faux gravelly voice serving him
well as he begins his own litany of "nigger" stereotypes"—from the refusal of
"extra bacon" from Mrs. Niggar ("I know better than to get between a niggar
and his pork") to the reminder to Mr. Niggar about the overdue balance on
their account ("I know how forgetful you Niggars are about paying your
bills")—even as he is performing an archetypal fifties "colored" character. As
Chappelle plays almost directly to the camera (in sitcom style) with a physicality
reminiscent of toned-down fifties "cooning" (a cross between Rochester and
Stepin' Fetchit), Clifton's knowing glee at throwing the name/term around in
stereotypical and contemporary vernacular terms—referring to the pater-
familias as "Mr. 'N' word"; reassuringly saying, "Niggar, please"; and finally leaving the house with "Peace, Niggar"—is juxtaposed with the critique of the
genre (and blacks' role in it).

The conscious mobilization of the phrase in this particular sketch also
seems an answer to critique about the series' use of the word—although Chappelle maintains that he and Brennan "just thought it was funny." When Clifton
and his wife, waiting to be seated at a fancy restaurant, take offense to the maitre
d's call for "Niggar, party of two," his anger is assuaged when the "Little Niggar"
appears with his date. Clifton's final set of lines put the final discursive cherry
on this subversive comedic sundae when he states, "I bet you get the finest table
a *niggar* has ever gotten at this restaurant"—as they all laugh uproariously, he
adds, "This racism is killing me inside." The absolute lack of acknowledgment
of his words by all the others (including his wife) is striking—particularly
because he continues to laugh. Unlike the Clayton Bigsby sketch, the use of the
word itself is more central to the sketch than the performance of race—
although one might argue that Chappelle's playing "colored" provides a dual
commentary on the historical and contemporary constructions of blackness in
the sitcom genre. I should also note that in various interviews with Chappelle
in mainstream media, the Niggar sketch is discussed with greater ease than
Clayton Bigsby—whether motivated by timeliness (many of the interviews
were done after season 2, during which the former was aired) or the genuine
discomfort/difficulty in the way *nigger* is repeatedly utilized in the Bigsby sketch
cannot easily be determined.

Undoubtedly, the politics of the *N* word have not gotten this much airplay
since the early nineties in discussions of a different type of creative text and
social context—namely, rap music and hip-hop culture. The liberatory potential
of the *Chappelle's Show*'s use of the *N* word, however, is complicated by another
wall over which the "aural wallpaper" is placed. In the first season DVD commentary during the "Mad Real World" sketch, Brennan calls attention to Tron
calling Chad a "nigger" in one of many hostile moments. The cocreators are in
agreement that white people are called nigger as much of the time as black

people are in the series' multiple narratives. Yet even as this indiscriminate use of the *N* word serves to lessen some of the historically based sting from the epithet, the rules of usage, unclear and situational, reflect a sense of ambivalence *and* indifference about the relationship between this particular *N*-word policy and presents a confusing model of racial awareness. Chappelle noted that if a white comic used the word, he would be "furious," but, with Brennan, in this instance, he shares ownership of the sociohistorically loaded term. This type of ambivalence carries over into readings of *Chappelle's Show*, when folks who have proclaimed themselves as "down" take fragments of the televisual text to places that I don't believe Chappelle had envisioned they would go.

## Conclusion

Through an examination of reading positions, cultural production, and the multiple layers of the text, the significance of the work done by both Chappelle and his show become clear even as the delineation of sociocultural imperatives within the work become muddied. As products of the network, netlet, and postnetwork era, respectively, *The Richard Pryor Show*, *In Living Color*, and *Chappelle's Show* navigate issues of race as best they could for their time. This assessment does not excuse, however, the ways in which other categories of marginalization are either elided or exploited. Nor does it explain how and why some of the most popular characters in the comic stables of these series, particularly the latter two, can be seen as fundamentally apolitical, bordering on minstrelsy.

The Men on Film series on *In Living Color* presented Blaine (David Allen Grier) and Antoine (Damon Wayans) as archetypal Snap Queens, whose double-entendre filled reviews inspired as much ire as fandom in the gay community—just as the previously discussed "Homeboys" did in their black fan base. Furthermore, those familiar with *Chappelle's Show* are undoubtedly aware that the two most popularly cited characters in the series—and their patented catchphrases—have not been discussed thus far simply because, ironically, I would argue they occupy the fringe of Chappelle's comedy. Like parsley on the *Chappelle's Show* discursive plate, the comic's portrayal of a cocaine-driven frenzied Rick James in Charlie Murphy's Hollywood Moment, which lampooned the salad days of the Super Freak and provided the oft quoted "I'm Rick James, bitch," as well as the nonsensical mimicry of the King of Crunk, Lil' Jon, utilizing his callbacks as his primary mode of expression, while undoubtedly funny—whether or not one knew the place these folks occupied on the continuum of black music—add color but little substance to the televisual meal. Regardless of their most quoted status (in spaces as varied as the control rooms of television stations to frat parties on State Street), these sketches provide little to no sociocultural context yet award the trappings of cultural cachet. While I doubt that knowing *Chappelle's Show* would be seen as a mark of distinction by the standards of Pierre Bourdieu's notion of taste culture (rarefied and certainly not televisual), I would argue that to a growing segment of our world, it is.

At a professional function that took place during the second season of *Chappelle's Show*, I met someone whose work is not connected to popular culture in any way. When he mentioned having seen *Chappelle's Show*, for a moment it was like he was flashing cultural currency—although admittedly, he thought Lil' Jon was just an outlandish fictional character in the series' troupe. The pervasiveness of these characters in the popular imaginary, although they play lesser roles than many more-complex figures in the series narrative, speaks to how televisual spectators across the demographic spectrum choose to privilege different aspects of the text. So after extensive discussion, research, screening, and examination of both this complicated televisual text and Chappelle's evolving comic persona, my initial intellectual quandary remains fundamentally unchanged, and while this is not necessarily a bad thing, it raises questions about how skillfully notions of race—in this case blackness and whiteness—can be made safe when narratives complicating those constructs are partially or superficially read.

Historian and cultural theorist George Lipsitz makes an unequivocal statement about the power and function of race in American society. "Race is a cultural construct, but one with sinister structural causes and consequences. Conscious and deliberate actions have institutionalized group identity in the United States . . . [including] the dissemination of cultural stories."[71] No doubt the way in which specific cultural stories are read can either contribute to or undermine hegemonic notions of race. One might also assert, however, that being in a position of media power—Chappelle as Comedy Central's $50-million man—would afford a space from which subversiveness could speak. The answer is yes and no. While ensconced at Comedy Central, on the fringes of the Viacom empire that includes media outposts the CW, CBS, BET, Showtime, and MTV, *Chappelle's Show*'s status, along with the equally irreverent but decidedly less political *South Park*, as the darlings of basic cable and the cash cows for the network, positioned it as marketable and center, not marginal and fringed. Given the biting and incisive nature of Chappelle's last stand-up special (2004), one would have predicted that season 3 of the series would continue to push boundaries—and buttons—for multiple audiences, as well as for the cable channel. One would have been wrong.

The much-anticipated and thrice-delayed third season of *Chappelle's Show* proved to be a battleground for Chappelle as a socially and politically aware person and his audacious and fearless comic persona. One of the concerns raised throughout this analysis of the series involved how it was being read by multiple audiences: in other words, what exactly were they laughing at? The cryogenic state of the series seems to be rooted in that concern with Chappelle questioning whether his series was exploding stereotypes or merely reinforcing them. As Dick Gregory stated, "When you mention his name among young folks, it's like mentioning Jesus in a Christian church."[72] The veracity of the civil rights era comic pioneer's statement, in many ways, contributed to the show's undoing. The comic's awareness of both the industrial and cultural cachet that his series had amassed was compounded by the pressure and responsibility that came with that coveted position.

As early as November of 2004 Gregory's reaction to the sketches that he had taped illustrated his comedic, intellectual, and, arguably, spiritual conflict. In Devin Gordon's *Newsweek* article he described watching Chappelle taping a sketch entitled "The Nigger Pixie." Chappelle, clad in the costuming of minstrelsy (blackface, white lips, gloves, red vest, and a Pullman Porter's cap), was the aforementioned pixie, a self-hating devil on the shoulder of prominent black men in American popular culture (like Tiger Woods and, of course, Dave Chappelle). The pixie exhorted them to react "naturally" and perform the stereotypical tropes of black masculinity. When Chappelle greeted journalists between takes, he apologized for his appearance, slyly adding, "Bet you never met a real live coon."[73] On *The Oprah Winfrey Show*, Chappelle's first televised interview since leaving his series, the comic provided a description of the sketch that differed from the one recounted in *Newsweek*: "The premise of the sketch was that every race had this . . . pixie, this racial complex. . . . The reason I chose blackface at the time was [because] this was going to be the visual personification of the 'N' word."[74] As with much of the work done on the third season, the comic's postperformance reaction to this sketch changed significantly once, one might hypothesize, he began to consider how the comedic critique was or was not being read. Chappelle would later state that it was the reception of "The Nigger Pixie" that led to his first flight from the series and his attempted hajj in late 2004.[75] Loud and long laughter from one of the white crew members gave the comic a moment of pause. "I know the difference of people laughing with me and people laughing at me—and it was the first time I had ever gotten a laugh that I was uncomfortable with." That sense of discomfort and the desire to meet the myriad expectations of insightful, incisive, and cutting-edge comedic discourse made the already arduous process of writing and performing in a weekly series overwhelming to the comic: "I felt like it had gotten me in touch with my inner 'coon.' They stirred him up. . . . When that guy laughed, I felt like, man, they got me."[76]

Comedy Central president Doug Herzog, Neal Brennan, and the comic himself maintained that network censorship was not an issue in the formulation of the comic content of *Chappelle's Show*: the last word on what would or would not play was Chappelle's. Brennan, who is no longer affiliated with either the series or the comic, bemoaned Chappelle's second guessing of the sketches, stating, "Dave would change his sketches so much and it got to the point that the show never would have aired if he had his way." In *Time* Brennan described a fractious creative process where a sketch that either he or Chappelle had pitched would be written and then taped, with the enthusiastic approval of the comic, only to be derailed later: "at some point, he'd start saying, 'This sketch is racist and I don't want this on the air.' . . . There was this confusing contradictory thing: he was calling his own writing racist."[77]

Despite the fact that both Brennan and Herzog have raved about the quality of the sketches that have been taped (only enough to fill four of the ten episodes of the series without the in-studio stand-up segments), Chappelle's questioning of his inner circle's assessments revealed his consternation about both the series' comic quality and his retention of his specific comic voice: "Everyone around me says, 'You're a genius! You're great! That's your voice!' But I'm not sure that they're right."[78]

Although "intense personal issues" were later cited as the reason for Chappelle's departure, the entertainment media mill spent much of the remainder of spring and summer cranking out speculative articles about the comic's disappearance after failing to report to the set in late April of 2005. Amid rumors of erratic behavior, possible drug abuse, and/or mental instability, the question "Where's Dave?" circulated freely throughout popular media. Comedy Central even capitalized on the unanswered query, using the phrase "Dave, phone home" in television advertisements for reruns of *Chappelle's Show*. Series regular Charlie Murphy spoke candidly about the impending death of the series: "It was like the Tupac of TV shows. It came out and got everybody's attention. It was a bright shining star and, for some strange reason, it burned out quickly."[79] During Chappelle's absence and his subsequent radio silence, Comedy Central adjusted its lineup to include other comics of color, Carlos Mencia on *The Mind of Mencia* and D. L. Hughley on *Weekends at the D. L.* The commercials for the latter series even directly addressed the cooling effect that Chappelle's disappearing act might have had on the position of black comics on Comedy Central, with Hughley stating, "You thought they wouldn't give another brother a show, didn't you?" Although the former, *Mind of Mencia*, has had decent ratings, it has not touched the widespread popularity of *Chappelle's Show*. Thus, it is not surprising that, despite Chappelle's walkout, the $50-million two-season deal remains in limbo—but the door is still open, according to Comedy Central.

"It was a clumsy dismount," admitted the comic in an exclusive interview with *Time*, in which he made it known that neither drug abuse nor mental breakdown had caused him to seek refuge with a family friend in Durban, South Africa.[80] The intensity of the media attention to his flight matched the level of popular cultural frenzy that his series had inspired. The comic maintained that his back-to-Africa movement had allowed him to gain perspective in a space where he could maintain his anonymity—so that he could stay sane. Chappelle broke his silence and stated on *Oprah*, in no uncertain terms, that he was not crazy. The comic also supported the validity of his paranoia regarding his series' inner circle as he recounted how deeply he had been injured by the claims made in the press about his self-imposed exile; particularly injurious was Neal Brennan's comment that his friend and writing partner was "spinning out of control." Amid these heartfelt admissions, Chappelle also quipped, "What is a black man without his paranoia."[81] While this line reflected his exquisite comic timing, it also spoke to his belief that when a celebrity of color "blows up," he or she faces different travails from other industry stars—and his or her missteps earn scrutiny that is rigorous at best and punitive at worst. At one of the many times that he spoke directly to the audience during his two-hour appearance on *Inside the Actors Studio*, he gave the budding artists a word of warning: "You guys are students now, so you're idealists. You don't know about where art and corporate interests meet yet. Just prepare to have your heart broken. . . . Get your Africa tickets ready, baby, because you have no idea."[82]

The tenuousness of Chappelle's position has been recognized in some journalistic corners. In her *New York Times* review of *Dave Chappelle's Block Party*, Manohla Dargis stated simply, "Turning your back on big money apparently means one thing: you're nuts. But Mr. Chappelle looked and sounded profoundly sane on James Lipton's "Inside the Actors Studio" . . . where, between cigarettes and jokes, he offered a mesmerizing, occasionally heart-melting glimpse into both the pressures of his fish-bowl existence and what it can mean for a black man when he makes white people laugh."[83]

I mourn the loss of *Chappelle's Show* as a contentious space for comedic social discourse. I also have to admit that the series' comic content, which was often full of sociopolitically informed declarations on the American (and particularly the African American) condition, was often lacking in ideological directives that did not seem vague and/or ambivalent, invite multiple readings—which is a good thing *and* a bad thing. When, in retrospect, Chappelle provided an assessment of the body of his television work, he seemed acutely aware of the problematic aspects of his show: "I was doing sketches that were funny but socially irresponsible. I felt like I was deliberately being encouraged, and I was overwhelmed. It's like you are cluttered with things and you don't pay attention to things like your ethics."[84]

One might also hypothesize that Chappelle's wariness about his series' comic content came as a result of internalizing questions about the roots of multiple audiences' laughter. The lackadaisical cheekiness of his comic persona seems tempered by a sense of introspection. No less witty after his time in South Africa, Chappelle returned to the stage with a sense of artistic renewal. The intimacy of the stand-up stage (particularly in comedy clubs), the ability to react to and interact with an audience, allows Chappelle a greater sense of comic autonomy—and a clearer sense of how they are reacting to the comedy as entertainment and as social discourse. Thus, the return of Chappelle to his show at Comedy Central seems highly unlikely.

Since Chappelle began instructing his fans not to watch whatever fragments of the abortive season 3 that Comedy Central might choose to broadcast (and to boycott any DVDs of said material), both the advertising for and the buzz about season 3 of *Chappelle's Show* have faded from popular media memory. In the closing moments of his time with Oprah, Chappelle admitted that he would like to do his show again (if a positive work environment could be created) and would try to "upload" his half of the DVD revenue to the *people*, through various causes (from those benefiting survivors of Hurricane Katrina to a fund for his old high school). Despite Winfrey's words of caution ("Be careful, you need boundaries. . . . You're on national television) Chappelle continued, "I would rather give the money to people other than the ones who were exploiting me. And if I could benefit the people, how awesome would that be? . . . So even if I say something socially irresponsible, it's going to a socially responsible cause."[85]

One could view Chappelle's saga as the morality tale of a young comedian who buckled under the pressure of being the hottest comic on the planet; however, that would oversimplify the complexity of the phenomena of Chappelle's persona in American popular culture. Chris Rock, who had been labeled the "funniest man in America," has progressively gained the ability to speak directly to the criticism of his controversial material, as exemplified in his *60 Minutes* interview and his responses to post-Oscar critique. By the time Chappelle returned from his "Durban retreat," the easygoing insolence of his early responses to the critique of his series' racialized parody did not come so easily. In an interview in February 2006, Chappelle concisely expressed his comedic and ideological quandary: "There is a line of people who will understand exactly what I'm doing and there is another group of people who are just fans, like the people—the kind of people who scream, 'I'm Rick James, b' . . . at my concert. They are along for a different kind of celebrity worship ride. They are going to get something completely different—that concerns me."[86]

While the series afforded him a national platform, as well as industrial and cultural cachet, it became a contentious discursive space in which he was uncertain how his work could be interpreted and mobilized. In hindsight Chappelle, who freely confessed that he loves his own jokes, became serious about the nature of the laughter that he was eliciting: Chappelle's statement, "I want to make sure that I am dancing and not shuffling," provides an uneasy inversion of the notion that originally drove the series.[87] No longer "dancing like nobody's watching," Chappelle's awareness of the reach of his comedic social discourse has made it difficult to dance at all.

Nevertheless, the significance of Chappelle's show, as well as his stand-up performance, cannot be underestimated: his comic persona is arguably the embodiment of the post-soul moment. In Chappelle's comic discourse one can hear a conflation of black comic voices: the cultural specificity of unabashedly black characters like those of Flip Wilson; the contentious commentary of *In Living Color*'s Homey the Clown, the radical black ex-con children's entertainer (created by Paul Mooney); the personal and social candor of Pryor, who made sly audaciousness a staple of black comedy in the post-soul era; the insolence of the Def Jam generation's politics of differentiation and moments of pointed sociopolitical critique reminiscent of Dick Gregory. Yet for all of the insolence and subversiveness that informs Chappelle's humor, there is also an innate quality of likability that enables multiple audiences to discern some aspect of his humor that speaks to and for them—and, at the same time, allows him great license to be as controversial as he wants to be. In one reflective moment on Lipton's show the comic said, "I don't know how this whole Dave Chappelle thing is going to end but I feel like I'm going to be some kind of parable—either what you're supposed to do or not supposed to do. . . . I'm going to be a legend or just that tragic (expletive) story, but I'm going to go all the way."[88] His statement made me think of Pryor and how his passing of the comic torch, as it were, to Chappelle made perfect sense.

In the end, when discussing Chappelle, using the word *persona* is a misnomer; we are always actually discussing personae. The performance of his comic discourse goes beyond inhabiting different character types for different sketches and connects with actually speaking to multiple constituencies in the process of articulating identity. While clearly blackness is privileged, Chappelle speaks to the skater, the slacker, the hipster, the "backpacker,"[89] and the aspiring cultural critic, like me, who longs to see a call to action in his comic discourse. The comic personae of *Chappelle's Show*—as well as his stand-up—embody an ambiguous and fragmented notion of blackness, which may well be the most accurate representation of this construct at this historical moment. The series occupied a space not easily mapped in theoretical terms. Neither the apolitical patchwork of Fredric Jameson's pastiche nor the purposefully intricate mosaic of Linda Hutcheon's postmodern parody, it stands as both representative text and idiosyncratic anomaly.[90] Norma Schulman discusses *In Living Color* in terms of Du Bois's notion of double consciousness—however, there are more than two constructs, identities, ideologies being fought on the discursive plane of this televisual text. I am also forced to examine my own point of annunciation, as a partial insider. Are my own ambivalent feelings toward the spectatorship of the series rooted in feeling as though *my* text has been co-opted? The promise and problem of *Chappelle's Show* and Chappelle's comic personae is that the inebriated frat boys yelling "Whuuuuuut" are as much Chappelle's constituency as I am. From differing reading positions we are both experiencing a televisual text that speaks to our historical moment—in ways that are clearer and yet more ambiguous than Chappelle's sketch comedy predecessors.

## Postscript

On March 3, 2006, I sat in the Paramount Theater in Vancouver, British Columbia. Although I was in town for an academic conference, I felt compelled to catch the late show of *Dave Chappelle's Block Party* on its opening day. As I scanned the enthusiastic crowd at the Cineplex, it was the demographic I might have predicted: overwhelmingly young, male, and white. I must admit to feeling a wave of mild dread as the batch of twenty-something males sitting behind me began a chorus of "I'm rich, bitch" and their rendition of Lil' Jon's "Whuuts."

Again, the question that had inspired this study came into my mind: "I know what I'm laughing at, but what are you laughing at?"

Once the film began, however, I was blissfully unconcerned with the reception of others. Drawn into the exuberance of Michel Gondry's cinematic representation of Chappelle's vision, his new millennial *Wattstax*, there was something both utopian and euphoric happening on the screen. In this instance the nonlinear structure simulated the sense of memories, Chappelle's memories, thus pulling us into Dave's subjectivity . . . Dave's world. The semishaky handcam moments on the streets of Dayton, Ohio, and its environs captured Dave, the post-soul Willie Wonka, handing out golden tickets redeemable for passage and entrance to the Brooklyn block party. He passed them out generously to his constituency—from two black teenaged boys, whose comfort with the camera allowed us to see the semigoofiness of their unabashed excitement to the two older white women, who work at the store where Chappelle buys cigarettes when he's at home, who confessed that they had known all along about his comic phenom status but had respected his privacy and let him make his purchases in anonymity.

Like the cinematic realization of what Chappelle had done metaphorically with the construction of his comic persona, the film, without prejudice and in the spirit of inclusion (but not without a knowing wink to the camera), gathered a diverse cadre of fans, drawn to the comic and transported to the "concert that [Dave] had always wanted to see." At once dreamlike and naturalistic, the movement between snippets of rehearsal sessions and the conversations between Chappelle and the Okayplayer virtuosos he had recruited (Mos Def, Jill Scott, Common, Erykah Badu, and The Roots) seemed less like a behind-the-scenes documentary than being backstage with friends of a friend who were doing a show. The only thing that separated the depiction of the conscious rap elite and those who were there to see them play was the fact that the former were seen performing on stage: no captions identified any of the speakers, whether it was Wyclef Jean or Brian Milsap, hip-hop legend and college band director, respectively. This democratizing sensibility is best illustrated when one considers that Ohio's Central State University Mighty Marauders, the band that earned a spot on the *Block Party* bill when it happened to be practicing as Chappelle shot the film's opening, had more individual and group screen time than Kanye West, the hip-hop superstar they accompanied on his song "Jesus Walks.".

Although I have already begun to look at *Dave Chappelle's Block Party* as media scholar, however, the impressions here are those of a spectator—in all honesty, a fan.[91] The film, like the recent interviews and appearances made by Chappelle confirmed many of the things I had theorized about the flight to Africa, the pedagogical impulses in his comedy and the liberatory potential of "dancing like no one is watching." The Block Party was a celebration of folks joining together to celebrate multiple articulations of black culture, hip-hop culture, post-soul culture. Chappelle, as the giddy yet cool host, had ushered us into his *worlds*. It was a glorious moment, when he was still Comedy Central's $50-million dollar man, before "The Nigger Pixie" and before the gnawing question about the nature of the laughter made it too difficult to dance. But even amid the celebration there were two moments that could be read as bitter-sweet: one was a conversation between Chappelle and ?uestlove Thompson of The Roots, explaining the affinity between Dave and many of the Okayplayers; the other was a semiconfessional moment, with Chappelle on the rooftop over-looking the Bed Sty block party site. Thompson's statement that "the thing that all [the folks performing at the block party] have in common is that our audi-ence doesn't look like us" directly speaks to the issue of having a diverse fan populace that may or may not be able or willing to read both the text and sub-text of the creative work. Chappelle comically redirected the conversation when Thompson began to talk about the shows full of "wild frat boys . . . inter-rupting [Dave's] narrative," yelling for Rick James, while Dave was trying to "tell stories," the circuitous series of jokes that often led to a punch line with a sociopolitical bite. However, the question of laughter and spectatorship across medium and across culture was, again, raised in connection with the legions of *Chappelle's Show* fans. It was even clearer on the rooftop, when Chappelle said, "There has to be a separation between the public image and the private image. I wanted to give something beyond that public image." The *Block Party* was his gift to his audiences. Euphoric, inclusive, and transient, it was the promise of a cross-cultural happening—it was a celebration. Yet fast-forward to the time of the film's release. On the talk-show circuit, promoting the movie (and telling his side of the "Where's Dave" saga), Chappelle, although candid, mischievous, and as funny as ever, was seemingly a bit nervous (as signified by the chain-smoking on *Inside the Actors Studio*). It seems that once you are aware of the power and the reach of your voice and your comic discourse and the impact of the repre-sentations in your comedy, a level of caution is inserted where the fearlessness once had been. I don't know whether that is good or bad. It just is.

As I left the theater and strolled back toward the hotel, I eavesdropped on a group of hipsters a few paces behind me (a black male, two white males, one Asian woman, and one white woman). One young woman raved about how fabulous Common and Erykah Badu had been. The other female said she thought Dave was hilarious when he was out with regular people, even repeat-ing one of his earliest comments to the camera: (after being warmly greeted by two elderly white people), he stated, "Old people fucking love me. You know you're doing something right when old people love you." One of the males was a big Blackstar (Mos Def/Talib Kweli) fan and remarked how "cool" it was when they brought Chairman Fred Hampton out during the song "Umi Says," with the bridge being replaced by Hampton's call for the freeing of political prisoners.[92] "Was that the song with 'I want my people to be free' in it?" a female voice asked. I smiled as I listened to the male voice confirm Hampton's identity and then proceed to explain who Hampton and four of the political prisoners he specifically named, the "New York Three" and "Mumia," actually were.[93] Finally, I heard the voice of a male that had previously not joined in on the conversation reply to the question, "What did you think?" His reply, "It was okay but not as funny as the show," revived the Greek chorus in my head: I know what I'm laughing at, but what are you laughing at? But by the time I could fight some sense of decorum, to turn around and glance at the speaker, I saw them entering a coffeehouse. There was a part of me that wanted to go back and question them, but in the end I just walked back to the hotel and listened to "Umi Says" on my I-Pod.

The title of this chapter describes Chappelle at this historical moment. The task of the provocateur is to incite dissension—to make people question things as they are—it's not necessarily his job to provide the answers. In the end I don't know what you're laughing at—and that's what worries me. Apparently, that is what continues to worry Dave Chappelle, too.

# *Epilogue*

## LAUGHING SAD, LAUGHING MAD

I BEGAN WRITING this epilogue days after Hurricane Katrina devastated the United States' Gulf Coast. The childhood hometown of my parents, Pass Christian, Mississippi, was devastated by wind, water, and debris—and relief was slow in coming. As my mother and the rest of my family awaited word from friends and relatives who lived in Katrina's path, all of whom survived and many of whom lost everything, it was difficult to think about comedy. Nothing was funny. Yet in the wake of Katrina, as the "the blame game" rhetoric was spun and as the stories of those who survived hurricane conditions only to be subjected to the danger and squalor of the Superdome and Convention Center came to light, one thing became clear: a majority of black and white Americans witnessed the same natural disaster but internalized the multiple tragedies and made meaning from the mediated images of Katrina and its aftermath in decidedly different ways.

According to a poll from the Pew Research Center for the People and the Press, "seven-in-ten blacks (71%) say the disaster shows that racial inequality remains a major problem in the country; a majority of whites (56%) say this was not a particularly important lesson of the disaster."[1] Similar statistics were generated by *Time*'s poll; when asked whether "the race or low income level of the victims slowed government relief efforts," 60 percent of white Americans believed that these were not mitigating factors as opposed to 73 percent of blacks, who felt that they were.[2] In the NBC/*Wall Street Journal* poll, seven of ten African Americans and three in ten white Americans were convinced the response would have been faster if "the victims had been in white suburbs rather than a predominantly black inner-city."[3] Perhaps what I found most disconcerting was that these numbers did not surprise me.

As myriad travesties and controversies emerged, I sat glued to the television, watching an American tragedy through the lens of blackness. It was impossible for me not to look at innumerable black faces and think, "That could be me; that could be my family." And while all natural disasters can elicit that response, my strong and uneasy identification was intensified by the gnawing feeling that race determined access to and quality of relief. The faces in the Superdome and the Convention Center were predominantly black: thus, the repeated references to violence, squalor, and danger in these "refuges" were tied to blackness. As Katrina survivors like Denise Moore described, after days of being "trapped" at the Convention Center, many felt as though they had "been brought there to die. . . . Without help. Without food. Without water. Without sanitary conditions—as though it's perfectly all right for these 'animals' to reside in a frickin' sewer like rats. Because there was nothing but black people back there."[4]

The fact that many of those who did not leave were not able to do so was lost on those who, as Illinois senator Barack Obama stated with indignation, "[were] so detached from the realities of inner city life in New Orleans . . . that they couldn't conceive of the notion that [residents] couldn't load up their SUV's, put $100 worth of gas in there and some sparkling water and drive off to a hotel and check in with a credit card."[5]

Furthermore, at a Black Congressional Caucus roundtable with invited members of the press, Democratic Representative from South Carolina James Clyburn candidly addressed the subject that few wanted to address directly: "Nobody wants to talk about poverty. Nobody wants to talk about race. Nobody wants to talk about the nexus of the two."[6] So at least for me there was a certain symmetry in the fact that President Bush jovially vowed that Trent Lott's lost mansion would rise again and that "we" would rebuild him "a fantastic house" on the same day that Kanye West called into question the "compassion" of the "compassionate conservative."

On September 2, 2005, West veered from the script, as he and (startled) comic actor Mike Myers made an appeal for contributions during NBC's live telecast, *A Concert for Hurricane Relief*. Beginning with his reflection on the racially coded use of the word *looting* ("I hate the way they portray us in the media. If you see a black family, it says they're looting. See a white family, it says they're looking for food")[7] and ending with what arguably became the most oft-repeated sound bite of the Katrina disaster: "George Bush doesn't care about black people." Although the remark was excised from the West Coast broadcast, West's comments brought the issue of race into the forefront of the discussion of multiple aspects of the relief effort. Ed Gordon, host of NPR's *News and Notes with Ed Gordon* (a program cosponsored by the African American Radio Consortium), emphasized that West "spoke for scores of Black people."[8] Gordon went on to elaborate on the crux of West's foregrounding of race in relation to Katrina relief: "There are those who suggest that the initially slow response had less to do with race and more to do with social class. Such comments miss the fact that it is virtually impossible to separate the color of your skin from the opportunities you are given to rise above the social and economic conditions you were born to."[9]

While the assertion of Morris Reid, Democratic strategist, that "it took a 28-year-old rapper, a popular culture figure, to get America talking about a real issue" might be an overstatement, one could argue that more Americans are aware of what West said than the fact that the Democratic National Committee Chair, Howard Dean, made a similar observation less than a week later.[10] The fact that West is a popular culture figure, hailed as "Hip-Hop's Class Act" on the cover of *Time* (Aug. 29, 2005), the week before his revelation about the media, Katrina relief, and Bush, raises the question of who has sway over the hearts and minds of the American populace. Which had more impact on Middle America, the *New York Times* articles on the travesty and tragedy of survivors in the Superdome and Houston's Astrodome or the episodes of *The Oprah Winfrey Show*, where Winfrey and celebrities in her Angel network (including Julia Roberts, John Travolta, and Chris Rock) went on location in the Gulf Coast? In a society fascinated by celebrity and the entertainment industry, the presence and/or the lived politics of these A-list performers draws the attention of the press and, in turn, the people. Just as Dick Gregory used his high profile (as a black comedian who had experienced crossover success) to draw attention to the civil rights struggle, when given the national forum of the benefit show, West used his industrial cachet and intense popularity with a racially diverse cross section of music consumers to make the American mainstream acknowledge what many blacks in the United States were feeling. And when Kanye spoke, for better or for worse, people listened. During his three-hour comic marathon at Eastern Michigan University on September 30, 2005, Dave Chappelle praised West's truth-telling as "courageous. . . . I'm proud. Proud," then adding (after a beat), with a shake of his head, "I'm gonna miss him." One might argue that Chappelle's bit underscores the (at least, spiritual) kinship between Gregory and West—hinting that there is often a price to be paid for public political candor.

Furthermore, when Bill Cosby came onstage at *Jazz at Lincoln Center's 'Higher Ground Hurricane Relief Concert' to Benefit the Salvation Army* on September 17, 2005, it seemed both ironic and appropriate that it was the conflation of his position as televisual icon and black comic legend that gave power and resonance to his appeal. One of many artists (black and white) who came out to support the relief effort for New Orleans, Cosby never used the word black in his five-minute seriocomic monologue, yet, whether intentional or not, the repeated use of the phrase "the people" seemed a synonym for "our people."

> This happened to the people. The Constitution says, "for the people, by the people, of the people." The people. And then in this United States, the people vote. The people that vote, vote people into office and those people are supposed to serve the people. [Pause] You see where I'm going? [laughter and applause] And their job is to serve the people. But the people who got into office, it appears, got into office, and forgot [a smattering of applause]—let me finish—the people. Now one might also think that those people who were slow coming may not have been the people who were supposed to be serving the people . . .

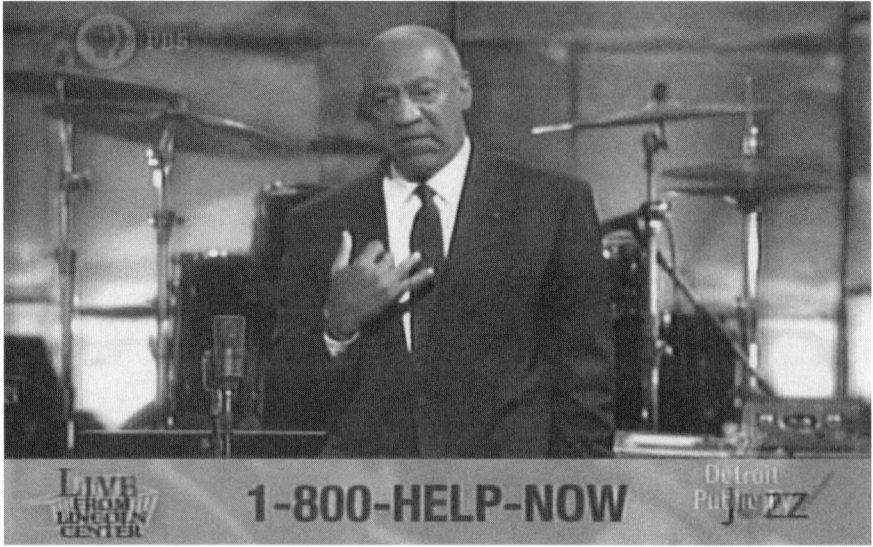

32. Bill Cosby talks about "the people" to the people at Higher Ground, a post-Katrina benefit at Lincoln Center. "Higher Ground Hurricane Relief Benefit Concert," *Jazz at Lincoln Center*, Sep. 17, 2005.

While Cosby also made an impassioned call for individual and institutional action based on "integrity, accountability and the fact that we are Americans," themes familiar to his often controversial discourse on the failings within the black community (particularly the black "lower classes"), the overall sensibility of his speech seemed to present a civil rights era ethos that more than fleetingly addressed post-soul thought—his urging to use the vote as a weapon was tempered by the acknowledgment that the government, as things stand, was not serving the needs of [black] people. While I willingly admit that this reading puts an optimistic spin on what I would call the mellowing of Cosby's rhetoric, it was, nevertheless, the power of his persona that affords him both the venue and influence to speak across lines of race and class.

Yet given both Cosby's iconic status and the disparate views of his directives for the black community, one must consider how the effectiveness of comedic discourse can be also diminished.

I came to this conclusion as a result of another, more personal discovery that came post-Katrina—one that also speaks directly to my work, albeit work not yet done. I was restless, irritable, and discontent over the positive spin generated by Bush's "army of compassion" and "urban homesteading act" and the fact that the questionable sensitivity of former first lady Barbara Bush's observations about how those folks in Houston's Astrodome, who were "underprivileged, anyway" were doing "quite well" (after being left displaced, uprooted, and traumatized) drew far less fervent media scrutiny that Kanye West's assessment of the president's investment in black folks' welfare.[11] I decided that I needed a bit of televisual solace before returning to my work. My TiVoed offerings did not seem sufficient, so I reached for a DVD I had not watched in a year: Steve Harvey's HBO *One Man* show (2001), filmed in Augusta, Georgia.

When Harvey came onstage in his double-breasted, yellow-suited glory, I eased back on the couch and sank into the comedy. My favorite bit offers a variation on his "White People vs. Black People" oeuvre:

> Black people handle getting fired different from white folks. You can't fire us the same. It ain't gonna go good. See, the difference between firing black people and white people is this: when you fire white people, they don't ever see it coming [in white voice] "What are you talking about? What are you, nuts? For crying out loud!" ... They got a whole list of things they go down when they think they ass is gone because they can't believe they're getting fired. Black people, on the other hand, we figure [with tired resignation], "Any day now, my ass is gonna be outta here." 'Cause we know if there's gonna be some firing going on: we're first. So, we pretty much expect it.

What follows is the tale of two terminations—of Bob, the amiable and oblivious white employee, and Willie Turner, a brother who "has been expecting it." Bob's denial over being "let go" is depicted as a product of disbelief that *he* could be "let go," and, while he bemoans his fate to the boss, he departs in quiet devastation. "But," as Harvey notes with mock severity, "Yeah, but when you go out there to fire Willie, it ain't gonna go like that." Replicating the exact process used to fire the Anglo employee, the boss attempts to fire Willie as amiably, privately, and quietly as he had Bob; this is not to be. After describing Willie's initial refusal to talk privately ("I got a desk right here. Whatever you want to say to Willie, you can say here."), Harvey shifts into the boss's point of view, who "knows that he needs to get this altercation behind closed doors right now because Willie is getting ready to show his whole ass. Willie's fixin' to act a fool." Harvey gesticulates madly (and thuggishly) as the angry wide-eyed Willie dares his boss to "Say it. Say I'm fired. I'll burn this mother down. . . . Say it. You better not say I'm fired. Say it. Say it. I'll kill your kids. I'll kill your kids." The bit culminates with Willie, having, indeed, "shown his whole ass," making the demand for his severance pay immediately: "Gimme my check," an insistent demand that induces the boss to summon the authorities.

I laughed like I had not laughed in a long time. I was laughing at differences of experience, as well as differences in perception. I found solace in the nuances of the regionalized black vernacular and the articulation of another African American comedic discursive, inflected more by the tone and meter of R&B balladeers than by hip-hop. While my viewing choice was undoubtedly based, in part, on the desire to lose myself in comedy that was not part of my current work, it also provided a space where there was no translation, explanation, or justification necessary. While others might have turned to more mainstreamed comedic fare, *The Cosby Show* or even *Chappelle's Show*, I chose what I referred to earlier as "For Us By Us" comedy. In moments when issues of race appear in boldface to people of color and are illegible to large segments of dominant culture, the burden of explanation always falls on the marginalized group, either directly or indirectly—and along with it comes the frustration over not being understood or heard or even acknowledged. One longs for either a literal or virtual safe communal space—an enclave. For me the comedic discursive space of Harvey's one-man show fulfilled that function. Catherine Squires asserts that "the enclave is signified by the utilization of spaces and discourses that are hidden from the dominant public . . . dedicated to Black interests and needs."[12]

A large swath of black comedy in post-soul America (and innumerable black comic personae including Harvey's) remained outside the sphere of this study: those who—by design *and* by default—remain ensconced within enclaves of black comedic discourse. As Squires also notes, "Enclaves provide the bedrock for marginal publics even when they benefit from increased political rights or friendlier social relations" and "the continued presence . . . of 'Black-only' spaces and media fulfill functions . . . that mainstream public arenas, institutions and media institutions have not."[13] However, no less complex or conflicted than the comedic discourse of those who have crossed over, there are ways in which For Us By Us comedy resonates as much with laughing to keep from crying as it does with laughing mad. Harvey's tale of Willie Turner acts as a comedic anecdote about anger, frustration, and resignation, telling it "like it is" rather than railing against why it *is* that way.

Furthermore, disparities arise when considering the gendered aspects of black comedy. Harvey's fellow "Kings of Comedy," Cedric the Entertainer, Bernie Mac, and D. L. Hughley, have gained varying degrees of mainstream success while remaining tied to their "roots" in the "Def Jam persona." However, while the names of black female comics, like "The Queens of Comedy" (Sommore, Miss Laura Hayes, Adele Givens, Mo'Nique)[14] draw audiences on the black comedy circuit (and some niched televisual spaces like *BET's Comic View*), access to the comic mainstream is not the only difficulty for the black female comic.[15] Cheryl Underwood's impassioned plea in her acceptance speech for "Best Stand Up" at the BET Comedy Awards (September 27, 2005)—"Black directors, hire us"—is reminiscent of Whoopi Goldberg's assertion that "they don't know what to do with me." These Original Kings and "Invisible" Queens assuredly warrant a volume of their own in which one can tease out the intricate construction of For Us By Us comedy—as an enclave public sphere and as an industrial as well as sociocultural construct. The study of this fluid segment of black comedy, inflected by region, class, and, of course, gender, which offers consternation and resignation along with solace, seems the next logical step in analyzing the significance of black comedic social discourse—and the nature of the laughter.

According to Antonio Gramsci, "Every social group . . . creates together with itself, organically one or more strata of intellectuals which give it homogeneity and an awareness of its own function not only in the economic but also in the social and political fields."[16] The black comics of *Laughing Mad* represent one or more strata of black organic intellectuals. Although the black comedy of both the civil rights era comics and post-soul comics, like the entertainment-based moments of philanthropy discussed earlier, might seem unlikely repositories for serious discourse on race and class, it is within spaces not marked as necessarily pedantic or particularly threatening that folks might actually become open to questioning their ideological presuppositions—whether during their spectatorial experience or in their postviewing musing. And the comic messenger makes a difference. Comedy is a powerful discursive tool; the notion (attributed to multiple sources from George Bernard Shaw and Joe Orton to my eighth grade English teacher, Mrs. Roshko) that if one gets an audience laughing, then while their mouths are open, you can shove the truth in, seems quite applicable here. I remained committed to the idea that the articulations of racial identity in black comedy speak to a multiplicity of reflections on the African American condition; the comic personae of Murphy, Rock, Goldberg, and Chappelle give voice to the jadedly hopeful, politically and pop culturally savvy, and media wary iterations of blackness in post-soul America. In the introduction to this book I inquired whether the comic players themselves, like many of us in the audience, are laughing mad. In the end the answer is yes and no, and my jaw is tight.

# Notes

Introduction

1. Langston Hughes, *The Big Sea*, 2nd ed. (New York: Hill and Wang, 1993), 237.
2. Wil Haygood, "Why Negro Humor Is So Black," *American Prospect* 11, no. 26 (2000): 26.
3. Dick Gregory, "Speech at St. John's Baptist Church," Birmingham, AL (May 20, 1963), http://americanradioworks.publicradio.org/features/sayitplain/dgregory.html (accessed March 28, 2006).
4. Nelson George, *Hip Hop America* (New York: Viking, 1998), xi.
5. The contemporary "sit-in" movement began on February 1, 1960, when four students from the North Carolina Agricultural and Technical College at Greensboro sat down at the segregated lunch counter in a Woolworth store and were refused service. One could even argue for setting the beginning of the era with those born after *Brown v. Board of Education*, like Bernie Mac, Steve Harvey, and, of course, Whoopi Goldberg.
6. Mark Anthony Neal, *Soul Babies: Black Popular Culture and the Post-Soul Aesthetic* (New York: Routledge, 2002), 3.
7. Michael Eric Dyson, *Open Mike: Reflections on Philosophy, Race, Sex, Culture, and Religion* (New York: Basic Civitas Books, 2003), 256–57.
8. M. M. Bakhtin, *The Dialogic Imagination: Four Essays*, ed. Michael Holquist, trans. Caryl Emerson and Michael Holquist (Austin: University of Texas Press, 1981), 159–60.
9. J. Fred MacDonald, *Blacks and White TV: African Americans in Television since 1948* (New York: D. McKay, 1992), 123.
10. Donald Bogle, *Primetime Blues: African Americans on Network Television* (New York: Farrar, Straus, and Giroux, 2001), 7.
11. Christine Acham, *Revolution Televised: Prime Time and the Struggle for Black Power* (Minneapolis: University of Minnesota Press, 2004), 3.
12. A statement made by Gray in the Marlon Riggs documentary *Color Adjustment* (1990).
13. Herman Gray, *Watching Race: Television and the Struggle for "Blackness"* (Minneapolis: University of Minnesota Press, 1995), 32.
14. Ibid., 88.
15. Ibid., 89.
16. Beretta E. Smith-Shomade, *Shaded Lives: African-American Women and Television* (New Brunswick, NJ: Rutgers University Press, 2002), 68.
17. Donald Bogle, *Toms, Coons, Mulattoes, Mammies, and Bucks: An Interpretive History of Blacks in American Films*, 3rd ed. (New York: Continuum, 1991), 280.
18. This chapter focuses on Goldberg's comedic work, although one might argue that, with the exception of her film debut as Celie in Spielberg's *The Color Purple* (1985), the same assertions can be made about the "integrated" nature of the filmic worlds of her dramatic works as well.
19. Neal, *Soul Babies*, 120.

CHAPTER I. FROM NEGRO TO BLACK

1. Dick Gregory, interview by Juan Williams, *Talk of the Nation*, Oct. 19, 2000, NPR, transcript.
2. Bruce Britt, "Leaping Barrier with Laughter: Flip Wilson, a Comic for the Times," *Washington Post*, Nov. 28, 1998, F1.
3. Phil Berger, *The Last Laugh: The World of Stand-Up Comics* (New York: Copper Square Press, 2000), 121.
4. Mel Watkins, *On the Real Side: A History of African American Comedy from Slavery to Chris Rock* (Chicago: Lawrence Hill, 1999), 497.
5. *Bell and Howell's Close Up! What's So Funny*, directed by Helen Jean Rogers, ABC, June 12, 1961.
6. Redd Foxx and Norma Miller, "Dick Gregory," *Redd Foxx Encyclopedia of Black Humor* (Pasadena, CA: W. Ritchie Press, 1977), 180–81. Mort Sahl also frequently played this hipster San Francisco night spot with a similarly politicized style of humor, prompting many to call "Dick the Black Mort Sahl and Mort, the white Dick Gregory."
7. *The Steve Allen Show*, directed by Steve Binder, written by Arne Sultan and Marvin Worth, syndicated, Jan. 9, 1964.
8. Ibid.
9. *The Jack Paar Program*, directed by Hal Gurnee, written by Marty Farrell, NBC, March 1, 1963.
10. Malcolm X, "On the Afro-American Problem as a World Problem," Dec. 13, 1964, http://www.brothermalcolm.net/mxwords/whathesaidarchive.html (accessed Nov. 10, 2005).
11. *The Ed Sullivan Show*, directed by John Moffit, CBS, Nov. 15, 1970.
12. Gregory received 1.5 million votes, and Democratic candidate Hubert Humphrey lost the election by a mere 510,000 votes.
13. Chris Weisman, "Dick Gregory: the 'Nightlife' Interview," *Nightlife*, Aug. 11, 1999, 22.
14. Berger, *The Last Laugh*, 192.
15. Dick Gregory, interview by Noah Adams, *All Things Considered*, NPR, Nov. 16, 1995.
16. Cedric Muhammad, "Political Mondays: Dick Gregory: A Valuable Man," BlackElectorate.com, June 20, 2005, http://www.blackelectorate.com/print_article.asp?ID= 1396 (accessed June 21, 2005).
17. The activities of COINTELPRO in the late sixties and early seventies were focused on "disrupting and discrediting" radical political organizations from SNCC and the Black Panthers to SDS and various components of the antiwar movement. Given Gregory's history with COINTELPRO and the revelations about the group's activities with Black leaders that has emerged in the past ten years (as public access to their files has increased), it is not surprising that the comic/activist would look warily at the group's activities and publicly encourage others to do the same: as early as 1968 the passionately nonviolent activist and then presidential candidate was included on the group's lists of "Black Nationalist Hate Group Leaders" along with Fred Hampton, Geronimo Pratt, and Stokely Carmichael (see Paul Wolf's Web site, www.cointel.org).
18. C-Span Coverage of the Million Worker March, Oct. 17, 2004. It should also be noted that Chappelle has stated in interviews that he grew up listening to Dick Gregory. Although this does not offer definitive proof of the elder comic's influence on the younger comic's choice of characterization for President Bush (as a "thug"), it does make clear that, unlike other post-soul comics, Dave Chappelle knows Dick Gregory.
19. Daniel Pike, "Activist Issues Bold Predictions during Press Conference," *Illinois Spotlight*, Copley News Service, Feb. 25, 2005.

20. Vic Sussman, "The Comic Who Broke All the Rules," *Los Angeles Times*, Oct. 22, 1998, Calendar sec., F55. The event was the evening honoring Richard Pryor as the first recipient of the Mark Twain Prize for Humor. When asked how it felt to see Pryor so honored, especially since Gregory had been one of the first black performers to attack racism and government corruption with slashing humor, the comic activist replied, "It's a great night. . . . I may have opened the door, but it was for a genius like him to go through."

21. Dick Gregory, interview by Juan Williams, *Talk of the Nation*, Oct. 19, 2000.

22. Quoted in "Biography: Kennedy Center Honorees," *Kennedy Center Honors*, Dec. 1998, http://www.kennedy-center.org/programs/specialevents/honors/history/honoree/cosby.html (accessed Sep. 5, 2000).

23. *The Jack Paar Program*, directed by Hal Gurnee, written by Marty Farrell, NBC, Dec. 11, 1963.

24. *The Jack Paar Program*, directed by Hal Gurnee, written by Marty Farrell, NBC, May 8, 1964.

25. There is a reference to his father's alcoholism in this bit—referring to the difficulty encountered when anesthetizing alcoholics. Cosby, as his father, counts backwards from 100, "4, 3, 2, 1. Now what do you want me to do?" No other reference is made in this routine.

26. This routine serves as an interesting counterpoint to Eddie Murphy's "Ice Cream" routine, which acknowledges how cruel children can be as it makes a superficial commentary about class.

27. Elvis Mitchell, "So Cool, He Sometime Stings," *New York Times*, Aug. 4, 2002, E1.

28. It should be noted that the construct of the "Super Negro" was an invention of white creator/producers and bore little relationship to the African American experience at that time.

29. This was also a time when Cosby was doing films that were not family friendly, like *Uptown Saturday Night* (discussed later in this chapter); its sequel, *Let's Do It Again*; and the gritty sex romp meets quasi-Altman seriocomic take on the ambulance industry, *Mother, Jugs and Speed*.

30. Bogle, *Primetime Blues*, 169.

31. Ibid., 169–70.

32. The logic, sensibility, and worldview of Cosby himself completely informed the construction of Dr. Huxtable. The line between the stand-up persona and the television character often blurred in the act-based sitcoms that followed *The Cosby Show* (Roseanne Connor/Roseanne Barr on *Roseanne*, Tim Taylor/Tim Allen on *Home Improvement*, Jerry Seinfeld/Jerry Seinfeld on *Seinfeld*); however, the conflation of Cosby and Huxtable exemplified the most skillful utilization of that blurry line.

33. The overwhelming success of *Bill Cosby: Himself* undoubtedly influenced Brandon Tartikoff at NBC to champion the Carsey-Werner series, although, reportedly, the working-class family suggested by Cosby was upscaled for media consumption during the Reagan years.

34. This (arguably) laudable quality in the construction of Cosby's comic persona masks some actual subversiveness in his comedy, particularly in the televisual comic persona in his landmark sitcom. For example, what other Black man, besides Bill Cosby, could play an OB/GYN with patients of a variety of races and ethnicities on prime-time television without significant ruckus on any front?

35. Bambi L. Haggins, "There's No Place like Home: The American Dream, African-American Identity, and the Situation Comedy," *Velvet Light Trap* (spring 1999): 29.

36. Gray, *Watching Race*, 80.

37. Linda K. Fuller, *The Cosby Show: Audiences, Impact, Implications* (Westport, CT: Greenwood Press, 1992), 69.

38. Issues of class and other less urbane constructions of the urban black experience were not directly confronted in the series—although some might argue that the

addition of Clair's cousin from Bedford-Stuyvesant (Erika Alexander) in 1990 may have been a response to the criticism over the fiscal insulation of the Huxtable clan.

39. Interestingly, the main signifier of wealth in this instance is the art in what has been previously constructed as the "Black middle class" decor of the Huxtable brownstone. In this episode Vanessa is seeking the acceptance of the "popular girls" and realizes the cultural cachet of their economic standing after the girls comment on the painting (Ellis Wilson's *The Funeral Procession*) over the fireplace. Vanessa admits that it cost $11,000 and explains that the artist was Clair's great-uncle. While this provides a forum for showcasing African American art and culture, one of the aspects of the series that was often lauded, it also establishes a sense of lineage—at least for Clair—a clear connection to the black cultural elite.

40. Quoted in Gray, *Watching Race*, 80.

41. Haggins, "There's No Place like Home," 30.

42. The series run was marked by personal tragedies. In 1997 Cosby's twenty-seven-year-old son, Ennis, was murdered, and in 2000 Madeline Kahn, a regular on the series, lost her battle with cancer.

43. Haggins, "There's No Place like Home," 29.

44. *Cosby* never broke into the Nielsen top twenty during its run; during its first and most-watched season, it reached its highest rating, twenty-first.

45. *Everybody Loves Raymond*, with comic Ray Romano as the series' central everyguy, was the highly rated centerpiece of the Monday night sitcom block on CBS. It is also interesting, however, that for a majority of the series' run the programming strategies of the netlets, UPN and the WB, may have also siphoned away the audience for *Cosby*: with the nontraditional family sitcom *In the House* (think *Who's the Boss?* with an injured NFL player as the nanny), starring actor, choreographer, and former *A Different World* producer Debbie Allen and Rapper L. L. Cool on UPN and the new millennial version of *The Waltons* (think a church instead of a mountain) in *7th Heaven* on the WB.

46. As I sat with my Gen Y surrogate son, Kevin, we were both relatively blasé about seeing Cosby onstage. Although I had grown up listening to his material and watching *The Cosby Show*, as a media theorist I had spent far too much time studying the representational politics of the televisual Cosby to see his work as unproblematic. Nonetheless, when he came onstage, in sweats and a U-Mass sweatshirt, both of us turned to each other and said (aloud, I am embarrassed to say), "That's Bill Cosby." Not being prone to celebrity awe, I was surprised by my reaction—but then again, it is not every day that one sees an icon.

47. Teresa Wiltz, "Bill Cosby in Vintage Form, No Lashing Out, Just Some Good Stories at Wolf Trap," *Washington Post*, July 10, 2004, C1.

48. The comic's controversial comments will be discussed further in the conclusion of this volume.

49. Watkins, *On the Real Side*, 521.

50. Foxx and Miller, "Flip Wilson," *Redd Foxx Encyclopedia*, 196.

51. "When You're Hot, You're Hot," *Time*, Jan. 31, 1972, 57.

52. Interestingly, long before there was Cheech and Chong or the boys from *Half Baked* (Dave Chappelle, Jim Breuer, et al.), there were comedic voices in the early sixties that had a hint of the countercultural wave to come, as exemplified by Jenkins's benignly constructed drug addiction.

53. In much the same way that comics have used (and continue to use) alcoholism and/or drug addiction as comic fodder, without addressing the sociological or sociopolitical ramifications or root causes of the disease, Wilson's junkie is sweetly inept—arguably the antithesis of either Lightnin' Bug or Junior, the protagonists of Pryor's "junkie and wino" routine, a version of which would later be performed on *The Flip Wilson Show*.

54. *An Evening with Flip Wilson*, Museum of Television Seminar, New York City, Sep. 23, 1993.

55. Dan Sullivan, "Flip Wilson Finds Comic Note in Nation's Long Hot Summer," *New York Times*, July 17, 1968, 37.

56. Ibid.

57. Josh Greenfield, "Flip Wilson: 'My Life Is My Own,'" *New York Times*, Nov. 14, 1971, D17.

58. Robert Hilburn, "Personality Means Flip Wilson," *Los Angeles Times*, Sep. 16, 1970, G17.

59. Watkins, *On the Real Side*, 522.

60. Quoted in Hilburn, "Personality," G2.

61. Ibid., G1.

62. Ibid.

63. Greenfield, "Flip Wilson," D17.

64. Christine Acham, *Revolution Televised: Prime Time and the Struggle for Black Power* (Minneapolis: University of Minnesota Press, 2004), 68–69.

65. In 1993 the comic recounted trying to slip unnoticed into a female impersonator show in Denver (he didn't want his presence at the performance to call his sexuality into question). Toward the end of the show the headliner called for the house lights to be turned up and thanked Wilson "for making what we do possible and thank you for your contribution to the well being of the gay community." Despite his wariness about the use of drag being equated with homosexuality, Wilson was touched by the impromptu tribute, stating, "That stopped me right in my tracks." Curiously, the series' producer Bob Henry followed Wilson's statement by asserting that Wilson was not doing drag: "Flip created such an honest work of art with Geraldine. . . . Some people, who are rather superficial, would say he's working in drag. Baloney! He created such a perfect, perfect characterization with Geraldine. Milton Berle . . . that was drag. He'd come out with big lipstick and the balloons and high heels. That was drag. But, in Flip's case, it was a work of art thank god a comedy work of art. That's why it sustained. Classic humor endures, things that are classic last forever. Geraldine got such big laughs . . . because it is indeed a work of art" (*An Evening with Flip Wilson*, Museum of Television Seminar, Los Angeles, March 12, 1993).

66. Greenfield, "Flip Wilson," D17.

67. Bogle, *Primetime Blues*, 181.

68. Acham, *Revolution Televised*, 73.

69. John Leonard, "Flip Wilson," *Life*, Jan. 22, 1971, 12. Leonard continues to assert "that [Wilson] doesn't frighten anybody . . . wouldn't hurt you anymore than . . . Carol Burnett or Ed Sullivan would hurt you" and that feeling "undeserving of [Wilson's] harmlessness . . . I know he wouldn't hurt me but maybe, just maybe, he should."

70. MacDonald, *Blacks and White TV*, 180.

71. *An Evening with Flip Wilson*, Museum of Television Seminar, Los Angeles, March 12, 1993.

72. Greenfield, "Flip Wilson," D17.

73. *The Tonight Show with Johnny Carson*, NBC, May 20, 1981.

74. Richard Pryor (with Todd Gold), *Pryor Convictions and Other Life Sentences* (New York: Pantheon, 1995), 93.

75. Watkins, *On the Real Side*, 544.

76. Pryor, *Convictions*, 113.

77. The ludicrousness of this exercise in seventies domcom relevance is exacerbated by the episode's B-line, in which Danny goes to the Pantheresque Afro-American Cultural Society—which yields the cringe-worthy result of the preteen red-haired hustler of the family being given a beret and being made an honorary member.

78. *Mo' Funny: Black Comedy in America*, written and directed by Yvonne Smith, HBO Films, 1993.

79. James McPherson, "The New Comic Style of Richard Pryor," *New York Times Magazine*, April 27, 1975, 242.

80. Ibid.

81. Ibid.

82. Pryor's revised recreation of the "Junkie and Wino" routine for *The Flip Wilson Show* (1973) provides yet another indication of what might have been had Pryor been able to survive on network television. In the sketch Pryor, as both Junior and Lightnin' Bug Johnson, presents the conversation between two dispossessed figures, both of whom have turned to "substances" to assuage sociohistorically specific pains, as they speak to each other across the generational divide.

83. MacDonald, *Blacks and White TV*, 193.

84. *Lily*, directed by Rick Wallace, written by Rosalyn Drexler et al., CBS, Nov. 2, 1973.

85. George, *Hip Hop America*, 36.

86. Watkins, *On the Real Side*, 562.

87. Pryor, *Convictions*, 6.

88. Nelson George, *The Death of Rhythm and Blues* (New York: Pantheon, 1988), 139–40.

89. *Wattstax*, directed by Mel Stuart, Columbia Pictures, 1973.

90. Jill Nelson, "Pryor Knowledge: The Rage, Vulnerability, and Painful Honesty of Richard Pryor's Comedy Changed America Forever," *Salon*, Nov. 24, 1998, http://www.salon.com/bc/1998/11/24bc.html (accessed Aug. 15, 2004).

91. This notion of Pryor being given representational and/or ideological passes is engaged further in the discussion of the cinematic constructions of his comic persona.

92. There were only two instances when the seven-second delay was utilized on *SNL* in its twenty-eight-year history: Pryor in 1975 and Andrew Dice Clay in 1990.

93. The original opening is now available on the DVD of *The Richard Pryor Show*.

94. James Brown, "Pryor Miffed," *Los Angeles Times*, Sep. 14, 1977, G4.

95. A more detailed textual analysis of the series will be undertaken in the book's final chapter in relationship to *In Living Color* and *Chappelle's Show*.

96. In the fall of 1977 Redd Foxx starred in a short-lived variety series on ABC.

97. It is interesting that much of the black culture overtly interjected into Pryor's show during its short run is not from contemporary popular culture but rather from a more distant black past. In one sequence the mise-en-scène of a postwar Harlem nightclub is meticulously re-created in style, music, and dance. In the twenty-minute seriocomic narrative passage Pryor is cast as a soldier returning from World War II to find his world and his girl have changed; in another, an extended performance of African dance by The Chuck Davis Dance Company quite literally brings in the African village set for the subsequent parody of the post-*Roots* commodification of African-ness. Yet another example can be seen in the special that spawned the series, where a bevy of beautiful black women, of varying hues, in a production number that crosses June Taylor with Alvin Ailey, celebrates black beauty to the sound of smooth jazz and each woman reciting the passage from Langston Hughes's "Harlem Sweeties" that describes her. While one might argue that the passage objectified the women, in a pageantlike manner, the assertion of non-Eurocentric beauty on prime time was, indeed, a rarity.

98. The day before the prize was presented to Pryor, in a lecture at the Kennedy Center the American Studies scholar Shelly Fisher Fishkin, who specializes in Twain, stated that the comic and the author "shared several essential elements: they use humor to point out the absurdities of the ruling class, they made their marks by recounting anecdotes from their lives rather than by telling jokes and they derive much of their style from African forms of storytelling." During the ceremony honoring the first Twain honoree another viewpoint was given when Chris Rock quipped, regarding a fictitious meeting between Twain and Pryor, "Richard would've said, 'I enjoy your work' and Twain would've said, 'Nigger, get my bag'" (Kevin Carter, "As Groundbreaking Comedian Richard Pryor's Health Declines, His Stature Grows," *Knight Ridder Newspapers/Star News*, Jan. 15, 1999, Arts sec., 1).

99. Carter, "As Groundbreaking," 1.

100. Nelson George, "The Rumors of His Death Have Been Greatly Exaggerated," *New York Times*, Jan. 17, 1999, A2.

101. Interestingly, in the latter the slyness of Gregory's humor also makes a cameo: the character takes great pleasure in challenging the Blackness of Reno's only male African American officer, Deputy S. Jones (Cedric Yarbrough), and in complimenting the only black female officer, Deputy Raineesha Williams (Niecy Nash).

102. Mark Reid, *Redefining Black Film* (Berkeley: University of California Press, 1993), 26.

103. Ibid.

104. Ibid., 19.

105. The same might be said of his portrayal of the down-and-out private eye in *Hickey and Boggs* (1972). Teamed with ex-*I-Spy* partner, Robert Culp, Cosby is not playing Alexander Scott here: Hickey is a contemporary, proud—and sometimes confrontational—Black Man. Although the film was neither a critical nor a commercial success, as Elvis Mitchell aptly describes: "Mr. Cosby's performance achieved a more fully realized brand of ghetto debonair" (Mitchell, "So Cool," E1).

106. Interestingly, when Cosby and Pryor next shared the screen, it would be in Neil Simon's *California Suite* (1978)—the duo play Chicago doctors on the vacation from hell.

107. Even Cosby, the cowriter and producer of *Leonard*, panned the film.

108. The issue of de facto prohibition on the Black comic leading man in mainstream comedy will be explored in more detail in the discussions of Murphy, Rock, and Chappelle.

109. Ed Guerrero, *Framing Blackness: The African American Image in Film* (Philadelphia: Temple University Press, 1993), 122–23.

110. This term, which refers to the adoption of any vestige of the racist stereotypes of the minstrel show into the popular entertainments that followed the genre's timely demise, is derived from perhaps the most patently offensive minstrel archetype: the "coon." As Donald Bogle notes, the coon was "the most blatantly degrading of all black stereotypes. The pure coons emerged as no-account niggers, those unreliable, crazy, lazy, subhuman creatures good for nothing more than eating watermelons, stealing chickens, shooting crap, or butchering the English language" (Bogle, *Toms, Coons*, 8).

111. Pryor, *Convictions*, 205.

112. Pryor contended that his firing of then Indigo president, former athlete/actor/activist Jim Brown (over creative differences on which projects should receive the green light) in 1983, had significant consequences for him: "The black film community was outraged. The NAACP turned on me" (Pryor, *Convictions*, 210).

113. Vincent Canby, "Screen: 'Jo Jo Dancer,'" *New York Times*, May 2, 1986, C9.

114. Rob Salem, "Pryor Conjures Up Ghosts, Comic Tries to Put Misspent Life into Perspective," *Toronto Star*, May 7, 1986, B1.

115. Canby, "Screen: 'Jo Jo Dancer,'" C9.

116. Paul Attanasio, "Jo Jo Dancer, Pryor's Tale," *Washington Post*, May 4, 1986, D1.

## Chapter 2. Murphy and Rock

1. The omission of Flip Wilson in this cavalcade of comic stars is rather telling in terms of how Wilson is viewed by black comics of the post-soul era. One might surmise that his contribution is minimized, to some extent, because of the Anglo-friendliness of both his persona and the content of his humor during the height of his popularity, which coincides with the zenith of the Black Power movement in the late sixties and early seventies.

2. The film begins with a sketch that establishes Murphy as one who has always rebelled against middle-class mores—as an eight-year-old telling a risqué kid joke

(with bodily functions as the punch line) to a stunned audience consisting of his family gathered for Thanksgiving dinner.

3. By 1987 Murphy could "open" a movie, something that only a handful of black actors before or since have been able to do. Along with that power—fueled by box office success—came the elevation of Murphy as the founding member of the "Black Pack," a term he coined at the press conference for *Beverly Hills Cop II.* Between the late eighties and early nineties Murphy and his "pack"—which included Robert Townsend (*Hollywood Shuffle,* 1987), Arsenio Hall (*The Arsenio Hall Show,* 1989–94), and Keenen Ivory Wayans (the future creator/producer of *In Living Color,* 1990–94)—were seen as the new wave of black comedy.

4. bell hooks, *Black Looks: Race and Representation* (Boston: South End Press, 1992), 112.

5. Donald Bogle, *Blacks in American Film and Television: An Encyclopedia* (New York: Garland, 1988), 230.

6. Stephen Holden, "Comedy's Bad Boys Screech into the Spotlight," *New York Times,* Feb. 28, 1988, Arts and Leisure, sec. 2, p. 1. Holden regards Murphy's comedy as the accompaniment to an age when "as the political climate turned more conservative and materialistic, hip irreverence turned sour, and the wink in the eye of comedy became a sneer."

7. Michael Sragow, "Eddie: What Happened?" *Salon,* Aug. 3, 2000), http://dir.salon.com/ent/col/srag/2000/08/03/eddie_murphy/index.html?pn=1 (accessed April 3, 2006).

8. Ken Tucker, review of *Chris Rock: Big Ass Jokes,* directed by Chris Rock, *Entertainment Weekly,* June 14, 1994, http://www.ew.com/ew/article/review/tv /0,6115,302712_3_0_,00.html (accessed May 3, 2004).

9. "White people say they'd vote for him because they think it's the cool thing to say . . . 'Sure, I'll vote for him' (punctuated with a dismissive 'yeah, right' chuckle)."

10. Malcolm X, "A Message to the Grassroots," quoted in Acham, *Revolution Televised,* 179.

11. Acham, *Revolution Televised,* 180.

12. Ibid., 182.

13. In *Bring the Pain* Rock's commentary on the O. J. Simpson case includes the discussion of alimony, Nicole Simpson's relationship to Ron Goldman, and the statement, "I'm not saying he should have killed her, but I understand," delivered with broad smile and a wink to the audience.

14. In fairness, Rock also takes to task the young fathers—"niggas [who] always want some credit for some shit they are supposed to do . . . [he says] 'I take care of my kids' . . . you're supposed to do that, you dumb motherfucker."

15. According to U.S. Census data from March of 2002, less than 25 percent of American families have single incomes, and less than 30 percent of families have a stay-at-home mom. United States Census Bureau, "Table FG1. Married Couple Family Groups, by Labor Force Status of Both Spouses, and Race and Hispanic Origin of the Reference Person: March 2002," June 11, 2003, http://www.census.gov/population/socdemo/hh-fam/cps2002/tabFG1-all.pdf (accessed Aug. 1, 2003).

16. Watkins, *On the Real Side,* 581.

17. W.E.B. Du Bois, *Souls of Black Folks: Essays and Sketches,* 3rd ed. (Chicago: A. C. McClurg, 1903), 615.

18. Chris Rock, interview by Ed Bradley, *60 Minutes,* CBS, Feb. 17, 2005.

19. For another aspect of premium cable outlet's African American–oriented programming see Christina Acham's analysis of HBO films and their representation of the historical black experience—from *The Tuskegee Airmen* to *Miss Evers' Boys.*

20. Renee Marcus, "Life in the Pop Lane; Mourning Late Night's Best Show," *Boston Globe,* Nov. 28, 2000, C1.

21. *Dennis Miller Live* (1994–2002) followed *The Chris Rock Show* on Fridays at midnight. Like Rock, *SNL* alum Miller was known for biting, heavily referenced politi-

cal and social commentary—and for his comedy's fluid position on the political spectrum.

22. In fairness, one must note that by the late nineties black comedy, in general, had begun to address social and political issues more directly. While Hall's persona was rooted in his "likability," which translates into being a nonthreatening figure for mainstream audiences—celebratory rather than critical—Rock's "equal-opportunity offender" persona is defined by confrontation, challenging rather than assuaging audience sensibilities.

23. Michael Griffith, a twenty-three-year-old African American, and two of his black friends, Cedric Sandiford and Timothy Grimes, had their car break down near a local pizza parlor in Howard Beach (Queens, New York). A group of white men spotted and harassed Griffith and his friends, yelling, "There's niggers at the pizza parlor. Let's get them" before beating them with baseball bats and tree limbs. Sandiford was knocked unconscious and Griffith was severely beaten, only Grimes escaped unharmed because he pulled a knife on his attackers. Griffith was fleeing from the attackers when he was struck by a car and killed. The Howard Beach incident set off a wave of protests and racial tensions in New York. The incident also acted as the inspiration for Spike Lee's *Do the Right Thing* (1989).

24. Acham, *Revolution Televised*, 188. The conclusion provides a thoughtful and thorough textual analysis of this sketch and several others from *The Chris Rock Show*.

25. Robert Bianco and Gary Levin, "Spike Prefers a World without Fox's 'PJs,'" *USA Today*, Jan. 18, 1999, D3.

26. Denene Millner, "This Isn't Comedy, It's Mockery—Ignorant and Deeply Unfunny," *New York Daily News*, Jan. 19, 1999, 28.

27. Howard Rosenberg, "*The PJs*: Equal Opportunity Satire; Much like Animated Spoof Series before It, This Spin on an African American Family Is Irreverent and Endearing," *Los Angeles Times*, Jan. 9, 1999, F1.

28. Ibid.

29. Like the "Supa's" name, there are multiple plays on black popular culture knowledge: the Hilton Jacobs projects are named after Lawrence Hilton Jacobs, the young black actor who played Freddy "Boom-Boom" Washington in the seventies sitcom *Welcome Back, Kotter*.

30. Neal, *Soul Babies*, 124.

31. Less than two years after his purported "good Samaritan" moment of giving a woman a ride home (picking up a transgendered prostitute, "Shalomar" Seluli, with outstanding warrants, on a Los Angeles boulevard known for male prostitution), Murphy was decidedly press shy. Despite his $5 million suit against the *National Enquirer* for its story on Murphy's alleged "secret life," the fact that the comic, whose stand-up monologues were repeatedly labeled as homophobic, was virtually "queered" might also explain in part why those among his faithful fan base, particularly his African American following, were not as outspoken in their defense of the comic.

32. Josh Wolk, "Chris Rock on Fire," *Entertainment Weekly*, March 19, 2004, 22.

33. Ibid.

34. Josh Wolk, "School of Rock," *Entertainment Weekly*, Feb. 4, 2005, 32.

35. Dyson, *Open Mike*, 258.

36. Ibid.

37. That distinction, one with which many of my students still struggle, Rock himself made when discussing African American spectatorship of black films with Spike Lee on his HBO late-night series. As Lee extolled the virtues of one particular film (John Singleton's *Rosewood*), Rock remarked that the "film was positive but that doesn't mean it was good."

38. Neil Strauss, "Confessions of Chris Rock," *Rolling Stone*, April 7, 2004, 64.

39. Ibid.

40. The act itself differed slightly from the set I had seen at Detroit's State Theater a few months earlier, but so did the audience. As comic Mario Joyner, Rock's opening act and former cast member on *The Chris Rock Show*, noted as he scanned the Detroit audience, "I see a lot of ambition, but I don't see a lot of black." While the act did differ slightly—with less of a focus on overtly political humor and more on sexual politics and jokes about "rims," it would be incorrect to assert that Rock made the act "Anglo-friendlier." Rather, he used the material that worked—broader, and less critical race- and sex-based, humor.

41. *Skeet* is slang for ejaculating on one's partner.

42. Grand Master Flash and The Furious Five's 1982 song "The Message" is considered the rap song to politicize the genre in its discussion about the realities of ghetto life.

43. This is in reference to the Bill Murray film with the central premise of one day being repeated ad infinitum until the central protagonist learns his lesson.

44. Fox already had *Malcolm in the Middle*, *The Bernie Mac Show*, and *Arrested Development*.

45. At a 2005 gathering of television critics, when asked about whether he intends to remain active in the series, Rock replied, "I've been working a while. I don't think I've ever done anything and walked out. I don't think there's any evidence of that. My name is Rock, not Chappelle" (Maria Elena Fernandez, "Rock Will Stand by New Show," *Los Angeles Times*, July 22, 2005, E2).

46. Paul Brownfield, "Finding the Humor in a Tough Situation," *Los Angeles Times*, Sep. 22, 2005, E8. Rock would have been thirteen in 1979 rather than in 1982, and the series' nuclear family of five is only half as large as the comic's actual family.

47. Fernandez, "Rock Will Stand by New Show," E2.

48. Chuck Crisafulli, "Q & A with Chris Rock," *Los Angeles Times*, June 5, 1996, F1.

49. Nathan Rabin, "Chris Rock," *The Onion AV Club*, Nov. 17, 2004, http://www.avclub.com/content/node/23281 (accessed April 3, 2006).

## Chapter 3. Post-Soul Comedy Goes to the Movies

1. Ed Guerrero, *Framing Blackness*, 126.

2. Ibid., 128.

3. Bogle, *Blacks in American Film and Television*, 18.

4. Guerrero, *Framing Blackness*, 132.

5. Intriguingly, some aspects of Murphy's stand-up act that had generated so much ire were excused within the context of a "guy" film. The misogyny that informed much of the material about women in *Raw* also found its way into *BHCII*—as exemplified by the repeated "it's a dick thing" ethos in the marital advice Foley offers to Taggart (a slightly sanitized version of Murphy's "Cumin' Hard" routine) and by Brigitte Nielsen's character, referred to simply as "the big bitch," whose shooting acts as a collective reassertion of masculine solidarity.

6. Rock's supporting role as Lee Butters in *Lethal Weapon 4* (1998), although not strictly an example of the fish-out-of-water film, offers a variation on how the black comedian can be utilized within the action comedy. While his role acts as a sort of narrative garnish to the already established interracial buddy paradigm, the character of Butters is constructed as a college-educated black detective who acts as an alternative to Riggs (Mel Gibson) and Murtaugh (Danny Glover), the old-school "cops who don't play by the rules." Cast as the "kid" with the veteran partners, Rock's role is a fairly thankless one, yet he still exhibits low dosage glimmerings of the comic's stand-up persona.

7. Gene Seymour, "'Bad Company' Isn't Good for Rock," *Los Angeles Times*, June 7, 2002, F2.

8. Elvis Mitchell, "Yes, He Looks like His Brother, but Does He Listen to Mozart," *New York Times*, July 28, 2000, E18.

9. In another independent film, Neil LaBute's *Nurse Betty* (2000), Rock's turn as the

sardonic hit man provides another example of a choice of role that—in terms of character voice, if not character construction—also exemplifies continuity between comic and screen persona. Even Rock's foray into the animated world is a bit edgier. In the title role of the Farrelly brothers' *Osmosis Jones*, he costars with a live-action Bill Murray in what can only be described as a conflation of standard animated heroism and live-action gross-out humor.

10. Elvis Mitchell, "So Cool," Aug. 4, 2002, E1.

11. In all likelihood, however, Murphy will dip into the generic well of action comedy again—*Beverly Hills Cop IV* is in the works as of this writing, scripted by Jason Richman, one of the writers of the Bruckheimer/Schumacher film *Bad Company*. Richman is also penning the third installment of the Jackie Chan/Chris Tucker *Rush Hour* franchise.

12. David Germain, "'X2' Proves That It Still Has the Power to Attract; 'Daddy Day Care,' a Family Comedy Starring Eddie Murphy, Lands in the No. 2 Spot," *Los Angeles Times*, May 12, 2003, E2.

13. The fact that Ice Cube, the veteran of the gangsta rappers par excellence, N. W. A, is now playing the role of father (or father in training) in lighthearted urban-suburban comedies like the *Barbershop* series or *Are We There Yet?* (2005), reflects not only a change in the rapper/actor/director's persona but also a different climate for black-oriented film. All of the aforementioned films experienced box office success. The circuitous path of Cedric the Entertainer's comic persona will be examined in future work focusing specifically on "The Original Kings and Queens of Comedy."

14. In 1983 Buchwald's story idea "King for a Day," in which an African potentate was deposed while on a trip to the United States, was originally optioned by Paramount as a vehicle to be reworked into a romantic comedy for Murphy. The comic claimed to have never seen the Buchwald treatment. In 1988 Murphy and movie producer Alain Bernheim waged a costly legal battle against Paramount Studios ($2.5 million) on charges that the studio denied them credit for, and profits from, the story on which *Coming to America* was based: in the end they were awarded $900,000. The film grossed $289 million worldwide.

15. David Ansen, "That Old Softie, Eddie Murphy," *Newsweek*, July 4, 1988, 58.

16. As early as 1987 the Black Pack creative community's collective efforts were making their way to the big screen—as exemplified in Murphy's *Raw*, to which Wayans and Townsend lent their writing talents and which Townsend directed.

17. Walter Leavy, "Eddie Murphy, Richard Pryor and Redd Foxx: Three Generations of Black Comedy," *Ebony*, Jan. 1990, 103.

18. Although far more affectionate, the verbal sparring between Benne and Vera is a touch reminiscent of the battles between Fred Sanford and Aunt Esther (veteran comic LaWanda Page) on the seventies sitcom *Sanford and Son*.

19. Hal Hinson, "Harlem Nights," *Washington Post*, Nov. 17, 1989, http://www.washingtonpost.com/wp-srv/style/longterm/movies/videos/harlemnights.htm (accessed March 16, 2004).

20. "Murphy and Others Lend a Hand in Getting Film Made," *Sentinel*, Feb. 25, 1993, B4.

21. Having initially viewed this film long before I began this area of study (and before falling in love with hip-hop), I remember thinking that the film was simply not as funny as I had expected it to be. I'd seen Rock on *Uptown Comedy Express*, on *SNL*, and even caught one or two of the eight episodes of *In Living Color* that he had done, and I was well aware of Nelson George's work as a music critic, who was an expert on the musical genre. Screening the film again, however, after myriad hours of hip-hop studies, I realized that there was much in the film that I simply did not get the first time around.

22. Another minor character, Eve, the reporter from the *Source*, puts Albert/Gusto in his place after he makes suggestive remarks and, when rebuffed, calls her a "groupie with

a pen." She states that she can write a "a puff piece" or an in-depth exposé that revealed the real nature of *CB4*: "Which would you prefer, Albert?" Although she is associated with Euripides/Dead Mike, after this sequence, Eve, as an intellectual black woman, is reduced to a fundamentally lineless existence.

23. Hal Hinson, "*CB4*," *Washington Post*, http://www.washingtonpost.com/wp-srv/style/longterm/movies/videos/cb4rhinson_a0a7fd.htm.

24. In the mid-eighties the Parent Music Resource Center, whose bipartisan leadership included Tipper Gore and Susan Baker, crusaded against "the growing trend in music towards lyrics that are sexually explicit, excessively violent, or glorify the use of drugs and alcohol." Arguably, their pressure on the Recording Industry Association of America, which eventually facilitated the "voluntary" record rating system, and their publishing of a list of the "Filthy Fifteen," which included songs from Madonna, Prince, and the Mary Jane Girls, as well as Judas Priest and AC/DC, provided a de facto branding system for young music consumers in the eighties and beyond.

25. The song parodies Kool G. Rap and D. J. Polo's "Talk like Sex."

26. *Big Ass Jokes*, the half-hour HBO special, which marked Rock's ascension into the higher echelon of stand-up comedy, premiered in 1993 (the same year as *CB4*), providing an inkling of the stand-up phenomenon that Rock would become.

27. Tyler and Gerard, respectively, as Marcus's trusted, comical, and socially inferior comrades in arms, serve as the bifurcation of the Tony Randall roles in *Pillow Talk* (1959) and *Lover Come Back* (1961).

28. Interestingly, Martin Lawrence's Tyler lacks any of the quasi-"playa-ness," which will later be mobilized in both his television program and his film roles. For Gerard, David Allen Grier's "countrified" (read lower-class, rural, black) buddy, his sensitivity—whether about his parents' behavior, which is neither urban nor urbane, or his desire for a monogamous, caring relationship—is a continual source for mockery.

29. The film's gross of $131 million was more than respectable.

30. Earl Calloway, "*Boomerang* Starring Eddie Murphy, Ecstatic with Humor," *New Philadelphia Courier*, July 22, 1992, B1.

31. Janet Maslin, "The Tables Are Turned on a Smug, Sweet Talking Don Juan," *New York Times*, July 1, 1992, C18.

32. Calloway, "*Boomerang* Starring Eddie Murphy," B1.

33. Peter Travers, review of *Boomerang*, directed by Reginald Hudlin, *Rolling Stone*, Aug. 6, 1992, http://www.rollingstone.com/reviews/movie/_/id/5949193 (accessed Dec. 6, 2004).

34. Kay Bourne, "Murphy Gets the Tables Turned in Fast Paced *Boomerang*," *Bay State Banner*, July 16, 1992, 14.

35. At just over $64 million in domestic and foreign box office, *Down to Earth* was Paramount's seventh-highest grossing film in 2001.

36. Kenneth Turan, "This Time 'Earth' Can Wait," *Los Angeles Times*, Feb. 16, 2001, Calendar sec., 1.

37. Elvis Mitchell, "*Down to Earth*: He May Be in Heaven but He's Dying at the Apollo," *New York Times*, Feb. 16, 2001, http://www.nytimes.com/2001/02/16/arts/16DOWN.html (accessed June 20, 2001).

38. On February 16, 2001, I was seated in a large theater in the local Cineplex with a crowd that was decidedly more integrated than it had been the previous summer when I saw the black comedian concert film *The Original Kings of Comedy* (Spike Lee, 2000) in the same venue. Although I did not have the opportunity to ask the young African American male what he meant, his comment seemed to speak to the "blanding" that the *Times* reviewers on both coasts address.

39. Manohla Dargis, "Chris Rocks, but Not as a Director; 'Head of State' Lacks Character Development and Great Camera Shots but the Leading Man Is an Expert at Searing, Topical Humor," *Los Angeles Times*, March 28, 2000, E14.

40. Ibid.

41. A. O. Scott, "Black Presidential Candidate Is Chosen so He Will Lose," *New York Times*, March 28, 2003, E16.

42. Character actor Nick Searcy plays Lewis as a cross between LBJ and George W. Bush.

43. Chris Rock, *Rock This* (New York: Hyperion, 1997), 224.

44. Manohla Dargis, "A Remake Files Down the Sharp Edges of a Prison Football Saga," *New York Times*, May 27, 2005, E1. Dargis further notes that "like the hip-hop heavy soundtrack these speaking roles [and the increased black presence in the film] are a mere calculation, a crude ploy to lure in black audiences and to make white audiences feel cool by proxy."

45. Wolk, "School of Rock," 32.

46. The audience for the Grammys was down 28 percent (18.8 million), and that for the Oscar precursor, the Golden Globes, was down by a startling 40 percent (16.8 million). Even with the 5 percent ratings slip, the Rock-hosted ceremony pulled 41.5 million viewers, more than the Grammys and Globes of the same year combined. See Scott Collins, "Oscar Viewers Down," *Los Angeles Times*, March 1, 2005, C1.

47. This assessment is based on the fact that each of the Best Picture nominations grossed less than $100 million domestically (before the March telecast), which, according to industrial conventional wisdom, is the marker of a "hit."

48. Lola Ogannaike, "This Oscar Host Is Willing to Call It as He Sees It," *New York Times*, January 2, 2005, E7.

49. Gil Cates, interview on *CNN Live*, CNN, Feb. 26, 2005.

50. Ogannaike, "This Oscar Host Is Willing," E7.

51. The "wardrobe malfunction" refers to the most TiVoed moment in television history. During the 2004 Super Bowl halftime, in a choreographed move, Justin Timberlake ripped off Janet Jackson's bustier "accidentally" revealing more than had been "intended." This "incident" spawned extensive discussions of "decency" on television in the press, the pulpit, and from the FCC. CBS was fined $550,000 by the FCC, Jackson's domestic sales on her new album sagged, and Timberlake emerged unscathed. The second, also football-related, controversy was a Monday night teaser, where Nicolette Sheridan, playing her *Desperate Housewives* character, Edie Britt, and clad only in a towel, seduces Philadelphia Eagles wide receiver Terrell Owens; the encounter ends in an embrace by the purportedly naked (shot from behind from the waist up) actress and the wide receiver. Despite complaints about the skit from Black NFL coaches like Tony Dungy to family-friendly media watchdogs, ABC was not penalized—although all those involved in the controversial segment of the skit apologized for "going too far."

52. Frank Rich, "Hollywood Bets on Chris Rock's 'Indecency,'" *New York Times*, Feb. 27, 2005, Arts sec., 27.

53. In "Chris Rock: The William F-ing Buckley of Stand-up," John Swansberg of *Slate*, the online magazine, asserted that both Drudge and Rock wanted the public to believe the rhetoric of "dangerousness" around the comic acting as host when in actuality, "Rock may speak in the irreverent language of blue comedy, but more often than not, his ideas are red state red" (Feb. 25, 2005, http://slate.msn.com/id/2113952/ [accessed March 5, 2005]).

54. Before presenting an award, Penn supplied an admittedly humorless retort, which began with "Forgive my compromised sense of humor" and ended with Jude Law "is one of our finest actors."

55. Paul Brownfield, "New Tune but the Song's the Same," *Los Angeles Times*, Feb. 28, 2005, E1.

56. Ibid.

57. Chris Rock, interview by Oprah Winfrey, *The Oprah Winfrey Show*, ABC, Feb. 28, 2005.

58. Alessandra Stanley, "If You Didn't Watch It, You Still Get to See It," *New York Times*, Feb. 28, 2000, E1.
59. John Anderson, "Dangerous? Edgy? Chris Rock Calls Himself Mainstream," *Cleveland Plain Dealer*, May 26, 2005, F1.
60. Jane Malanowski, "Not to Say This Is a Better Movie Than Beatty's," *New York Times*, Feb. 11, 2001, Arts sec., 27.
61. Chris Rock, interview by Ed Bradley, *60 Minutes*, CBS, Feb. 17, 2005. In the same segment Rock further responded to Driver's comments, challenging the writer to "tell me one opportunity that was denied to you because I told a joke." Interestingly, almost a decade ago there was a mitigated controversy with Rock's *Vanity Fair* cover (August 1998), which depicted the comic in a circus milieu. Some bristled at what could be seen as a minstrel-like quality to the way that Rock was depicted, dressed as a clown (including baggy pants, red and white checkerboard shirt, red bowtie, black and white spectators [shoes], and white gloves) and red cheeks and nose, clown white on his lips and eyes. Although, one could also argue that his costuming and pose (arms and legs akimbo sitting on top of a barrel), the accompanying headline, "Chris Rock to Be Young, Gifted and the Funniest Man in America," and Rock's serious (perhaps, incredulous) look into the camera, are knowingly at play with the minstrel tropes.

CHAPTER 4. CROSSOVER DIVA

1. Valerie Smith, *Not Just Race, Not Just Gender: Black Feminist Readings* (New York: Routledge, 1998), xiv.
2. See chapter 1 (000).
3. As a black woman, who is also "Bambi from Southern California," I can understand, on an empathetic level, the pleasure of defying expectations generated by one's name.
4. Robert Hurwitt, ed., *West Coast Plays*, no. 21–22, California Theatre Council, 1988.
5. Quoted in Enid Nemy, "Whoopi's Ready, but Is Broadway?" *New York Times*, Oct. 21, 1984, E2.
6. Nemy, "Whoopi's Ready," E2.
7. Her first HBO Special was *Whoopi Goldberg: Direct from Broadway* (1985), a filmed version of her one-woman Broadway show, with the monologues shot as individual vignettes rather than as a theatrical performance.
8. The first swirl of controversy around the film ensued when white director Steven Spielberg, known for his blockbusters (*Jaws*, *Raiders of the Lost Arc*, et al.), was chosen to direct the film version of Alice Walker's book, a decision questioned by many in the black community. The second flurry came when, after receiving eleven Oscar nominations, including Best Actress, Best Director, and Best Picture, *The Color Purple* was shut out completely, raising questions about whether a predominantly black-cast film could garner the industry's highest award.
9. On February 13, 1984, the *Washington Post* reported that Jesse Jackson refers to Jews as "Hymies" and New York City as "Hymietown" in private conversations with journalists.
10. AIDS was first reported in the medical and popular press in 1981. In October of 1987 Reagan publicly spoke, for the first time, about the epidemic in a major policy address. By the beginning of January 1988, almost sixty thousand AIDS cases had been reported and almost twenty-eight thousand of those diagnosed had died.
11. Watkins, *On the Real Side*, 565.
12. Quoted in Patricia Hill Collins, *Black Feminist Thought: Knowledge, Consciousness, and the Politics of Empowerment*, 2nd ed. (New York: Routledge, 2000), 81.
13. This is not to say that this was the only cause in which Goldberg has been involved—it is just her highest-profile activism, aside from Democratic presidential campaigns.

14. Darryl Gates was the controversial police chief of Los Angeles. His fourteen-year tenure included both the Rodney King beating and the LA uprising following the court case that acquitted the officer involved in the King beating. In July 1991, some four months after the King beating, the Christopher Commission report was published. The commission, headed by attorney Warren Christopher (who later became U.S. secretary of state), was created to conduct "a full and fair examination of the structure and operation of the LAPD," including its recruitment and training practices, internal disciplinary system, and citizen complaint system. The commission found, among other things, that a significant number of officers in the LAPD repetitively use excessive force against the public and persistently ignore the written guidelines of the department regarding force.

15. Kam Williams, "Whoopi Goldberg: The *Kingdom Come* Interview," *Washington Informer*, April 18, 2001, 21.

16. Smith, *Not Just Race*, xxiii.

17. Dorothy Gilliam, "The Puzzle of Pearl Bailey on Her Philosophy of Life," *Washington Post*, Oct. 17, 1989, C2.

18. Watkins, *On the Real Side*, 392–93.

19. Elsie A. Williams, *The Humor of Jackie "Moms" Mabley: An African American Comedy Tradition* (New York: Garland, 1995), 78, 76.

20. Watkins, *On the Real Side*, 514.

21. In 1969 Mabley even scored a top-forty hit with her heartfelt version of "Abraham, Martin, and John."

22. Williams, *The Humor of Jackie "Moms" Mabley*, 89.

23. Before the age of fifteen Mabley had been raped twice and forced into an arranged marriage.

24. Williams, *The Humor of Jackie "Moms" Mabley*, 81.

25. In *Engel v. Vitale* the Supreme Court held that the idea of the state to mandate prayer in schools was contrary to the First Amendment's ban against the establishment of religion. This case remains controversial in regard to the definition of what "freedom of religion" means today.

26. Although Mabley did note that Lady Bird tried to let her in the back door, whereas Caroline (JFK's daughter) had always let her in the front.

27. Mabley died within a year of the film's release in 1975.

28. Quoted in the *Tri-State Defender*, "Amazing Grace Opens . . . 'My Picture Different': Moms Mabley," Aug. 10, 1974, 10.

29. I refer to the violence surrounding the desegregation of the Little Rock schools, as a result of *Brown v. Board of Education* in 1955, and the similarly intense social upheaval caused by school busing for purposes of integration in Boston in 1976.

30. Bogle, *Toms, Coons*, 329.

31. Ibid., 332.

32. Janet Maslin, "Goldberg on the Run Disguised as a Nun," *New York Times*, May 29, 1992, C1.

33. Bogle, *Toms, Coons*, 332.

34. CBS Cable, "Pearl Bailey, Pt. 2," *Signature*, Aug. 1982.

35. Liner Notes, *Pearl Bailey Sings for Adults Only* (Roulette Records, 1954).

36. Gilliam, "The Puzzle of Pearl Bailey," C2.

37. Ibid.

38. It is interesting that Bailey's advocacy was never seen as a liability, whereas Goldberg's became significantly less prized by the campaign she had so ardently supported.

39. CBS Cable, "Pearl Bailey, Pt. 2."

40. Whoopi Goldberg, *Book* (New York: Avon, 1997), 123.

41. Neal Lester notes that the song "'The Right to Love' (1950s) was written for Lena Horne and her white husband Lennie Hayton when they made their marriage public after three years of keeping it secret. Here, the couple whose love is 'wrong'

and 'shameful' becomes 'indifferent to the cold, unfriendly stares, / indifferent to the whispered talk'" (Neal A. Lester, "Black/White Interracial Intimacies in Popular Music," *Interracial Voice*, Guest Editorial (2001), http://www.webcom.com/~intvoice/lester.html (accessed April 6, 2006).

42. CBS Cable, "Pearl Bailey, Pt. 2."
43. Jacqueline Genovese, "Whoopi Goldberg Again Reaching the Top: Up from Drugs and Welfare, Black Actress Now Highest Paid Woman in Hollywood," *WE MBI*, June 13, 1993, 10.
44. Ibid.
45. Bogle, *Toms, Coons*, 333.
46. Jay Carr, "Made in America: Don't Buy It," *Boston Globe*, May 28, 1993, E2.
47. Janet Maslin, "A Man, a Woman and a Sperm Bank Yield a 90s Romance," *New York Times*, May 28, 1993, C3.
48. Bogle, *Toms, Coons*, 334.
49. Yuseef Salaam, "Whoopi Goldberg's *Made in America*, another Hollywood Hoax," *New York Amsterdam News*, June 5, 1993, 25.
50. Abiola Sinclair, "Whoopi and Ted's Excellent Adventure," *New York Amsterdam News*, June 12, 1993, 32. Sinclair also notes, in response to Salaam's argument, that "not once in any film produced by a Black male has a Black woman worn her hair in a natural or in braids. Black women who were in braids are laughed at via *Martin*. . . . When he [the black film producer] dreams, apparently he dreams of women with long straight hair who can pass the paper bag test."
51. Founded in 1904, the Friar's Club is a fraternal organization whose members have included scores of the biggest names in show business of the past century, from Irving Berlin and George M. Cohan to Frank Sinatra, George Burns, Jerry Seinfeld, and, of course, Whoopi Goldberg. Besides being involved in philanthropic activities, the club is best known to the general public for the legions of comic/comic actors in its membership (e.g., Billy Crystal, Drew Carey, and Bill Murray), as well as for its uninhibited and notoriously harsh "roasts" of its celebrity members.
52. "Whoopi Goldberg Defends Actor Ted Danson's Blackface," *Los Angeles Sentinel*, Oct. 14, 1993, A1.
53. "Whoopi Goldberg: No Slapstick Comedy," *New Pittsburg Courier*, Oct. 20, 1993, A5.
54. Ibid.
55. Abiola Sinclair, "Ted and Whoopi Part Deux," *New York Amsterdam News*, Oct. 16, 1993, 26.
56. "Whoopi Goldberg Defends Actor Ted Danson's Blackface."
57. Ibid.
58. hooks, *Black Looks*, 76.
59. Jawn Murray, "Talking Whoopi," *BVBuzz*, March 21, 2005, AOL Black Voices, http://bv.channel.aol.com/entmain/bvbuzz/20050321 (accessed March 21, 2005).
60. Marc Warren, "Whoopi Goldberg Receives the Kennedy Center's Mark Twain Prize for American Humor," *Afro American Red Star*, Oct. 16, 2001, B4.
61. MSNBC, *Hardball with Chris Matthews*, January 14, 2005.
62. Quoted in Jeffrey Resner, "10 Questions for Whoopi Goldberg," *Time*, Nov. 22, 2004, 8.
63. Williams, "Whoopi Goldberg," 21.
64. Ibid..
65. Stephen Holden, "'Kingdom Come,' Off to the Cemetery with Laughter, Tears, and Belches," *New York Times*, Nov. 11, 2001, 11.
66. Goldberg's first foray into the sitcom world was the short-lived CBS show *Baghdad Café* (1990), costarring Maureen Stapleton.
67. The acronym, WWF, for World Wrestling Federation, was changed to WWE (World Wrestling Entertainment) in 2005 to avoid confusion with the other WWF, World Wildlife Foundation.

68. Charles Isherwood, "One Woman, Uh-Huh, but So Many Guises," *New York Times*, Nov. 18, 2004, E1.

69. Ibid.

CHAPTER 5. DAVE CHAPPELLE

1. Lola Ogunnaike, "Nothing's Out of Bounds for Dave Chappelle," *New York Times*, Feb. 18, 2004, E1.

2. Dave Chappelle, interview by Terry Gross, *Fresh Air*, NPR, Sep. 2, 2004.

3. Ibid.

4 . Tricia Rose, *Black Noise: Rap Music and Black Culture in Contemporary America* (Hanover, NH: Wesleyan University Press, 1994), 21.

5. The animated series *South Park*, created by Chappelle's Comedy Central brethren Trey Parker and Matt Stone, often parlays in gross-out humor, as well as popular culture parody. *Boondocks*, however, Aaron MacGruder's syndicated cartoon strip—which chronicles the lives of prepubescent Black radical, Huey; his younger brother, gangsta wannabe, Riley; and their grandfather, as they move from the city to the suburbs—engages in incredibly incisive cultural and political criticism.

6. *And You Don't Stop: 30 Years of Hip Hop*, directed by Richard Lowe and Dana Heinz Perry, VH1, 2004.

7. Ogunnaike, "Nothing's Out of Bounds."

8. George, *Hip Hop America*, 94.

9. MTV News, "Fugees—Yes, Even Lauryn—Reunite for Dave Chappelle's Block Party," Sep. 20, 2004, http://www.mtv.com/news/articles/1491206/20040920/fugees.jhtml (accessed Nov. 7, 2004).

10. The concert documentary, directed by Michel Gondry (*Eternal Sunshine of the Spotless Mind*), was the object of a bidding war after its screening at the 2005 Toronto Film Festival. The victor was Rogue Pictures, a subsidiary of Universal's Focus Features, which released the film in 2006.

11. MTV News, "Fugees."

12. MTV News, "Dave Chappelle: The Reason Grandmas Know Who Lil Jon Is," June 6, 2004, http://www.mtv.com/news/articles/1488068/20040601/lil_jon_1.jhtml (accessed Nov. 8, 2004).

13. Gray, *Watching Race*, 138.

14. Beginning in the sixties, Cosby broke ground by taking that well-traveled comic's route: from spots on Jack Paar and Steve Allen to starring television roles on *I-Spy*, *The Bill Cosby Show*, *Fat Albert and the Cosby Kids*, to his most successful film work to date, *Uptown Saturday Night*, to the status of "America's Dad" on *The Cosby Show* to *Leonard Part 6* (proving that, for a multiplicity of reasons, the movement between media is not always the easiest . . . even for a television icon).

15. When one looks at Chappelle's role in *You've Got Mail* and Jamie Foxx's in *The Truth about Cats and Dogs*, the similarities are striking.

16. This appears to transpose the Black men of the Tuskegee Syphilis experiments (1930s–1970s) and the Tuskegee Airmen.

17. Ron Glass on *Barney Miller*, John Amos (briefly) on *The Mary Tyler Moore Show*, and Tim Reid on *WKRP in Cincinnati* exemplify the "integrated" workplace comedies common in the seventies. One could also discuss *The Flip Wilson Show* as a venue for Black comics in the seventies; however, for the most part Wilson's variety series served as a showcase for already established Black comics who had either achieved varying levels of mainstream success, like Cosby and Pryor, or his older contemporaries, like Redd Foxx and Slappy White, who had yet to cross over in a medium other than stand-up.

18. Anare V. Holmes, "Up Close and Personal with Dave Chappelle," *Indianapolis Recorder*, Apr. 20, 2001, A1.

19. Here I am faced with a certain quandary in terms of this discussion. I consider myself neither expert nor particularly enamored with many aspects of the *Def Comedy Jam* personae. This sentiment is due in part to the fact that, during the original run of *Russell Simmons' Def Comedy Jam* on HBO (at a period in my life when premium cable was still considered a luxury), I had watched barely a dozen episodes of the series. I also found the borderline misogyny of the gender politics in many of the acts that I had seen to work in unlikely tandem with the "family values" rhetoric of those days. Both aspects of the series seemed to operate as (disparate) fronts on the assault on feminism.

20. Rudy Ray Moore, the X-rated comedian who delivers his raunchy rhymes to jazz and R&B accompaniment, has had an influence on both Black comics and rappers. While non-Black audiences were not aware of Moore until the resurgence of interest in blaxploitation in the early nineties, Moore had a loyal cult following in the Black community. Moore's recordings were for Black audiences in the seventies what Redd Foxx's "party records" (adult-oriented, sexually explicit comedic fare) were in the fifties and sixties. "Dolemite" has influenced hip-hop artists ranging from 2 Live Crew to Ice-T to Big Daddy Kane (who featured Moore on his 1990 "Big Daddy vs. Dolemite"). From his first "party record," *Eat Out More* (1970), to the cinematic embodiment of Moore's alter ego, "Dolemite," the super stud pimp daddy (based on a raunchy version of a "toast," of rhyming tall tales of one-upmanship) in the self-produced blaxploitation cult classic, the self proclaimed "Godfather of Rap" carved out a comedic niche but took a much more shocking approach to his comedy by filling his act with profanity and sex, as well as his "toasts." Along with his "colorful" characters (pimps, players, hustlers, and prostitutes), Moore produced decidedly "blue" versions of toasts, folklore, and Black narrative traditions that had dominated African American street culture since the early twentieth century, like his iteration of the trickster tale "Signifying Monkey."

21. Alexander starred with Eddie Given in arguably the most odious examples of televisual minstrelsy, *Homeboys from Outer Space*.

22. Kristal Brent Zook, *Color by Fox: The Fox Network and the Revolution in Black Television* (New York: Oxford University Press, 1999), 105.

23. A. J. Jacobs, "Black to the Future," *Entertainment Weekly*, June 14, 1996, http://www.ew.com/ew/report/0,6115,292941_7_0_,00.html (accessed Aug. 5, 2003).

24. The 2006 merger between UPN and the WB began a new chapter in netlet history. While the CW (*C* for CBS, UPN's parent company, and *W* for Warner) came together in hopes of following Fox's path into network status, it retains vestiges of both the teen and "urban" niches—arguably more of the former than the latter. In the fall of 2006 the CW will still have black shows, most of which will be part of the netlet's Monday "black block" of comedy: with family fare like *Everybody Hates Chris*, the sitcom standout of the class of 2006, based on the adolescence of Chris Rock; *All of Us*, the Will Smith–produced blended family sitcom; and the single-folk sitcoms *Girlfriends*, the UPN six-season veteran, and its spin-off, *The Game*, both products of Kelsey Grammer's production company.

25. *Jacksonville Free Press*, "Comedian Chappelle Accuses Fox of Racism for Show Fumble," July 15, 1998, 13.

26. Cho details this experience in her first concert film, *I'm the One That I Want* (2000).

27. MTV News, "Dave Chappelle: The Reason Grandmas Know Who Lil Jon Is."

28. Dave Chappelle, interview by Terry Gross, *Fresh Air*.

29. Allison Hope Weiner, "Funny Business," *Entertainment Weekly*, Aug. 20, 2004, http://www.ew.com/ew/report/0,6115,681698_3_0_,00.html (accessed Aug. 21, 2004).

30. Kam Williams, "Outrageous Comic Calls His Show a Hip Hop Masterpiece Theater," *Recorder*, Jan. 17, 2003, sec. C.

31. Ibid.
32. This is Chris Rock's reassurance to white audience members in his *Bigger and Blacker*.
33. An interesting reversal of this notion is used on the second season of *Chappelle's Show* with a game-show parody, done with actual New Yorkers off the street, called "I Know Black People."
34. On February 4, 1999, Amadou Diallo was killed in the entrance hall of his Bronx apartment building when undercover officers, who said they mistook his wallet for a gun, fired forty-one shots, hitting the street vendor from Guinea nineteen times and making the killing an international symbol of police brutality. See "USA: Amnesty International Calls for Review of New York City Police Shooting Tactics," March 3, 2000, http://www.amnestyusa.org/countries/usa/ document.do?id= 76035D7F4FBED5958025689A00477247 (accessed Nov. 7, 2004).
35. One must also note that this show was taped in 2000. In this pre-9/11 context it was all right to criticize the NYPD and police in general. Even the comedic climate has changed a bit on that front with some comics, black and white, defending the practice of racial profiling for the sake of "national security."
36. Unlike the payoff of the archetypal Def Jam joke, there was a bit of an edge embedded in the shtick with the statement about the impact and anger over social services being cut during the early Bush years.
37. In *Passenger 57* an ex-cop, played by Wesley Snipes, gives a signal (that may have been a thumbs-up) to other passengers when he is ready to make his move against the hijackers.
38. This bit also features an impersonation of a slightly naughty Ed Bradley asking Katherine Wylie if Clinton "was aroused" during their alleged encounter, which in turn gives way to a rather predictable series of masturbation jokes.
39. The props he gives to San Francisco—"they are a savvy" audience—clearly seems a commentary on the other California city, Sacramento, where *stupid*, not *savvy*, was the word he used to describe the crowd.
40. Dave Chappelle, interview by Jay Leno, *The Tonight Show with Jay Leno*, NBC, Aug. 30, 2004.
41. I refer to the decision made during the Reagan years to have ketchup count as "vegetable" for the federally subsidized school lunch programs designed to serve the nutritional needs of underprivileged children in American public schools.
42. I refer to the differing responses that the black and white communities have to the not guilty verdict in the O. J. Simpson trial: voicing a black Simpson supporter's response to white outrage, Chappelle exclaims, "It burns don't it. . . . That justice system burns. Welcome to our world."
43. Among other things, this can be used to describe sexual play with urine. Kelly is accused of relieving himself on a fifteen-year-old girl as a part of their sexual encounter.
44. Quoted in Hillary Atkins, "Chappelle's Show," *Television Week*, May 31, 2004, 36.
45. Neal Brennan and Dave Chappelle, interview by Charlie Rose, *The Charlie Rose Show*, PBS, April 28, 2004.
46. Weiner, "Funny Business."
47. Neal Brennan and Dave Chappelle, interview by Charlie Rose, *The Charlie Rose Show*.
48. Tom Shales, "The New Season: Pryor's Angry Humor: The Savagery of 'Soap,'" *Washington Post*, Sep. 13, 1977, sec. B.
49. *Mo' Funny: Black Comedy in America*, written and directed by Yvonne Smith, HBO Films, 1993.
50. Kristal Brent Zook, "The Fox Network and the Revolution in Black Television," in *Gender, Race, and Class in Media: A Text-Reader*, ed. Gail Dines and Jean M. Humez (Thousand Oaks, CA: Sage, 1995), 522.
51. Gray, *Watching Race*, 138.

52. Norma Miriam Schulman, "Laughing across the Color Barrier: *In Living Color*," in *Gender, Race, and Class in Media: A Text-Reader*, ed. Gail Dines and Jean M. Humez (Thousand Oaks, CA: Sage, 1995), 439.

53. The absurdity of this statement is a direct response to the premature exit of David Edwards on *The Real World LA*. Edwards, with whom Chappelle grew up, was the first cast member to be kicked out of the house. On the DVD commentary Chappelle remembers (with what seems like a trace of anger) his response when the same phrase was used when David was asked to leave: "Don't feel safe . . . the guy weighs maybe a buck-twenty. It was ridiculous."

54. Lerone Bennett Jr., *Ebony*'s executive editor, interview by Tavis Smiley, *The Tavis Smiley Show*, PBS, June 18, 2003.

55. Gray, *Watching Race*, 144.

56. This is the case in the "Intervention" sketch when the white liberal couple, who took in Tyrone so he could improve his life by becoming a real estate agent, describe how, when they were away, he sold their house and had a "Tyrone $450,000 Crack Party" with the proceeds. Outlandish? Yes. Sympathetic to crackheads? No.

57. Dave Chappelle, interview by Bob Simon, *60 Minutes*, CBS, Oct. 20, 2004.

58. Todd Boyd, *Am I Black Enough for You? Popular Culture from the 'Hood and Beyond* (Bloomington: Indiana University Press, 1997), 31.

59. Dave Chappelle, interview by Bob Simon, *60 Minutes*.

60. Neal Brennan and Dave Chappelle, interview by Charlie Rose, *The Charlie Rose Show*.

61. Ibid.

62. Dave Chappelle, interview by Terry Gross, *Fresh Air*.

63. Neal Brennan and Dave Chappelle, interview by Bob Simon, *60 Minutes*.

64. The story of his grandfather as inspiration for Clayton Bigsby is drawn from the director's commentary on episode 1 of the *Chappelle's Show* Season 1 DVD, 2003.

65. Ibid.

66. According to their DVD commentary, the black friend in question was Say Adams, African American, feminist, vegetarian artist, who did cover art for some of Def Jam's biggest artists—"a bright, sharp, cutting edge dude." According to Brennan the sketch made Adams feel the same way he had felt when Adam Horowitz (Ad-Rock of the Beastie Boys) said the *N* word at the Apollo—the implication being that it just felt *wrong*.

67. The head of one supporter, played by Neal Brennan, explodes, splattering blood and flesh all over the predominantly white book covers of the Bigsby-authored volumes.

68. Hazel V. Carby, "The Multicultural Wars," in *Black Popular Culture*, ed. Michele Wallace and Gina Dent (Seattle: Bay Press, 1992), 193.

69. Boyd, *Black Enough*, 30.

70. Chappelle fielded questions on the "Niggar" sketch on NPR (*Fresh Air*), PBS (*Charlie Rose*), and CBS (*60 Minutes*).

71. George Lipsitz, *The Possessive Investment in Whiteness: How White People Profit from Identity Politics* (Philadelphia: Temple University Press, 1998), 2.

72. Quoted in Christopher John Farley, "Dave Speaks," *Time*, May 23, 2005, 68.

73. Devin Gordon, "Fears of a Clown," *Newsweek*, May 16, 2005, 60.

74. Dave Chappelle, *The Oprah Winfrey Show*, directed by Joseph C. Terry, Feb. 3, 2006.

75. Chappelle, a Muslim since 1998, attempted to make a hajj, the required pilgrimage to Mecca, but did not have the required visa to enter Saudi Arabia.

76. Chappelle, *The Oprah Winfrey Show*.

77. Quoted in Farley, "Dave Speaks."

78. Quoted in ibid.

79. Sun Wire Services, "End of Chappelle's Show No Joke," *Ottawa Sun*, Aug. 4, 2005, 26.

80. Quoted in Farley, "Dave Speaks."

81. Chappelle, *The Oprah Winfrey Show.*

82. Dave Chappelle, *Inside the Actors Studio,* Feb. 12, 2006.

83. Manohla Dargis, "A Comedian's Ultimate Goal: Rock the Block," *New York Times,* March 3, 2006, E1.

84. Chappelle, *The Oprah Winfrey Show.*

85. Ibid.

86. Ibid.

87. Quoted in Simon Robinson, "On The Beach with Dave Chappelle," Time.com (Web exclusive), May 15, 2005, http://www.time.com/time/arts/article/ 0,8599,1061415,00.html (accessed May 17, 2005).

88. Chappelle, *Inside the Actors Studio.*

89. This is a term often used for folks who listen to and embody the underground hip-hop lifestyle.

90. Linda Hutcheon's notion of postmodern parody states that "through a double process of installing and ironizing, parody signals how present representations come from past ones and what ideological consequences derive from both continuity and difference.... Parody is doubly coded in political terms: it both legitimizes and subverts that which it parodies" (Linda Hutcheon, *The Politics of Postmodernism* [New York: Routledge, 1989], 93, 97). Jameson likens pastiche to parody as "the imitation of a peculiar, unique or idiosyncratic style" but establishes it as "a neutral practice of such mimicry, without any of parody's ulterior motives" (Fredric Jameson, *Postmodernism or the Cultural Logic of Late Capitalism* [Durham, NC: Duke University Press, 1991], 17). As previously stated, neither definition seems *completely* applicable to *Chappelle's Show.*

91. I am currently writing an article comparing *Block Party* and *Wattstax* as celebrations of black culture and, markers of its mainstream consumption.

92. Chairman Fred Hampton Jr., political activist and poet, is the son of Fred Hampton, who was assassinated in an FBI COINTELPRO operation in Chicago on Dec. 4, 1969. The junior Hampton was a community organizer working with the National People's Democratic Uhuru Movement before being arrested on charges of aggravated arson during the LA uprising. Hampton was convicted and sentenced to eighteen years in prison. An international campaign to free Hampton was launched, and on Sep. 14, 2001, he was released from prison. Hampton remains politically active in a variety of ways, including touring the country with hip-hop artist Mutulu Olugabala from the rap group Dead Prez.

93. Undoubtedly there are similarities between the ongoing legal woes of the "New York Three" and "Mumia." Jalil Abdul Muntaqim (Anthony Bottom) and Albert Nuh Washington were arrested in San Francisco in 1971 and Herman Bell in New Orleans in 1973 for the killing of two New York City police officers in May 1971. The first trial ended in a mistrial, but despite defense allegations that eyewitness testimony had been coerced in the second trial, the "New York Three" were convicted and sentenced to life in prison. Each of the New York Three was named in COINTELPRO documents as members of the black liberation movement who had to be "neutralized," and each has served almost thirty years, with all appeals exhausted and clemency or parole the only paths to release. Albert Nuh Washington died from liver cancer in 2000; Jalil Abdul Muntaqim and Herman Bell continue to serve their life sentences.

   Only recently has the picture become less bleak for Mumia Abu-Jamal. From July 1982 until December 2001 Abu-Jamal had been on Pennsylvania's death row for the killing of police officer Daniel Faulkner. In December of 2001 the sentence of the journalist, Black Panther, MOVE member, and outspoken critic of police brutality and racism was commuted to life (although the conviction was upheld). During his incarceration Abu-Jamal, who has repeatedly proclaimed his innocence, has produced articles, radio commentaries (thru the Prison Radio Project and *Democracy*

*Now!*), and several books, including *Live from Death Row* (1996) and *We Want Freedom: A Life in the Black Panther Party* (2004). With the status of cause célèbre, Abu-Jamal has attracted high-profile supporters such as filmmakers Spike Lee, John Landis, and Oliver Stone; actors Ed Asner, Alec Baldwin, Samuel L. Jackson, and Tim Robbins; hip-hop artists The Beastie Boys, Public Enemy, and Rage Against the Machine; and cultural critics/political activists Noam Chomsky, bell hooks, Dick Gregory, and the Reverend Jesse Jackson. In December 2005 the United States Court of Appeals for the Third Circuit, Philadelphia, agreed to review the defense's claims of judicial bias (in relationship to jury selection and instruction, as well as the exclusion of determination of fact and new evidence during both the trial and appeal). As of the spring of 2006 Mumia Abu-Jamal remains in prison.

EPILOGUE

1. Pew Research Center for the People and the Press, "Two-in-Three Critical of Bush's Relief Efforts: Huge Racial Divide over Katrina and Its Consequences," *Pew Research Center*, Sep. 8, 2005, http://people-press.org/reports/display.php3?ReportID=255 (accessed Sep. 20, 2005).
2. "For Bush, the Storm after the Storm," *Time*, Sep. 19, 2005, 45.
3. Marc Sandalow, "Katrina Thrusts Race and Poverty onto National Stage," *San Francisco Chronicle*, Sep. 23, 2005, A13.
4. On National Public Radio's *This American Life*, the September 9, 2005, program, "After the Flood," was dedicated to allowing those who endured Hurricane Katrina and its aftermath to speak out. Denise Moore talked of her experiences in the Convention Center: from her anger with the authorities for lineups every four hours in the blistering heat for buses that never came to her gratitude to some of the so-called "looters" and those who in pre-Katrina life she would have labeled "gangsters" and "thugs," who acted as Robin Hoods, procuring water, juice, and diapers, etc., and who "got together, figured out who had guns and decided they were going to make sure that no women were getting raped because we did hear about women getting raped in the superdome and that nobody was hurting babies. And nobody was hurting these old people."
5. Clarence Page, "Obama Points to Danger of Passive Indifference," *Baltimore Sun*, Sep. 16, 2005, 15A.
6. Terry M. Neal, "Race, Class Re-Enter Politics after Katrina," washingtonpost.com, Sep. 22, 2005, http://www.washingtonpost.com/wp-dyn/content/article/2005/09/22/AR2005092200833.html?referrer=emailarticle (accessed Sep. 25, 2005).
7. West's reference to the media's construction of posthurricane looting was also explored in countless blogs and in Aaron Kinney's "'Looting' or 'Finding,'" Salon.com, Sep. 1, 2005, http://www.salon.com/news/feature/2005/09/01/photo_controversy/index.html (accessed Sep. 6, 2005). Kinney's article details the blog-driven controversy over two photographs (and captions) posted on Yahoo News, both depicting individuals wading through chest-deep water and carrying food items that came from a nearby grocery store. Dave Martin's Associated Press photograph, in which the person shown was a young black man, bore a caption that describes the man's actions as looting, while Chris Graythen's photo for AFP/Getty Images, which shows a white male and light-skinned woman in a similar activity, uses the term *finding*. As Kinney notes, for better or for worse, bloggers were "quick to raise allegations about insensitivity and racism regarding the disparity of the two captions."
8. Ed Gordon, "Now Is the Time for Us to Talk about Race," Newsday Wire Services, *Passaic County (NJ) Herald News*, Sep. 25, 2005, B7.
9. Ibid.
10. Morris Reid, interview with Brooke Anderson, "Rapper's Comments on Race Fuel Nationwide Debate," *Showbiz Show*, CNN, Sep. 8, 2005. This segment also featured

a sound bite from Howard Dean's commentary on racism and Katrina: "Skin color, age and economics played a significant role in who survived and who did not."

11. Bob Moon, "Houston, We May Have a Problem," *Marketplace*, PRI, Sep. 5, 2005, http://marketplace.publicradio.org/shows/2005/09/05/PM200509051.html (accessed April 10, 2006). This segment captured the comments of Barbara Bush during a goodwill visit to the Astrodome.

12. Catherine R. Squires, "Rethinking the Black Public Sphere," *Communication Theory* (Nov. 2002): 458.

13. Ibid., 459.

14. Mo'Nique, with her starring role in UPN's *The Parkers* (which ended its five-year run as the highest-rated series with the African American audience), a starring role in *Hair Show* (2004), an (almost) straight-to-video comedy, and supporting roles in questionable comedic fare such as *Three Strikes* (2000) and *Soul Plane* (2003), has been able to generate a screen presence that is (somewhat) akin to her stand-up comic persona.

15. *The Original Kings of Comedy* (2000) was the Spike Lee–directed concert film that brought the comic talents of Harvey, Hughley, Cedric, and Mac to the attention of a wider (mainstream) audience, while the Showtime concert equivalent, *The Queens of Comedy* (2001), solidified but did not expand the fan bases for Miss Laura Hayes, Adele Givens, Sommore, and, the most industrially successful black female of this court, Mo'Nique.

16. Antonio Gramsci, *Selections from the Prison Notebooks*, trans. and ed. Quintin Hoare and Geoffrey Nowell Smith (New York: International Publishers, 1971), 3.

# INDEX

# About the Author

BAMBI HAGGINS, the director of graduate studies and an assistant professor of Screen Arts and Cultures at the University of Michigan, teaches about television history and representations of class, ethnicity, gender, and sexuality across media. Haggins has begun work on a second volume focusing on "for us, by us" black comedy and the nature and significance of insider laughter.